PATRICK & BEATRICE HAGGERTY LIBRARY

W9-AQU-596

ditor: Claudia M. Wilson
r: Holly D. Gordon
: Ron Gross
Kewal K. Sharma
ComCom Division of Haddon Craftsmen, Inc.
Binder: R. R. Donnelley & Sons Company

neurial Nutritionist

1987 by Harper & Row, Publishers, Inc.

served. Printed in the United States of
part of this book may be used or reproduced
er whatsoever without written permission,
case of brief quotations embodied in critical
reviews. For information address Harper &
hers, Inc., 10 East 53d Street, New York, NY

Congress Cataloging-in-Publication Data

y King.
preneurial nutritionist.

ohy: p.
ndex.
cs—Practice.   I. Title.
45   1987   613.2′068   86–14890
-043662–X

89   9   8   7   6   5   4   3   2   1

THE ENTREPR
NUTRITIONIST

Kathy King Helm

Sponsoring
Project Edit
Cover Desig
Production:
Compositor:
Printer and

The Entrep

Copyright (

All rights r
America. N
in any man
except in th
articles and
Row, Publi
10022.

Library of

Helm, Kat
    The entr

    Bibliogr
    Includes
    1. Diete
RM218.5.
ISBN 0–06

1817

HARPER & ROW, PUBLISHERS, New York
Cambridge, Philadelphia, San Francisco, Washi
London, Mexico City, São Paulo, Singapore, Sy

86 87 8

613.2
H36
1987

Contents

Preface

The first person to write about an idea is an innovator, the second is a plagiarist, the third is drawing on common knowledge, and the fourth is doing research (1). Information on how to start your own business or become an entrepreneur fills the bookstore shelves and lay reading journals. It is becoming common knowledge.

How then will this book be different? Although much of what businesspersons describe may apply to the problems facing a dietitian who starts a private practice, applied knowledge specific to the nutrition arena is lacking. By drawing on our own experience, the knowledge of how our peers think, and our research into practice management, my contributing authors and I hope to give a dietitian's view of private practice and entrepreneurialism.

Dietitians' initial business exposure often shapes the future of their private practices and greatly influences their probability of success. It is important, therefore, that the practitioner be prepared for the venture and that all decisions be well thought out.

This book follows the practical and logical stages that usually occur in the development of an entrepreneurial venture. It is designed for easy reading. Actual experiences of practitioners, as well as questions commonly asked at over 60 private practice seminars and lectures conducted since 1979, are highlighted.

The opinions are obviously those of the author and contributors and should provide only a starting point or option for the business owner's personal research. In very few cases are there absolute right and wrong ways of doing things. It is the practitioners who must make the best decisions in their own settings and live with the consequences.

This is not a how-to book that guarantees success because your business is well run. There are elements such as the dietitian's personality and attitude that can destroy the best of financed and organized businesses.

For practitioners and students who think that one day private practice may be their chosen mode of practice, this book should help define what skills and resources will be needed to succeed. Many of the ideas will be beneficial to the individual wanting to become an "intrapreneur"—an employed dietitian interested in innovation and generating income (2). Established private practitioners may recall many of their own frustrations and exciting moments and may even find new ideas.

Acknowledgments go to my editors at Harper & Row, especially Earl Shepard and Claudia Wilson who continually gave encouragement. I would like to thank all of my authors and practitioner reviewers for the contributions that broadened the focus of this book. Thanks to Edna Jones Hunter who typed the majority of my manuscript. A special acknowledgment goes to my family for its continuing support, guidance, and cheerleading over the years as each new project was invented.

REFERENCES

1. McCue, Jack: *Private Practice: Surviving the First Year,* The Collamore Press, MA, 1982.
2. Mescon, Michael, and Timothy Mescon: "Breeding the Corporate 'Intrapreneur' " in *SKY,* July 1984.

Introduction

Becoming an entrepreneur even on a small-time basis is a temptation. Today, nutrition's "window of opportunity" in marketing is wide open. Public interest in nutrition is greater than ever before. We dietitians are qualified to lead the way, but the process of using our scientific information and developing it into a business is foreign to most of us.

Starting a business may be one of the most challenging and difficult ventures you ever undertake. Trial and error are part of every new business's growth. Becoming skilled requires study, practice, evaluation, more study, more practice, and more time and money.

Successful private practitioners usually are creative individuals with good clinical backgrounds and communication skills. They commonly have mature personalities and adequate financial backing. Business acumen and position in the community improve and evolve with time.

Dietitians who are thinking about private practice often want to try it "on the side" instead of as their only income. It is only natural to want to minimize the risk and expense. The effort can still be financially and professionally successful if quality output, commitment to clients, and perseverance are high priorities. To succeed, part-time commitment cannot mean lower quality or less intensity when it is called for.

According to the Small Business Administration figures in 1985, there were 3 million women who were self-employed. This is a 75 percent gain in 10 years, and women represent the fastest growing segment of small business (1). Because over 97 percent of the members of The American Dietetic Association are women, it should be noted that owning a business and being successful at it is a growing option for women.

The earliest known private nutrition practice was begun by Eloise Treasher in 1949 in Baltimore, Maryland. As Eloise retired from work at The Johns Hopkins Hospital, many physicians wanted to continue sending their patients to her, and her business began. Eloise has stated that "private practice is not for everyone and not everyone will be good at it. But, if you offer quality, you will be in demand" (3).

In 1953 Norma MacRae began her business in Seattle, Washington. Today she has a full-time partner, is an author of several books, and consults to the food industry. When asked about her success, Norma stated, "I knew 'I had arrived' when physicians started coming to see me as patients" (3).

Other pioneers include Virginia Bayles, R.D., a Consulting Nutritionist in Houston, Texas, and author Dorothy Revell, R.D., from Fargo, North Dakota. Carol Hunerlach, R.D., of Maryland is credited with spearheading the movement to teach dietitians about private practice and in organizing the Consulting Nutritionists, a dietetic practice group on the Council on Practice of The American Dietetic Association. These are the dietitians who have identified private practice as an area of professional interest, and members often use the title Consulting Nutritionist.

The contributing authors all have areas of specialty that distinguish them, and their chapters provide new insight to the readers:

Olga Dominguez Satterwhite, R.D., began her private practice, Nutrition Consultant Services of Houston, in 1976. She is bilingual and first marketed her services to the Spanish surname physicians in and around the Texas Medical Center area for their local and foreign patients. Before opening her business doors, she had contacted over 200 physicians and had enough signed consultant contracts to equal her monthly salary. She secured a personal loan and opened a well-financed, full-fledged office with a part-time secretary in a medical complex. Today she subcontracts to fifteen other practitioners. Much of Olga's time is spent in negotiating contracts and in the management of accounts and people. She is the publisher of a successful weight loss program and other teaching booklets. Her clients include private patients, corporate health programs, restaurants, HMOs, renal dialysis units, and medical clinics. Olga also conducts seminars on private practice and marketing.

Marilyn Schorin, M.P.H., R.D., is past chairman and cofounder of the Sports and Cardiovascular Nutritionists Dietetic Practice Group of The American Dietetic Association. She has worked with the MR FIT program and is coauthor of a booklet, "A Recipe for Fitness," for Best Foods. In 1980–1981 she designed and produced a program for nutrition and sports for Johnson & Johnson's "Live for Life" program. In 1982 Marilyn was a scientific consultant for "Upjohn Healthworks."

Becky McCully, M.S., R.D., has been a popular private practitioner in Oklahoma City since 1978. She writes a weekly nutrition column for the *Daily Oklahoman* newspaper and appears as a guest on local radio and television. Becky's major client account is with a group of ten cardiologists, teaching cooking classes and instructing patients. Becky began her business as an independent practitioner subleasing space in a physician's office building. As she became known, other physicians wanted her to see patients in their offices. Eventually she contracted with the group where she presently works. Recently, she was elected chairperson of the Consulting Nutritionists Dietetic Practice Group of The American Dietetic Association.

Jan Thayer, R.D., is an accomplished businesswoman, media personality, and community leader from Grand Island, Nebraska. She is coowner of Wedgewood Nursing Home and is a Licensed Nursing Home Administrator. She works as a consultant dietitian, and is a member of the Volunteer Faculty for the University of Nebraska College of Medicine. For nine years Jan produced a daily radio segment entitled "Food for Thought." At present she is featured on regular interview segments on KOLN-KGIN TV. Jan is past president of the Nebraska Dietetic Association and past chairman of the Consultant Dietitians in Health Care Facilities Dietetic Practice Group of The American Dietetic Association.

Paulette Lambert, R.D., has a very successful private practice in Tarzana, California. She specializes in using behavior modification techniques with patients who have eating disorder and weight control problems. Paulette's clients include a predominance of executives and professionals and their families. She began her business in space sublet from a physician but now has her own office. Today she has three associates, and the four see more than 250 clients per week in group and individual consults. Paulette is past chairman of the Consulting Nutritionists of Southern California dietetic practice group.

Susan Tornetta Magrann, M.S., R.D., is a published writer, lecturer, and consulting nutritionist in private practice in California. She is the editor of a monthly nutrition newsletter for Vons supermarkets and an instructor for workshops on publishing produced by Health Update. Susan has been a contributing writer to *Sporting Times, Women's Track World, The Jogger, Gemco Courier,* and *Muscle Digest.* She is past president of the Orange County, California, Dietetic Association.

Cecilia Helton, M.A., R.D., is a college instructor in Idaho and a participant on their College of Education Microcomputer Team. Her chapter on computer applications in nutrition is meant to acquaint the practitioner with the terms and major functions of computer hardware and software. Cecilia has teaching experience, has been a consultant dietitian to nursing homes, and worked as a clinical dietitian. Her major area of interest is in education media.

I began my business in 1972 in Denver, Colorado. I was frustrated with the lack of patient teaching in the hospital setting at that time and excited by the future of preventive nutrition. I decided to keep my investment and overhead low, work day and night, try private practice for one year, and then reevaluate. These decisions were not hard to come by since I was single and had nothing of value to borrow against—but I had the time and dedication.

My business was located in several physicians' offices in the blue-collar area near the hospital where I had worked. One physician paid me a retainer two days per week and I consulted at six other medical offices by appointment. I spent a lot of time in transit and trying to market my services to physicians.

The first year I charged $7 for the initial visit and $2 for revisits—and still had complaints about fees! I supported myself from the start, supplementing my income with cleaning houses and sewing. For every hour of generated income, I usually worked three hours on paperwork, marketing, or projects with no guaranteed income.

Before one year was up, I knew the concept worked. I decided to borrow $1000 (not a sufficient amount even then) and opened an office in a new local medical building. I loved it. Patients came to me.

I raised my prices a little to cover the increased overhead and it started to look like a legitimate business. I carried malpractice insurance, but I wanted to incorporate to better protect my business from lawsuits. Lawyers told me not to worry because I wasn't financially worth suing (that was a low blow). I finally incorporated my third year in business.

During my third year I decided to sublease the office two days per week to a speech therapist. That freed me to take consultant positions on the side and start a masters degree in exercise physiology to broaden my expertise. It also gave me a change of pace from constant weight loss and therapeutic counseling.

To promote my business I gave one to three free talks per week. I appeared weekly on NBC KOA TV and monthly on KMGH TV for a total of seven years. I also started volunteering with the state dietetic organization and as a sports nutritionist to the exercise physiology department at the University of Denver.

Sports nutrition, media work, paid public speaking, and more fun jobs started to come my way as my expertise grew and I became known. My approach to nutrition was from a wellness point of view, so when the trend finally hit Denver, I was ready to grow with it.

From my business experience, I have learned that when the tough decisions have to be made no one can do it better than I. I have stopped looking for that expert on a white horse. From consulting to more than 4000 patients I have readjusted my thinking about counseling techniques, human physiology, and weight loss. I and the entrepreneurs I know continue private practice because we love the chance to be creative, to work with people, and the freedom. The difficulty of the challenge makes us appreciate the rewards even more.

REFERENCES

1. *The Kiplinger Washington Letter,* Washington, D.C., June 21, 1985.
2. "A New Look at the Profession of Dietetics," Report of the 1984 Study Commission on Dietetics, The American Dietetic Association, 1985.
3. King, Kathy: "Starting a Private Practice," Study Kit 3, The American Dietetic Association, 1982.

Kathy King Helm, R.D.

About the Author

Kathy King Helm, Registered Dietitian, graduated in Food Science and Nutrition from Colorado State University and completed a dietetic internship at Beth Israel Hospital in Boston. In 1972, after practicing two years as a clinical dietitian, she began her private practice in a north Denver suburb. Today she and her family live in Lake Dallas, Texas, and she works as a consultant to The Greenhouse Spa and The Lewisville Sports Medicine Center.

Ms. Helm specializes in preventive nutrition, weight loss, and sports nutrition. In addition to consulting with private patients, at spas, for sports' teams, including the Denver Broncos, and for wellness programs, she has been a lecturer, writer, and media spokesperson.

Ms. Helm's entrepreneurial activities include developing a natural sports drink, publishing a consumer booklet, "Let's Get To Know Vitamin Supplements," and coproducing seminars for dietitians on marketing and private practice.

She is a past president of the Colorado Dietetic Association, and chairperson of the Council on Practice and on the Board of Directors of The American Dietetic Association.

one

ENTREPRENEURIALISM

chapter 1

The Entrepreneurial Spirit

The 1980s have seen a renewed interest in fostering the entrepreneurial spirit in America—that desire to develop new ideas, generate income, and assume more control of one's own work. Increasing numbers of people are realizing that entrepreneurship is a vast, untapped source of personal and career fulfillment. Many dietitians recognize that this spirit is the catalyst needed to generate new ideas and new jobs that will instill vigor into the dietetic profession.

Historically, innovative, risk-taking individuals had to leave their employee settings to be able to use their talents. Dietitians chose private practice for its freedom and excitement. They had to accept its uncertainties. Initially, the majority of practices involved therapeutic counseling or consulting for nursing homes. Practitioners today write, publish, lecture, and appear in the media. Others develop software, consult to wellness and athletic programs or drug rehabilitation and penal institutions. Some practitioners own their own eating disorder clinics, computer companies, marketing firms, or fitness programs.

Today, you do not have to be in private practice to have an entrepreneurial spirit, but private practice still represents the ultimate level of independence. Changes in attitudes and expectations by employers, however, are making the workplace more receptive to new ideas and more assertive individuals. The new term *intrapreneurial* has been coined to describe an innovative employee or work setting (1). Concurrently, dietitians who once avoided private practice because it involved "too much risk" are now looking at it differently. At many of their "stable" jobs, employers are cutting staffs and budgets.

Presently, the marketing *window of opportunity* for nutrition is wide open. Nutrition has never been a "hotter" topic and it will remain so for some years to come. How fortunate and exciting that this should happen during our professional careers! However, as with all great ideas and trends, it too will fade as the market becomes saturated with nutrition information, fads, and programs. Already practitioners report that their clientele and medical communities are more educated and more aware of the basics of nutrition. Underlying all of this marketing opportunity is the realization that few dietitians have known how to tap into it. It is still not to late to learn!

THE QUALITIES OF AN ENTREPRENEUR

We hear about individuals who start private practices "to fill a need for counseling outside of the hospital" or "to concentrate on wellness"—but what makes these individuals want to do such a thing in the first place? What drives some to do it, while others only talk of it? What character traits distinguish entrepreneurs from employees? How do you tell if you're one of them?

There are few universal criteria that are common to all successful entrepreneurs. The personal qualities, experience, or financial resources that were necessary for one entrepreneur's success may be less important for another.

With a few notable exceptions, experience is a key factor in private practitioners' success. Private practice is not an employment avenue usually recommended for the new graduate. It is, instead, for the individual with skills and expertise beyond what is considered normal schooling experience. The individual also needs adequate financial backing. However, it is recognized that encouraging potential entrepreneurs merely to have years of experience in dietetics without regard to the type and quality of experience is not well founded.

A successful entrepreneur has numerous areas of expertise that should be developed. They include a thorough working knowledge of how a business operates, an appreciation for marketing and financial management, practical knowledge in working with clinical nutrition and counseling patients, and expertise in communication skills, to name a few. It is important that a businessperson develop his or her own unique areas of specialty.

The character of entrepreneurs is also extremely important. They need a fierce dedication to achievement and perseverance. They must not be afraid of risk taking. Enthusiasm is essential. Successful entrepreneurs know how to be tough, how to accept criticism, and how to make quick decisions and yet be flexible. Personal integrity is crucial. They must be able to accept responsibility and stick by commitments. As nutrition counselors it is also important to be people oriented, empathetic, and exceptionally good in communicating with others.

There is no guarantee that a private practice will show an immediate profit. Individuals starting their own business cannot be prone to discouragement or boredom. A successful entrepreneur is a realist as well as a dreamer—reaching for the stars, while maintaining a firm, earthly footing.

Successful entrepreneurs also share the ability to learn from others. Many will set up informal mentor relationships, then learn from and consult with that person on major decisions. Others will *network* and share ideas and problems with other entrepreneurs.

WHY CHOOSE PRIVATE PRACTICE?

Dietitians on the verge of leaving employee status for that of private practice find that being an employee no longer gives them what they need. They want a chance to really see what they can do with their skills and verve. It is as if they have come to the end of a certain passage. They can no longer grow in the present environment. Venturing into the unknown becomes necessary in order to continue personal and career growth.

Other reasons for starting a private practice are to gain flexibility of time, to be your own boss, to be better able to follow patient care, to create and implement programs, to do a variety of challenging work, and communicate yourself for profit and for recognition.

The potential exists to make it in a big way and if successful, to make much more money then you ever could as an employee. There is a tremendous swelling of pride in your work and in yourself as you bring to fruition projects that you originate. In society as a whole, entrepreneurs receive the approval and respect of many people who realize the commitment and effort entrepreneurship exemplifies.

What Price Is Paid?

Many of the benefits granted the employee, for example, regular paychecks, paid sick leave, pension plans, health insurance programs, regular working hours and vacation time are no longer givens when you are your own boss. It may dawn like a revelation for the new entrepreneur that if he doesn't work a day, he doesn't get paid. There are no benefits when self-employed except what you provide for yourself.

MEGATRENDS FOR DIETETICS

Since publication of John Naisbitt's book *Megatrends* there has been great interest in applying his information to one's own life setting (2). Through his company's research he has forecast the major social, economic, political, and technological movements taking place and expected in the future. An advisory committee of the American Dietetic Association identified the megatrends that are affecting our profession and those that will continue to play a large role in our entrepreneurial future (3):

1. The marketplaces where dietitians make their livings are changing at astounding rates, requiring new skills (3). A larger percentage of Americans is living longer, which results in more people with chronic illnesses. Home health, retirement communities, and programs for the elderly will become more prevalent. The interest in physical fitness, wellness, and eating good foods is still growing. The food industry is recognizing that good nutrition is now a legitimate concern of the buying public and is trying to produce items that appeal to it. Ethnic groups are becoming larger, especially the Spanish-speaking segment, increasing the need for bilingual materials and dietitians.

The changes in funding for medical patients through the use of Diagnose Related Groups (DRGs) will no doubt eventually be used by all insurance purveyors (4). It is expected that there will be staff cuts and hospital closings that will greatly affect the number of dietitians, who will lose formerly "stable" clinical positions. At this same time hospitals are looking to new areas for revenue generation. Some are trying outpatient nutrition clinics, wellness programs, corporate outreach, storefront emergency clinics, and publishing—all areas where dietitians could act as employees or consultants.

Only aiming for the status quo—what has worked well in the past—will only drop the dietitian behind in today's market. To remain current each of us must acquire new or advanced skills. If a dietitian is threatened by the work being done by a dietetic technician, pharmacist, or nurse, maybe it is because the practitioner isn't doing the level of work he or she should be. That feeling is unsettling to us all but should be used as a catalyst for change.

The skills and knowledge now becoming necessities for most practitioners in their work settings are (3):

- Management skills so that practitioners are more involved in policy making and revenue allocation.
- Communication skills (writing, speaking, media work, and scientific publishing) so that practitioners can be recognized more readily as experts in their field.
- Marketing know-how to be involved more effectively with the "buying" public who inevitably supports us.
- Resource and fiscal management skills to help the practitioner become familiar with the "numbers" of his business and speak the language of business.
- Networking can expand the practitioner's influence, power, resources, and professional and personal fulfillment. Nutrition cannot be seen as a single narrow field, but one of many dynamic ones.
- Negotiating skills should be improved for power and effectiveness.
- For counselors, their level of humanistic care can be expanded through more expertise in behavioral and social sciences.
- Learn how to effect public policy and become active in the process.

2.   The use of high technology is growing, especially the use of computers (3).   Where there is high tech there must be high touch or we as humans will reject it (2). This means that we should have an appreciation for the use and timesaving capabilities of the computer, but we must never underestimate the importance of our interpersonal counseling skills.

3.   The quality of practice can be assumed no longer; we must generate proof of effectiveness and accountability (3).   No longer will our clients, let age, seniority, title, or education be the sole reason to hire a person—they want to see results.

4.   Wellness and the private sector will be the greatest areas of future job growth (3).   There are more people who are well and want to stay that way than there are ill people. Acute care will always be important, but more people are interested in good eating, healthy foods, sports nutrition, preventive nutrition, weight loss, eating disorders, and nutritional changes through the life cycle. Individuals are being encouraged to take more responsibility for themselves. Marketing to reach this public sector will become our professional challenge.

　5.　The age of information is with us (3).　Medical care is changing from curing the passive patient to offering information for self-help. The media wants information in nutrition as never before. Practitioners with speaking skills are in demand. The need for creative communication is paramount.

　6.　Competition to our "specialty" is growing (3).　Because of nutrition's new-found popularity, many other specialists and the lay public are looking to nutrition for their livelihood. Normal nutrition information is readily available. We must offer more. Our challenge today and in the future is to assume the roles that best use our expertise while we continue to learn and upgrade. Interpretation of nutrition information and application of food knowledge to the needs of the individual still seem to be our best professional niche.

　No amount of legislation, third party recognition, and marketing by the American Dietetic Association will make as much impact on competition as will our individual efforts where we work and live.

　Perhaps by recognizing these trends and thoughtfully evaluating our strengths and weaknesses, we will be able to participate more actively and mold our own futures.

THE FUTURE OF PRIVATE PRACTICE

Career avenues for dietitians in private practice who distinguish themselves will abound. The private practice career specialties that are considered up and coming include writing and speaking, consulting to hospitals on clinical specialties and in wellness programs, acting as sales representatives in business and industry, offering nutrition assessments in private offices, consulting at eating disorder clinics, consulting for corporate and commercial fitness programs, consulting on media, marketing, and food technology for food industries, consulting on kitchen design and management and the development of computer software. This is just a sampling of what diverse avenues the entrepreneurial dietitian can pursue. It can be recognized easily from this listing that experience and education outside of the required nutrition curriculum and traditional career settings may be needed to compete successfully in the future.

REFERENCES

1. Mescon, Michael, and Timothy Mescon: "Breeding the Corporate 'Intrapreneur,'" *SKY,* July 1984.
2. Naisbitt, John: *Megatrends,* Warner Books, New York, 1982.
3. Minutes, April 1983, Practitioner Continuing Education Advisory Committee to the Council on Practice of The American Dietetic Association.
4. Williams, William, insurance expert, Third Party Task Force Meeting, Chicago, IL, June 1983.

chapter 2

Is Private Practice for You?

A private practice exists when a nutritionist decides to work as an entrepreneur instead of as an employee. The concept includes a variety of diversified businesses, all with the same purpose in mind—to promote nutrition and to generate a profit.

In his article, "Private Practice: On Our Own," Rodney E. Leonard states that his research found,

> Nutritionists who develop counseling practices in their community are independent-minded workaholics who believe nutrition is preventive health. They enjoy being around people and don't like working for someone else. They will speak on nutrition at the drop of a hat. They also are good managers who plan carefully, or they likely would not have survived the three to five years it often takes to develop a successful practice (1).

COMMONALITIES IN PRIVATE PRACTICE

Although there is wide diversity in private practice businesses, the majority of practitioners support themselves, especially initially, with one-to-one counseling. In private practice there is a shift in the type of nutrition information that is used most—from medical diets to "normal" or preventive nutrition with special emphasis in weight control. Many practitioners report that at least 70 percent of their clients have weight loss as a primary or secondary diagnosis. Other diets that are commonly seen include fat controlled heart diets, diabetic, and allergy diets (1).

Practitioners find that this business is seasonal with slack times occurring over the holidays and in late summer. It is important to remember that these times do exist. They are great times to plan your own vacations but good times to avoid when planning group classes, mailouts, and grand openings of offices.

A common feeling shared by private practitioners is that as their businesses grow, their relationships with other health professionals begin to mature to true members of the "health care team." The fact that the patient is being treated more for chronic problems instead of acute, life-threatening ones is surely one reason the interrelationships are less strained and more cooperative. As an entrepreneur, a dietitian can also devote more time to patient instruction and follow-up than is traditionally available as an employee and, therefore, the results with the patient may be far more impressive. Referring physicians, office nurses, and other employees become very supportive of effective nutritionists.

Another common idea shared by practitioners is the conclusion that the beginning pace can't be kept up forever. Therefore, the need arises to develop projects that will continue to bring in revenue without the consultant's constant input, such as in publishing, or by developing copyrighted programs and selling them or by hiring other professionals to help cover contracts.

Not for Everyone

A major point that needs to be made at this time is that you can't just assume that because you have good ideas, money, lots of energy, and the right credentials you *should* start your own business. If you have the above, you might also think about going into business and industry, sales, management, and other nontraditional employment avenues. As mentioned, good progressive corporations are starting to recognize the value of hiring more creative individuals who are looking for other career alternatives, but want regular pay checks and benefits.

Successful private practitioners agree that the positive aspects of being an entrepreneur far outweigh the negative ones. However, most people who have tried it and then stopped, state that, looking back they did learn a lot, but that the commitment had been too great for what they had to show. Starting a new small business is *certainly not for everyone* and it is *not* the only answer for professional happiness.

The negative aspects of starting a private practice are very real but certainly not insurmountable when a nutritionist does careful research, and develops well thought-out solutions. The fear of the unknown is often more paralyzing than what really happens.

In logical and practical terms the possible risks of being an entrepreneur can include financial and emotional insecurity (at times), a large time commitment, no paid benefits (retirement, vacation, sick leave, etc.), a financial investment ($10,000–$40,000 or more initially), family patience, and the need for more assertiveness, which is not comfortable for everyone.

MAJOR REASONS WHY BUSINESSES FAIL

The major reasons businesses fail include:

1. Not borrowing or saving enough capital to run the business and pay living expenses (2)
2. Not conducting a market survey or conducting a poor one that results in starting a business in a weak market or one where the competition is too strong; however, even a good survey cannot guarantee success
3. Not advertising or promoting enough to start sufficient money coming in (2)
4. Joining forces with the wrong business partner—the average partnership lasts less than two years. Partnerships take special understandings concerning time and money commitments, duties, and other shared aspects of running a business (2)
5. Lack of political and business acumen so that poor decisions are made that hurt your good efforts
6. Lack of hard work necessary to produce top quality output and rise above the competition
7. Especially for women, negative interference by the spouse or family disapproval can jeopardize their commitment to their business venture

FEARS

Dietitians who are about to start their own business report that one of their greatest fears is of "failure"—not reaching the degree of success that they feel would be considered respectable. If this is of great importance to you then some soul-searching to distinguish between what determines your self-worth and what constitutes an entrepreneurial venture needs to be made. Some of the most successful business people alive have had numerous business ventures that didn't succeed as they were originally planned. The mark of a good business person is knowing how to change in midstream and when to get out. A successful tool that business people and counselors suggest when fear has you worried is, ask yourself what is the worst thing that could possibly happen? If the business fails, you may have to get a job again and maybe pay back a loan. Is that so bad?

Other fears commonly shared by newcomers to private practice and some possible solutions include:

Marketing won't bring in patients.

   Solution: Conduct a good feasibility study to see if the service is needed. Talk to one or more marketing or public relations professionals for suggestions and for evaluation of your marketing program. Marketing professionals are familiar with how to "package" an idea or service so that it is attractive to your potential market. Traditionally, health professionals have looked at promotion, advertising and marketing as "commercialism" instead of a necessity for survival. Marketing should be aggressive, but tactful and in good taste. It is essential that adequate *money* and *time* be invested in marketing.

Q & A

Traits of Successful Nutrition Practitioners

What types of persons have succeeded best in their own businesses?

From my observation there are several similarities among the individuals who do best in private practice:

- They like working for themselves—that freedom is a high priority and overrides many drawbacks to working alone and financing projects themselves.

- Not only were they excited about what they wanted to try in their own business, but they were dissatisfied and disenchanted with what they had been doing.

- They are usually risk-taking, creative, self-confident, self-motivated individuals. The most successful ones do not blame anyone for what hasn't happened, and they feel in control of their abilities and potential.

- Most successful practitioners are intellectually curious and open to new ideas and methods of doing something better. They strive for short-term excellence on every project or they don't agree to do it.

- Probably most important is that the person has a strong desire to persevere and be successful. He or she is willing to wait through lulls and disappointments that discourage the less committed individuals.

Competition from weight clubs, spas, clinics, medical, and chiropractic offices is fierce in my area.

   Solution: In this situation you have no choice but to get to know the competition *well.* Find out what they have to offer, who actually does the nutrition counseling, and what they charge. Then, offer services that are *different* and *better.* Be distinctive: don't follow the leader. Market well, but don't ever feel that you can compete dollar for dollar—give public speeches and use the media. Also, very importantly, look at the competition differently—not as the enemy, but as allies that have (at their expense) educated the public to the value of nutrition. Your job is to establish yourself as a resource for *good interesting* nutrition information.

How do I know if I am being ethical and not committing malpractice when I am on my own?

Solution: Ethics and malpractice are not that nebulous. Ethics, honesty, and standards of practice don't change just because you are an entrepreneur instead of an employee. Simply, if you state the truth, do not misrepresent, and follow your patients nutritionally as your peers would in similar situations, you have little to worry about. (Look at Chapter 13 for more detail on these topics.)

I am afraid that I won't keep current without the input of other professionals around, for instance, in the hospital.

Solution: This can be a problem. However, since your livelihood will depend upon staying up with, if not leading, the times you must develop some solutions. First, join a local nutrition journal club or start one. Start subscribing to nutrition newsletters and journals or use a personal computer to do searches or access databases. Read the newspaper regularly and begin browsing through more business-related magazines and other resources. Start networking with other nutritionists both in the local area and on a national basis with the dietetic practice group, Consultant Nutritionists in Private Practice of The American Dietetic Association.

I've always had difficulty with getting organized.

Solution: This problem is extremely important, and it will take care of itself. You will either have to hire someone to organize for you or learn to do it yourself, if you want to stay in business. As a self-employed person you alone are responsible for your output; there isn't an employer or supervisor looking over your shoulder telling you what to do and when to do it.

Good time management is essential. Start a notebook and begin writing lists of things to do and then *prioritize* them and *date* them. Many people write lists, but fail to do the most important things on time because other items are easier or more fun.

I'm afraid people won't think I am worth what I charge.

Solution: The first consideration is to ask yourself what you think you are worth. Choose fees that you are comfortable with and ones that are equitable for the patient. Realize that you will be "worth more" as you become established and your reputation for good service grows. Constantly strive to improve your expertise, skills, and knowledge. When you are comfortable and self-assured, it won't matter if someone disagrees with you.

Will I be able to make a living in private practice?

Solution: You can give it a great try! It is strongly suggested that you become familiar with the problems of starting a small business and study small business management before taking the plunge. Also, allow plenty of time for planning, researching, and introducing yourself to prospective clients. Take time to save money before you quit a full-time job or commit yourself to the high overhead of business life. Many new practitioners find it beneficial to have several consultant contracts in addition to their therapeutic endeavors to help generate a more steady income.

I am afraid about having to contact physicians to build the business.

Solution: We are all afraid at times. But keep in mind that you are creating a service for the benefit of the physician's patients—you both have a shared common cause. Discuss your services in these terms with physicians. Look at business differently—as a game—you will win some and lose some. Not every potential client will be interested in your services, nor will every physician. To distinguish ourselves as true nutrition specialists we cannot afford to see ourselves as merely an auxiliary service only available to patients on the whim of a physician. Consider marketing directly to the public. Many practitioners feel that to see private practice only in terms of physician-referred, one-to-one counseling is outdated and self-limiting. We have important information that the patient/client needs and wants. Patient-centered care is our primary function.

ASSESSING WHETHER PRIVATE PRACTICE IS FOR YOU

As the saying goes, "If it's worth doing, it's worth doing well," so goes the effort put into starting a private practice. Just wanting to try it may carry you far, but how far and how well you go can be dependent upon how well you plan, organize, and carry out your "ideas."

Right now you may feel somewhat overwhelmed by the concept of private practice. The best way to overcome that feeling is by breaking down the whole into manageable tasks and smaller, simpler goals. Don't take time to worry right now about the business name or the color of your calling cards—that will come soon enough.

Philosophically, any dietitian or nutritionist can go into private practice, but the extent of your education, expertise, initiative, and personal abilities will be the deciding factors. You can develop the areas of business in which you are qualified, that you like to do, and that will "sell." Since you will be investing a lot of time in this project, it will make the time pass much faster if you choose projects that are "labors of love."

Evaluating Your Strengths and Weaknesses

It is important that *you* look at your strengths and weaknesses objectively. You need to know what your strengths are because you will want to capitalize on them and base a lot of your business decisions on them. Knowing your weaknesses will show you where you could be vulnerable. You can seek outside help to supplement or retrain your weaker areas, such as typing, public speaking, marketing, writing, etc. The less you are able to do for yourself, the more it will cost to operate a business. The cost of delegating responsibilities and retaining office staff must be weighed against the value of a professional practitioner's time in generating income.

Q & A

Private Practice Challenges

What is the most difficult part about starting a private practice?

The answer to this question varies with each individual, but some of the most common difficulties are:

- The fear of leaving the security of employment with its regular paychecks, fringe benefits, and close working relationships.
- For young people without assets or connections to obtain a loan, trying to start a business while underfinanced is frustrating and limiting.
- For practitioners who desire physician referrals, it is a common complaint that trying to get appointments with physicians is time-consuming, difficult, and sometimes frustrating.
- Time management is sometimes difficult for practitioners. Balancing income-producing activities (counseling, consulting to organizations, writing diet manuals, etc.) with the need to continually market and promote the business (interviewing for new consultant positions, working with the media, writing for exposure, public speaking, etc.), with the need for a good personal life is difficult.
- Some practitioners state that acquiring the discipline necessary to do the unfamiliar and uncomfortable things necessary to run a business is very difficult for them. Being assertive in negotiations, taking back printing that is not done well, handling difficult patients and physicians, firing poor assistants, and trying to please unhappy clients are not easy tasks, but must be carried out.
- The frustrations from the inconsistencies of private practice are sometimes more than a person likes to bear. Patients don't always show up for appointments, after you have driven across town to see them. Snow storms and holidays can keep you from earning a penny some weeks. Contracts come and go without much warning. Good referring physicians move or hire their own dietitians and stop sending clients.

Education   Whether or not a dietitian's nutritional education is adequate to function in private practice is dependent upon the individual's level of competence and continued learning. What seems to be lacking in our educational experience are business, psychology, and communication courses.

In a survey of successful practitioners conducted by editor Rodney Leonard, *The Community Nutritionist,* he found that

> Several of the nutritionists seemed to view their own educations with mixed emotions. All were aware of the importance of nutritional science courses, . . . but each expressed a feeling that academics left them poorly equipped to enter private practice. . . . If they had to do their schooling over again, they would choose a curriculum heavily weighted toward building communication skills and acquiring a basic knowledge of business practices. They would take public speaking, journalism, marketing, public relations . . . bookkeeping or accounting, economics. . . . (1)

As with most areas of study, nutrition students are taught a broad common core of information. At this time specialization is seen as a post-graduate endeavor. The challenge to the graduate is twofold: first, to glean and apply the learned information and, second, to continually improve and update knowledge and apply the new information. To help with this process, it is imperative that educators and The American Dietetic Association remain abreast of the changing needs of the practitioner.

Graduate education should open more varied doors in business and improve a nutritionist's marketability. Besides in nutrition, dietitians are taking advanced degrees in exercise physiology, communications, health promotion, food technology, or marketing, to name a few.

Practitioners do not agree on the exact role that an advanced degree will play in an entrepreneur's career. Some feel that it is "an absolute necessity" that provides an edge in today's professional world and competitive market. Others feel that advanced degrees are perhaps only important in clinical settings, academia, and government positions. Everyone agrees that a Master's or PhD will not compensate for a lack of ability, skill, or personality traits needed to succeed in business.

Reeducation is important when a dietitian has not remained current in the areas of nutrition that will be used in practice. Due to the growing nutrition awareness of the public and the sophistication of the competition, new business owners cannot afford to be outdated.

For dietitians who have not practiced for some time, do not underestimate what you know. However, you should consider taking updated dietetic courses, qualifying for dietetic registration (if you aren't registered), and perhaps working in a teaching or therapeutic setting for a while to refresh your education and improve your counseling skills.

Experience/Expertise   Experience and expertise can be gained in a variety of ways—from working in a family-owned business, working as an employee, working as a volunteer, or trying a business venture of your own. The quality of the experience and the degree of involvement are usually as important as the number of years, but adequate time and exposure are necessary.

Dietetic experience past the internship or master's level is all but mandatory to gain composure and practical nutrition knowledge and also to better understand those things not taught in school. People presently in practice have recommended two years to ten years of experience in a variety of dietetic positions before starting out on your own. In a report published by the New York Academy of Medicine, "Statement on Physicians in Private Practice and Referrals to Consultant Dietitians" it was recommended that consultant dietitians be registered or meet the educational requirements to be registered, plus have a minimum of four years of recent clinical experience (3).

Young dietitians should use their time wisely as they wait before starting a business. The time spent gainfully employed can be utilized to develop and refine programs and skills that can be marketed later. Organizations offer greater opportunity to work with well-financed programs, more printed literature, larger libraries of resources, and better client referral systems than you will likely have when you start your own business.

Commitment Limits   You will need to decide on the amount of personal commitment you want to have to private practice. Small business owners find that when they make the decision to start a business it affects everyone around them, as well as their normal household routine, their recreation, conversation, and family life.

There are some major questions to ask yourself and decisions that need to be made. Will you work at private practice full- or part-time? Will you try to keep your other job? Will you have an office in a medical or commercial building, share or sublease space, or try to work out of your home? How much debt can you handle? How comfortable are you with risk taking? If you have a family, how will you juggle your responsibilities there? Can you hire household help?

When determining your limits, recognize that having support for your venture from your family and friends can be very helpful on your road to success, but it is not impossible to succeed if you don't have it. Involving other people in your decision making may help solicit their support for your projects.

MARKETING YOU AND YOUR CAREER

Seldom will leaving your career to chance produce the results you want. Much effort has already gone into your education and jobs you've held, and now thought must go into deciding where to go next.

We often assume that successful people fall into all the good opportunities. Wrong! Successful people make their own luck and recognize an opportunity when it comes their way. Not every new venture works out. For every one that works, there may have been two or three that were only "seminars," training you for the "real" opportunity that will come along later. The key is to learn from each experience. Through trial and error private practitioners learn what works well for them, and their practices change accordingly.

In an article, "Managing And Marketing Your Career," Chicago employment agency president, Art Ritt, notes that,

> It is basic that you start from the beginning with the premise that you are not only going to develop a product that is highly marketable (your credentials), but [also have] a plan to enhance the value of that product as it progresses. As with all products, you must control the quality and quantity of the ingredients, package it properly, and determine who would be most interested in buying the package you are developing (4).

Take the time to plan the steps you want to achieve and then evaluate if you need to improve your experience or education.

Once you have an idea of where you are going and how, develop an attitude of short-term excellence as a means to your end objective (4). People and their businesses are highly valued when they continually produce work of high or excellent quality. Never look upon a job that you do as a "stop-gap" until your "big break" comes along. The opportunity to do something bigger or better often comes along because of the reputation you have for doing any job well.

On packaging your skill, Art Ritt states,

> Many excellent products have not sold because of unimaginative and inferior packaging. Your individual packaging will be made up of many variables, including personal appearance, personality, attitudes, etc. Your resume and credentials will get you in front of your consumer, but the packaging attributes will close the sale (4).

You are the only one managing your career. Its growth will come from your use of sound judgement and aggressive marketing. (See "Becoming a Consultant," page 290.)

PREPARING FOR PRIVATE PRACTICE

If you decide that private practice is for you, you must prepare to meet the challenges ahead. Changing from being an employee into an entrepreneur and adventurer can create excitement, as well as stress. Understanding some of the changes that will occur may make them less stressful, and you more productive. Doing your homework so you are ready to confront the project of starting a business will improve your chances for success.

The Stress of Innovation

Trying something different, whether good or bad, creates stress. Stress is not negative or positive except in terms of how each person chooses to handle it. Some individuals thrive on change in their lives and will put up with the accompanying stress just to have the change. Others like the status quo, and work very hard *not* to allow change to disrupt their routines. Most of us are somewhere in between—we want some change to add variety to our lives but not so much that we feel we have lost control.

Common changes that are shared by private practitioners follow:

- Money takes on a new meaning. New business owners learn that to survive they must generate income in excess of expenses. In the beginning you may have to do boring consultant jobs just to keep money flowing regularly. Fun, creative work with great future financial potential may have to take a backseat to immediate revenue producing projects. Or, if you have the collateral, a loan could be obtained to finance the business while the creative project is completed and readied for marketing.

    Dietitians who have trouble asking people to pay a fee for services soon learn to ask. Responsible people expect to pay an equitable price for goods or services. They often ask what the arrangements for payment are if you don't offer the information, so don't shy away from the subject.

- Family and friends may feel threatened by the loss of time and attention given to them. Starting a private practice is time consuming. And more significantly, as you become excited about what you are creating, you will want to work more. Families and friends don't always understand nor are they always empathetic to your new-found work. In your excitement it may be important to reevaluate your priorities and the amount of time allocated to each so that you are able to work without undue pressure from outside.

    Speaking of pressure, it is a good time to bring up the fact that sometimes well-meaning spouses and friends act like stage mothers to the new entrepreneur. They want to live out their dreams of success through you. Their lists of suggestions and projects can be so numerous and sometimes so grandiose that you can become overwhelmed or rebellious.

- New business owners soon learn to research all angles and ask for a lot of advice before making a decision. Pride should not stop someone from coming up with the best solutions. No one expects a person who is new to business not to make any mistakes. But, there is no excuse for repeated blunders when there are so many people and resources available to help the new business person.

Looking for Resources

Research your local area to see what resources and counseling services are available to you. Continuing education courses and business-oriented classes are available at colleges, universities, adult education, the Internal Revenue Service, banks, and the YMCA or YWCA. You may consider seeing a career counselor, going to a testing service, or consulting with another private practitioner (see Chapter 24).

The Small Business Administration also offers classes, materials, and counseling services through their two programs SCORE (Service Corps of Retired Executives) and ACE (Active Corps Executives). These two programs will work to match you with a retired or active business person who will be available to answer your business questions. You may keep requesting new advisors until you are satisfied with the match-up, and many entrepreneurs are very happy with the quality of the help.

The American Dietetic Association and the Consulting Nutritionists Practice Group have developed seminars, study kits, and publications to help the practitioner develop new career avenues. ADA is becoming more active in pub-

PATRICK & BEATRICE HAGGERTY LIBRARY
MOUNT MARY COLLEGE
MILWAUKEE, WISCONSIN 53222 **19**

lishing or copublishing materials written by members. As an added bonus, it is usually possible to apply for continuing education credits for much of the course work and the seminars you attend in preparation for starting a business. The opportunity to network is invaluable.

The local Chamber of Commerce can give you demographic information about your office area. Realtors can advise you concerning rental space, city areas of new growth, and going property costs. Local professional groups of business owners often sponsor meetings, offer network systems and good referrals for reasonable legal work, printing, accounting, etc.

In looking for financial resources, consider the following: using your own money, borrowing against your savings or other collateral, taking out an unsecured loan, borrowing from a silent partner, friend, or family member, or bringing in a partner with money, or finally, incorporating and selling stock. Several of these options are not highly recommended, but they do exist (see Chapter 7).

Use Your R.D. and L.D.

The major competition to a private practitioner's business is not from the ranks of our own profession. It is from the public sector and from other professionals with letters after their names, such as Ph.D., N.D., D.O., M.S., R.N., M.D., etc. Some of these individuals are qualified in nutrition, but most are not. Most have legitimate degrees, but some do not. No wonder the public is confused about whom to go to with their nutrition questions!

The one trademark that no one else can use, except a qualified individual is R.D. for Registered Dietitian. It denotes a level of competency past the college level, passing a competency exam, and maintaining a certain level of continuing education. As the public becomes more aware of how to determine whether a person is qualified in nutrition, it will not be unusual to be asked if you are a Registered Dietitian.

The letters L.D. for Licensed Dietitian can also be used by legally licensed practitioners. Licensure is being passed by some states to help protect the public from unqualified people giving out nutrition advice.

The use of the letters C.N. for Consulting Nutritionist is not recommended by The American Dietetic Association. Since there are no standards of practice at this time to determine or control the use of the letters, anyone can legally use them, and their use cannot be legally protected. Using additional letters after your name connotes credentials, advanced degrees, or competence of a certain level— paying dues and belonging to an organization is not recognized as sufficient criteria for using letters.

Talk to People/Start Improving Visibility

When starting a business it helps to let other people know who you are and what you are planning to do. Word of mouth is one of the best sales tools you can have. To help generate good will and curiosity in people, offer to give public speeches and seminars. Contact the local media and offer to be available for programming (see Chapter 22 on this subject first, however). Visibility and credibility can be established in your community without risking your present position or committing yourself to much overhead expense.

Improve Your Resume

A private practice may take you into unfamiliar territory and you will need to be able to advise people of your credentials and experience—a resume or curriculum vitae can help.

A resume is more than a chronological listing of your job experience. It should also help the reader understand your career objectives, the highlights of your professional life, and what skills you have developed because of the experience. The resume should be neat, well typed and reproduced by a high quality machine. A resume must not require intense concentration, but be easily understood.

To write a compelling resume requires making decisions in a logical order:

1. Boldly at the top of the resume, state your name, address, and phone number (both office and home can be included).
2. Next determine if you want to state a professional *Objective*. If you do, write it in one clean phrase. For example, "Seek to develop a private practice in Nutrition." An objective is not mandatory and you may feel it is too limiting or not specific enough for a desired position. You may decide that it will take more than one resume to cover your different career interests. For example, one to highlight your counseling experience and one your media expertise.
3. Next, for people who have had several uninterrupted years of experience in the same field, simply state the objective and show the appropriate *Experience*. But for people who are changing their career emphasis or who have intermittent experience it may work best to provide a *Summary* first before mentioning experience (5). The *Summary* would include what you would like to emphasize from your entire years of experience. The term *Relevant Experience* would follow appropriately, and you simply choose and describe those jobs which are applicable. Describe your special skills and abilities in a way that will highlight your uniqueness (6).
4. "If you are straight out of school, the *education* section should come before the *experience*. However, if you have some solid work years behind you, put the *experience* first," suggests Randy Ring in an article "Resumes Revisited" (5).
5. Experts state that the *Personal* section of a resume should not contain information that may bring out personal biases in the reader. It can work against you. If you feel so inclined, add a *Personal* section that includes your date of birth, 'Excellent health,' 'Willing to travel or relocate' (if that's true), and possibly your availability date (5, 6).

There are no hard and fast rules on the length of a resume, but it is strongly suggested that it be condensed to one to three pages. (See Figure 2.1 for a sample resume.) A Curriculum Vitae can run more pages and is specialized for the

Figure 2.1　Sample Resume

RESUME

Sandy Ritter　　　　　　　　　　　　　　Home Phone: (216) 597-6620

47 Maple Avenue　　　　　　　　　　　Office Phone: (216) 432-4321
Cleveland, OH 44111

OBJECTIVE

To start a private practice in nutrition and specialize in weight loss programs, sports nutrition, and consultation to corporations.

SUMMARY

Have a background in programs for the public. Situations include the development of an outpatient nutrition clinic while at St. Anthony Hospital, consulting for a local cardiology and fitness center, and conducting weight loss classes at the YMCA and Sporting House.

PROFESSIONAL
EXPERIENCE

Outpatient Clinic Dietitian, St. Anthony Hospital, Cleveland, Ohio, February 1982 to present.
　　Duties have included full responsibility for the coordination of the clinic nutrition program. This involves scheduling of patients, diet instructions, writing reports, budget design, and working closely with physicians.

Nutrition Instructor, Howard Cardiology/Fitness Center, Cleveland, Ohio, June 1983 to present.
　　Duties include interpretation of nutrition data, prescription of diets, and client instruction. Also conduct monthly nutrition seminars for new clients.

Nutrition Instructor, Central YMCA and Sporting House, Cleveland, Ohio, August 1984 to present.
　　Duties include conducting ongoing weight loss classes two nights a week along with a psychologist and exercise specialist.

Therapeutic Dietitian, Harlan City Hospital, Harlan, Illinois, March 1979–February 1982.
　　Duties included instruction of patients on medical diets, supervising meal service on floors, and conducting prenatal classes in nutrition.

EDUCATION

Internship, Beth Israel Hospital, Boston, Massachusetts, 1978.
B.S., Federal City College, Washington, D.C., 1977.

AWARDS

Recognized Young Dietitian of the Year, Illinois, 1981.

Figure 2.1 *(Continued)*

MEMBERSHIPS   The American Dietetic Association
               Ohio Dietetic Association (Community Nutrition Chairman,
                  1984–1985)
               Cleveland Dietetic Association
               Nutrition Education Society
               Consulting Nutritionist Dietetic Practice Group, Council on
                  Practice of the American Dietetic Association

References and additional information available upon request.

---

academic fields. For purposes of introduction when you speak, it may be beneficial to write a one page, double spaced, typed narrative about yourself (see Figure 2.2).

Take Time to Be Creative

A final exercise that may be beneficial to develop before starting private practice is taking time to let your mind be creative. Creative people are sometimes perceived by others as wasting time and energy, and as being "different." Creativity helps a small business owner to compete in the marketplace and to enjoy the labors of the business more fully.

Some suggestions on how to develop your creativity include:

1. Don't allow barriers, such as money, time, resources, etc. stop your free flow of ideas on how a project could be developed—reality can be dealt with later after the full potential of the idea has come forth.
2. Associate yourself with other creative people who encourage you to try new ideas.
3. Keep a note pad with you so you can write down any new idea as it comes to you.

Figure 2.2 Sample Personal Summary

MARY JONES, R.D.
PERSONAL SUMMARY

Mary Jones is a Registered Dietitian who is a graduate of Georgia State University and St. Mary's Hospital in New York City. She lives in Baltimore, MD, where she is known as a specialist in cardiac nutrition and as an innovator in the field of fitness. She is the author of two booklets on nutrition and fitness and is presently working on a book for young women athletes. Ms. Jones is a member of the Maryland Governor's Council on Physical Fitness and the Sports and Cardiovascular Nutritionists dietetic practice group of the American Dietetic Association.

4. If you get "stuck," change your pace, or the room where you work—go do something fun and let the project drop for awhile (7).

Creativity does not come on demand. Nor will it usually come when you leave time aside for it. However, it is beneficial to take time for yourself—even a few minutes a day—to relax and develop free-flowing ideas.

LEAVING YOUR OTHER JOB

How you leave your present job or how you handle your job while you start a private practice on the side can be very important professionally. Your reputation either will precede or follow you in your new venture, so the past is never really gone. Try to leave as amicably and cordially as you can.

If you are starting a business on the side it is definitely suggested that it be "on the side." Do not create hard feelings or get fired because you used the photocopier to print all of your diets or solicited patients up on the floors of the hospital. Also, be aware that many employers consider starting a private practice after hours as moonlighting, or conflict of interest, and it may jeopardize your job. Several clinic dietitians have found that their employers were less than understanding when they established part-time private practices in the same community and offered services that competed with their clinic services. That is not a smart move. Put yourself in the employer's spot—wouldn't you make the dietitian decide which job she or he wanted more? It would have worked better to be in a different community or to offer excellent, but noncompetitive services, such as group weight loss classes with a psychologist and exercise specialist or diabetic cooking classes. Your reputation and goodwill toward you will grow as you become known for your private practice services, and your identity, separate from your employer, will grow.

A common question dietitians ask when they quit their jobs is "What is mine when I quit?" Generally, the rule of thumb is: intangibles probably are yours (including the names of your contacts); tangibles (patient records, the Rolodex, etc.) probably are not. If you invented something on your salaried time, it belongs to your employer usually, unless you have another agreement. If you have written materials that you want to use later in your private practice, rewrite them, improve on them, and print them differently.

A former employer cannot keep you from practicing your profession—unless you signed a noncompete contract—and that must still be within reason. One practitioner reported that the food service company she worked for had her sign a contract when she first started. It stated she could not work as a dietitian for anyone for five years within a 100-mile radius of the large metropolitan area where she lived. That may be considered a restriction of trade, and it may not stand up in court for two reasons: First, it is an unreasonable length of time and geographical area for the employer to assume a former employee could compete with the company's business; second, usually a former employee can be asked not to solicit business from his former employer's accounts, but can't be asked not to solicit from every account in the entire area. A good suggestion would be to

Q & A

Business Option

Is there any way I can go into business and not "jump in with both feet"?

Yes, you can work for someone as a consultant or sublease space and never establish your own freestanding office. The other person can take phone calls, schedule appointments, collect the fee, and pay you a percentage, a flat rate, or a retainer fee.

To make the business grow you will still need to introduce yourself to the staff and market constantly. Also, market to the potential clients and never let anyone forget that you consult there. Try to get exposure in the local community and in the media. Don't assume that someone else will do this for you.

Q & A

Increasing Revenue

How can I make the most money in private practice?

There are four major ways to make more than average in private practice:

- Most obvious is to have the right personality, services, and "gimmick" to attract and satisfy a large segment of the market. In other words develop a high volume business.

- When you have the contacts, skills, and business volume to do it, subcontract accounts to other professionals.

- Produce something to sell that will continue to bring in revenue, such as, a book, teaching materials, computer programs, new food product, etc.

- Consult to industry instead of the medical community. If you have marketing or media experience, kitchen layout, or equipment design expertise, management savvy and reputation, or food technology know-how, use it as a consultant.

avoid signing such unreasonable contracts in the first place and thus avoid future problems.

REFERENCES

1. Leonard, Rodney E.: "Private Practice: On Our Own," *The Community Nutritionist,* Washington, D.C., July–August, 1982, 1:4.
2. Mancuso, Joseph: *How to Start, Finance and Manage Your Own Small Business,* Prentice-Hall, New Jersey, 1978.
3. New York Academy of Medicine: "Statement on Physicians in Private Practice and Referrals to Consultant Dietitians," 1979.
4. Ritt, Art: "Managing And Marketing Your Career," article from Ritt and Ritt Employment Agency, Chicago, 1981.
5. Ring, Randy: "Resumes Revised," *Women's Work,* New York, July–August, 1979.
6. Perry, Ellen: "Resumé Makeover," *Working Woman,* New York, June, 1985.
7. Hoffer, William: "Innovators at Work," *Success,* New York, 1985.

two

STARTING YOUR BUSINESS

Steps in Starting a Private Practice

Successful private practices have been started in many different ways and under a variety of circumstances. Some have been handed to the nutritionist by a physician, clinic, or client, while others were outgrowths of jobs, and still others were started without contacts or encouragement from anyone.

There are some basic stages and decisions that are common to most private practices. Those include: developing the scope of the business, determining resources, establishing an office, marketing, and determining client policies. The following chapters will discuss the topics in detail.

DEVELOPING THE SCOPE OF THE BUSINESS

Write a business concept about the business you want to start. It could be a one page, typed statement in narrative style that crystallizes your thoughts about what you want your business to do. You can use it to educate and inform your bank, lawyer, accountant, and anyone else about your venture. Not everyone is aware that dietitians can go into business for themselves. They are also unaware of where clients will come from and what the market potential is.

Conduct a market survey to help determine the needs and potential of your proposed business area. A formal survey can be conducted by mail or by interview, or you can talk to people informally and learn from the media. The major purpose for conducting a survey is to tailor the services you provide to fill the needs of your clientele. Other benefits that often accompany taking a survey

CHECKLIST FOR STARTING A BUSINESS

Date Completed

1. Business concept   _____

2. Market survey   _____

3. Business plan   _____

4. Lawyer: _____ Phone: _____

5. Accountant: _____ Phone: _____

6. Business consultant: _____ Phone: _____

7. Public relations: _____ Phone: _____

8. Financial backing: _____

9. Location: _____

10. Plan for large expenses: Amount/Source

    Furniture   _____

    Scale   _____

    Calipers   _____

    Stationery   _____

    Printed material   _____

    Insurance   _____

    Telephone installation _____

    Answering service   _____

Date Completed

11. Establish fees   _____

12. Develop promotion campaign   _____

13. Develop appointment schedule   _____

14. Devise chart system   _____

15. Collect and/or write teaching tools   _____

include generating interest in your future business, or you may find an office space or develop contacts that will be invaluable in the future.

Prepare a business plan or business prospectus, a comprehensive evaluation of your business's potential, including strong and weak points. It will help you better decide the direction of your energies, the ranking of your priorities, and your immediate and long-term business goals. This is a necessary tool for making financial agreements with investors, banks, or other lenders.

DETERMINING RESOURCES

Interview professional advisors to ascertain whether they would be of benefit to you and your business. Advisors should include a lawyer who would advise you of any legal needs for your business. An accountant can set up or review your proposed bookkeeping and tax procedures. A public relations specialist could advise you on brochure and calling card design and promotion ideas. A small business advisor may be of benefit to you for overall guidance and direction. Don't be afraid to interview several professionals from each specialty.

Financial backing to start your business will be necessary. It can be your own money or someone else's. Inadequate capital is one of the major reasons that businesses fail. Poorly financed businesses usually take more time, effort, and commitment before the owner sees a profit. The amount of money needed to start a business can vary greatly depending mainly upon the office space chosen, the marketing budget, the quality of handout materials, as well as the type of telephone coverage.

Collect materials and write instructional forms and booklets that you will use to distinguish your services or business. Subscribe to lay periodicals or nutrition/health newsletters that may be of benefit to you. Order booklets, pamphlets, or other handout materials in modest amounts until you know which ones you will use regularly.

ESTABLISHING AN OFFICE

Evaluate office locations to determine the financial commitment you want to have and the image you want to portray. You will have to decide whether you want to work out of your home, rent a full- or part-time office, or share space with another professional. Numerous other decisions can be made after your office locale is determined.

Establish office policies such as your fee schedule, office hours, and the days of the week you will see patients and those you will use for marketing. A telephone can be ordered and arrangements made for either an answering service or recording machine to cover the phone when you aren't available.

Legalities involved in setting up an office and business include checking zoning, signing a lease, obtaining any licenses for your local area, and filing a Trade Name affidavit or Fictitious Name form, if needed. Other decisions include whether to incorporate or not and the types and amounts of insurance to carry, including malpractice, office liability, health disability, fire, and theft.

MARKETING

Determine the marketing plan for your business. Another major reason businesses fail is that they don't market themselves enough. Just opening up your doors for business and telling a few doctors about it will usually not work. An organized program of ongoing promotion and advertising directly to your target markets should be developed for your business. The budget needs for marketing may be as high as 15 percent of your total budget the first year and 5–10 percent or more of the total each year thereafter.

Print promotion and marketing materials could include business cards, brochures, letterheads, and envelopes. Many private practitioners have logos printed on notebooks to hand out for the patients' diets, introductory letters printed to send out to physicians and clinics, and "thank you for the referral" letters to send back to physicians. A business card should be routinely enclosed with all correspondence. Brochures and cards should be offered at all speaking engagements and to your patients.

Announce you are open for business. Send out announcements to physicians, clinics, health agencies, or other potential referral agencies or clients, as well as other dietitians. Join speakers' bureaus in your area through your dietetic organizations, womens' clubs, libraries, or other agencies. Offer to speak for community and church groups. Contact the local media to see if you could offer your expertise.

DETERMINING CLIENT POLICIES

Establish office procedures to ensure that appointments can be made easily. Try to impress patients with the nondietetic functions of your office. Phone coverage for your business must be efficient and callbacks should be timely. Personalized care must begin when the client first calls to either inquire about your services or make an appointment. Charts on patients should be available at each visit. Billing should be at the time of the patient's visit. Bookkeeping can be very simple, especially for a small business.

Instruct patients or consult with clients and work to let them know that they are important to you. Produce the extra effort for them so that your services are well respected and your reputation grows. A nutrition instruction, speech, project, or other item you produce should include not only the common information, but also some of the lesser known facts and some definite flair.

Follow patients or clients well and try to always keep doors open to them. Network not only with other dietitians, but also with persons in related fields. Networking allows you to learn from others with more expertise or similar problems. Whenever a client or patient is referred to you, be sure to acknowledge the referral and encourage more.

Assess your business regularly and determine what ideas and programs are selling, which ones you want to keep because they are satisfying, if not profitable to you, and which items must be changed or dropped. Sometimes it may be that more time, effort, or money must be given to a project to make it work. However, putting more money into a poor idea has been a problem many businesses have had to recover from. The marketplace is constantly changing, therefore to compete you must evaluate and improve what you have to offer.

CONCLUSION

The best rule of thumb in determining what your business should offer and how, is to ask yourself and others, "what would impress you?" Which office location would be the best considering all the pros and cons? Do you think an answering service is worth the extra money? How fancy do the business cards and brochure need to be? What kind of advertising best projects the image you want your business to have?

chapter 3

Writing a Business Concept and Plan

Business consultants agree that before a potential business owner goes far he should first put his plans in writing and then do some research on the feasibility of his future venture. These tools are often called the *business concept* and the *business plan,* respectively. Their purposes are to share information, find problems, organize the business development, and raise capital.

Unfortunately, it is not rare for a future entrepreneur to be so sold on an idea for a new business that he is totally blind to quite obvious reasons why the idea will have a poor chance at success. Some examples are locating the business too far from the *buying customer* or too close to the strongest competition—a nationally known hospital with a free clinic—or wanting to become a nutrition consultant to only Greek restaurants. Although these ideas have a chance of working, they may take too long before adequate income is generated.

An experienced business person or professional advisor could look over the concept and plan and perhaps find overlooked problems. Having your ideas clearly stated will also help reduce the amount of time needed by paid advisors to assess your business needs. Many banks and all potential venture capital investors will request this information when considering a loan. All in all, business people take the time to prepare these documents because they are useful, provide insight and give the appearance of having one's act together.

BUSINESS CONCEPT

The proposed scope of your business—what you will sell, to whom, where, how, when—can all be stated briefly in the business concept. Ordinarily, one typewritten page is sufficient to convey a business overview (see Figure 3.1).

Figure 3.1 Sample Business Concept

Diet Control is designed as a profit-making counseling service created by Jill Smith, R.D., to help improve the dissemination of good, sound nutrition information to the public.

Nutrition consultations with clients and contracts with wellness programs at corporations will be Diet Control's major sources of revenue. Other services will include group weight loss classes, cooking demonstrations for special diets, and public speaking. Educational materials and teaching programs will be developed and published for use with the clients and for sale to other consulting nutritionists. All materials will be copyrighted and owned by Diet Control.

Market research has indicated that the local public is very interested in nutrition. Also, 23 physicians in this area will regularly send patients for nutrition counseling. Comprecare Health Program has signed a letter of agreement for nutrition consultation 15 hours per month (copy enclosed). Negotiations are pending for two industrial wellness programs that want nutrition services for their employees.

To promote this new business, the *Daily News* has agreed to write an article. Interviews have been scheduled on KOA-TV and KDEN radio. Weekly advertising will be purchased in the *Sentinel* paper. When the office is ready for business, an announcement, along with a brochure and calling card, will be sent to 300 local physicians, wellness program directors, and community centers. The proposed grand opening is set for March 1, 1988, in the Brook Medical Complex, 1400 Jefferson Boulevard, Denver, CO 80214.

When writing the concept, think of it as a promotional description of your venture. Avoid unnecessary details and concentrate on the strong, salable points.

A concept is used successfully not only for a new business but also for new projects, for example, a proposed eating disorder class, a new food service concept for drug rehabilitation centers, or whatever. As a communication tool, the concept can actually serve many of the functions of a brochure at a fraction of the cost.

BUSINESS PLAN

A business plan is a document written to raise money for a growing company. It is a detailed document that evaluates the business potential and is used to interest lenders (1). By the time the plan is researched and written, you should have enough information to evaluate whether your business concept is viable and to better estimate how much the venture will cost. Again, like the concept, the plan can be used not only for new businesses but also for established ones and for new projects. The marketing survey (Chapter 4) will be needed to fill out the plan and to make a more accurate assessment of what will "sell."

Business consultants will charge from $3,500 to $15,000 or more to research and fill out a business plan, but you can do it yourself. A CPA can be very helpful with much of the information. Typically, a plan will be 5 to 30 pages long, but consultants report that they have seen ones with hundreds of pages when the project necessitated it. The important point is to cover the subjects well with pertinent information. The plan should be updated and changed as needed.

A banker or venture capitalist uses a plan to evaluate whether he wants to invest in your business. Your plan can help you organize your venture and set priorities for better time management.

In his book *How to Start, Finance and Manage Your Own Small Business,* Joseph Mancuso goes into great detail about what a plan should and should not include and highlight (1). He also shares results of his research on what items "sell" a venture capitalist or banker on a plan. For readers who seriously want to raise their business capital through outside financing, please refer to the more extensive explanations and examples in that book.

How a Business Plan Is Read

Although a business plan needs to be complete and thorough, the average investor only spends five minutes looking it over. Therefore the plan's layout and high-lighted information are extremely important. In his research Mancuso found that there are typical steps in that five minutes of reading (1,2,3).

Step 1. Determine the characteristics of the industry and company. Is this a growing market of interest to the public? Is competition doing well? Is anyone making a lot of money in this field? Could this company do well?

Step 2. Determine the terms of the deal. What is being offered in return for the money? How much is needed, and how will it be used?

Step 3. Read the latest balance sheet. Is the company making a profit or just scraping by? Are the income projections reasonable considering the balance sheet?

Step 4. Determine the caliber of the people in the deal. This step, most venture capitalists claim, is the single most important aspect of the business plan. The founders, board of directors, current investors, and professional advisors' names are scanned in hopes of finding a familiar name. The reputation and quality of the team are important.

Step 5. Determine what is different about this deal. This difference is the eventual pivotal issue for whether an investor chooses to back a business venture. Is there an unusual feature in the service or product? Nutrition is "hot" but are your programs designed to take advantage of it, are they exciting? Does the company have a patent or a significant lead over competition? Does the company's strength match the skills needed to succeed in this industry? Does the inexperienced owner recognize his limitations and have good advisors? Or is there an imbalance? An investor is seldom intrigued with companies that hold a marginal advantage over competing firms or products. Good ideas or products that are better than others will attract capital.

Step 6.   Give the plan a once-over lightly.   After the above analysis, the final minute is usually spent thumbing through the business plan. A casual look at product literature, graphs, unusual exhibits, published articles, and letters of agreement or recommendation support the argument for unusual enclosures. Although additional items seldom make a difference to the final outcome, they can extend the readership.

If the plan is rejected, it is customarily returned to you. When trying to interest a banker in your venture, it is not out of line to ask why it was rejected. If the banker wants to work with you, he may give you ideas on how to improve the plan or ask you to request a smaller loan or increase the collateral to secure the loan.

When an investor looks at the packages of business plans, Mancuso found that four elements determine which one is the chosen first: (1) company name, (2) its geographic location, (3) length of business plan—shorter ones are read first —and (4) quality of cover—interesting but not necessarily expensive (1).

Writing a Business Plan

A business plan is a personal document. Yet there are some common ideas that should be considered when writing a plan. The different segments of the plan can be written in narrative form, as an outline, or in numbered, highlighted points. The easier it is to read and grasp the significant numbers or unique features, the better.

The Table of Contents   The first step is to write a table of contents; a sample table follows (1,3):

  I. Introduction
 II. Goals and objectives
III. Action strategies
 IV. Business summary
  V. Marketing and sales
 VI. Competition
VII. Research and development
VIII. Management
 IX. Financial reports and accompanying explanations

The order of the table is not so important as what information is included and how the information is highlighted. Adding too much detail can be a mistake. All of the following points of explanation do not have to be included; choose those that fit your needs.

Supporting facts and figures
  I. Introduction (a paragraph or two)
     A. In a sentence, what is this business venture?
     B. What is the public's probable interest in this idea? How big is the market?
     C. What is unique about your idea?

II. Goals and objectives of your venture. What are your professional and financial reasons for starting this business? What accomplishments do you want to strive for? What objectives will help you reach your goals?

III. Action strategies. List the stages of growth and development needed first to open the business and then lead it toward achievement of its objectives and goals. What should be accomplished or completed by the first month, third month, and so on?

IV. Business summary
   A. Principal products or services. What are you going to sell? List your areas of strength as well as potential fields from the market survey that you would consider entering because they will sell well.
   B. Describe the unique features of the business and its services.
   C. Describe patents, trademarks, copyrights, or other trade advantages.
   D. Describe any trends within the business environment that might be favorable or unfavorable to the company.

V. Marketing and sales
   A. Describe the market. History, size, trend, and your service's or product's position in the market. Identify sources of estimates and assumptions.
   B. Who is the end user of your services? Describe demographically. How will they be reached?
   C. Who are intermediate referral agents (physicians, clinics, corporations, hospitals, etc.)? How will they be reached?
   D. Advertising: annual budget and media used.
   E. Is business seasonal?
   F. Customer primary motivation to purchase your services: price, performance, health reasons, and so on.
   G. Are any proposed government regulations expected to affect your market (DRGs, third party payment, etc)?

VI. Competition
   A. List major competition: their location, probable percent of the market, and strength and weaknesses. (It can actually be more impressive that other businesses are doing well. Your challenge is to do it differently and better.)
   B. Is new competition entering the field?
   C. Compare your prices with those of the competition.

VII. Research and development
   A. State any new field your firm contemplates entering. Is it complementary to what you presently offer? Are you planning to expand to health clubs or offer computer analysis of menus?
   B. Are you developing any new booklets, programs, or food items for sale?

VIII. Management
   A. Are resumes included?
   B. Are references included?
   C. List Professional Advisors.

IX. Financial reports (Ask a banker which reports he needs.)
   A. List projected start-up costs.
   B. Present pro forma balance sheets giving the effect of the proposed financing. What is your repayment plan?

    C. Show present and past balance sheets, tax returns, and profit and loss statements, if already in business or purchasing an ongoing practice.
    D. Yearly projections of revenues and earnings for five years.

This business plan should be considered a working tool, one that is just as valuable for internal audit as external promotion or fund raising. A well-thought-out business concept outlining your expectations for a private practice and a plan to implement those concepts are invaluable in translating your ideas into a successful business.

REFERENCES

1. Mancuso, Joseph: *How to Start, Finance and Manage Your Own Small Business,* Prentice-Hall, New Jersey, 1978.
2. *Guidelines for Raising Venture Capital,* from Corporate Financial Counseling Department of Irving Trust Company, 1976.
3. Brown, Cyrus: *Business Plan Package,* Technimetrics, New York, 1973.

chapter 4

Marketing

Too often we assume that with our good education and quality information, people who need nutrition advice will automatically come to a nutritionist. Private practitioners know that is not true! We need good packaging and promotion just like every other service or product on the market.

The biggest mistake most nutritionists make when it comes to marketing is that we don't do enough of it. Marketing includes finding out what people want or need and then filling that need. "Spend energies on making sure you have what people want!" (1). The goal is consumer satisfaction.

Successful practitioners report that it takes time for people to know you and your business. Later, when you are established, as much as 50 percent or more of your patient and business referrals will come from your past marketing efforts and growing reputation (2).

WE ARE NUTRITION EXPERTS

Nutritionists and dietitians are highly qualified professionals who have the right and responsibility to educate the public on nutrition matters. We are certainly more qualified than most trade book authors, magazine writers, and physicians to discuss nutrition. Letting other people know about your nutrition expertise may require more assertiveness than you are accustomed to using, but it may also assure you of future recognition, income, and personal satisfaction.

> People who are well want to stay that way. Since more people are in good health than ill health, our marketing direction and emphasis must change to recognize that fact.

The public both ill and well is very excited about nutrition and what it can do. People want accurate information. Marian Burros, former consumer reporter for the *Washington Post,* stated in an interview,

> When it comes to the really controversial subjects, like junk foods, empty calories, sugar-deceptive commercials, cupcakes and school breakfast programs, where are most nutrition educators? Talking about zinc and magnesium. By not speaking out, you make matters worse. How desperately we need you to stand up for what you know is right (3).

Sue Calvert Finn, Ph.D., R.D., marketing expert with Ross Laboratories, Columbus, Ohio, states that "a major reason dietitians seem to delay marketing is because we keep trying to refine or improve our product (our education and expertise) instead of using what we have while it's still useful and ahead of the field." Ms. Finn also adds, "Don't just create the opportunity and awareness for nutrition. . . . Go after or create the paying job to use the information. There is no right way to market, yet, there are a lot of successful people who know how to market" (1).

RECOGNIZING MARKETING OPPORTUNITIES

You may hear a successful person described as lucky, being in the right place at the right time, or knowing the right people. Some of these statements may be true, but there are people who have all the good things but are not successful, or had nothing, but did succeed. The mark of a successful person is one who recognizes opportunity when it appears and uses it to show excellence. He or she also turns obstacles into opportunities through hard work and innovation (4).

The most obvious method of recognizing a marketing opportunity is when you see needs not being met. If present nutrition services do not cover all needs, explore ideas to fill the void. Another common method is to identify situations where you could offer services that are better and different than those presently available. Opportunities also come knocking at your door, usually disguised as hard work. Given enough time, effort, money and innovation, an opportunity may blossom into an "overnight success" (4).

Timing is crucial to the evolution of new ideas. Given a fantastic idea, but the wrong time, you will be met with development resistance, high costs, and marketing barriers. Learning when and how to introduce new ideas is what businesses spend millions of dollars on each year in market research, public relations and sales training (4).

COMPETITION

No amount of legislation in the form of certification, licensure, or threatened lawsuits will ever be able to eliminate the mammoth amount of nutrition-related businesses that have sprung up in the last 15 years. A segment of the public is willing to pay for the promise of good nutrition and health, for quick weight loss at any cost, and for miracle disease cures. Nutrition products and services are a multibillion dollar operation. These companies have the money to circumvent or fight most legal battles. Many will, however, fail because of poor business management or poor products and fraudulent claims.

The point to remember is that these companies will probably always be a fact of life in our professional careers. The most effective way to handle them is to know as much as you can about them—their claims and their weaknesses. Listen to your patients who have used them and store the knowledge for possible future use.

Equally as important to recognize is the fact that many of the nutrition-related companies in America that do not employ qualified Registered Dietitians still give out very good, sound nutrition information. Some also do a fantastic job of developing materials and programs that educate the public. We don't own the only corner in the market!

The field of nutrition is becoming a very popular professional avenue for many health specialists, including pharmacists, chiropractors, nurses, dentists, and health educators. A Denver biochemist stated several years ago that he gave physicians five to ten years before they "invent" nutrition and start specializing in the field. An article by June Stevens, R.D., in the March, 1982, *Journal of the American Dietetic Association,* "The Coming Physician Surplus," notes that by 1990 there will be 70,000 "surplus" physicians looking for a way to support themselves (5). Even today a popular topic at medical conventions and in medical schools is new career avenues in wellness, sports medicine, nutrition, and preventive medicine.

Our professional uniqueness will suffer because of competition by other soon to be qualified and experienced professionals. This should not be discouraging news but instead a challenge! All it means is that we need to reexamine our education, our continuing competency, and the way we market nutrition.

Traditionally, clients have come to us upon referral, and since that may not be effective in the future, *consulting nutritionists should think about going directly to the consumer.* If a referral is needed for a medical diet, the physician could be called for his or her okay.

A private practitioner in Connecticut advertised weekly in three local newspapers for the eight years she was in business before retiring. She had so many patients that she worked six days a week just to see everyone. She, however, only averaged five patients per year who were directly referred by physicians. Professional referrals were not necessary for this practitioner to have a successful business. Of course other practitioners may have different experiences.

Local Competitors

Before doing a marketing plan, you will need to know something about your competition: Who is your competition? Whom are they selling to? How well are they doing? How strong are they in the market? What do they offer? Can you do it better or differently? A word of advice, don't always look at competition as negative. Their action in the marketplace, good or bad, may have increased the public awareness about nutrition and may make your job easier. That awareness also was given to you free of charge, but probably at great advertising expense to them.

MARKETING STRATEGIES

It is extremely important to the eventual success of a business that the owner decides upon long-term marketing strategies as well as short-term tactics (6). Short-term tactics lead you into the day-to-day decisions on whether you decide to consult at a renal unit or at a corporate health spa. Long-term strategies are a mixture of solidly reasoned projections and intuitive guesses about where your business should go in the future. What trends will grow and take your business along with them? What current nutrition trends and medical treatments will cease to exist in five or ten years?

Three major reasons why long-term strategies fail to lead a business into areas of growth and success are because the chosen strategy was for too narrow a market (consulting only to Greek restaurants), the competition was too well established (try starting another low calorie weight loss franchise), or the strategy was not flexible or did not adapt to the new marketplaces, and the services did not sell (6). Reevaluation of the market is a continuous process that will help keep the business operating and open doors to future opportunities.

The following five steps can help entrepreneurs in mapping out a total marketing strategy (6):

- Define the target market area(s).
- Research the customers' needs.
- Develop and/or redevelop your service(s) to meet the customers' needs.
- If subcontracting or expanding your staff, recruit and/or train personnel to deliver the service to the defined market.
- Develop the sales approach and advertising support necessary.

MARKET SURVEY

A market survey is conducted for a new or ongoing business in order to help determine the customers' needs. Many of us coming from medical backgrounds are uncomfortable when we say customers—it sounds so commercial. The truth is, it is commercial. This is a business—created to make a profit. To do that people must be willing to buy what you have to sell.

After completing the survey you should be better able to evaluate your business potential and refine your services to fit the potential markets. Because most small businesses do not have the capital to flood the media to create a "need"

Q & A

Marketing Components

I have observed that so many public nutrition programs sponsored by private practitioners, hospitals, and health departments are very poorly attended. What can I do to avoid that happening?

When developing a service or product to fill a particular consumer's need (your identified target), experts suggest that you analyze the four marketing components: product, price, place, and promotion.

Programs that attract large audiences are usually considered successful because their marketing components fit their intended target. The opposite is assumed (that one or more components did not fit), if the program or service didn't attract the target market.

I can use some personal experiences to illustrate these points. I was once paid to speak on sports nutrition to the members of a Nautilus fitness center in Ft. Collins, Colorado. The speech was scheduled for 7:30–9:00 P.M. on a Thursday evening in February at the center. Two months before the speech the person in charge of the presentation requested a 5″ × 7″ black-and-white photo, copies of sports nutrition-related newspaper articles that mentioned me, and my resume.

These requests and arrangements weren't unusual, but the results were. When I arrived I saw a program banner across the doorway and my newspaper articles on several posters. The staff was excited about the program and the local newspaper had run an article to promote the program.

The room was packed. There were no chairs so everyone sat on the floor or leaned against the walls and exercise equipment. As uncomfortable as it was, the program ran overtime because of the volume of questions.

The price was included as a member benefit, guests were $15 each. The place was convenient, but not especially comfortable; there was adequate space for free parking. The product (speech format, topic, and speaker) were of interest to this audience. And finally, the promotion was excellent in that it attracted attention, created excitement, and reached the intended target.

I once promoted a program for the public on normal nutrition at a local hotel meeting room and had dismal attendance. I wanted to see if the concept could work and I certainly found out.

The program was entitled "Preventive Nutrition" and offered a one-hour presentation by me followed by questions. Numerous handouts were offered. The fee was $15 per person. I encouraged preregistration, but people could register at the door (a big mistake because I had no idea if 5 or 500 were planning to attend).

The program was promoted each week for three weeks at noon during my nutrition segment on NBC-TV "Noonday" in Denver. I had been on the program every week for three years and had good response to any recipe offers or call-in segments. Over one million people watched the program daily. In addition I purchased a $300 one-eighth page ad in a large local newspaper and sent flyers to recent speaking engagements and other groups. Less than 30 people attended.

In my evaluation I felt the price and place were appropriate. However, the timing was poor because it conflicted with the first run of "Roots" on television. The promotion did not generate excitement. The program had a nebulous title and lacked a marketing "hook" or "handle" to attract the audience's attention such as a controversial speaker or topic.

In order to avoid these problems, carefully evaluate the marketing components for your projects. Evaluate each program and how it could be improved to attract and excite the target market. Develop promotion that exposes the target market to your message multiple times and through the use of different promotion tools. Make the promotion exciting, interesting, creative, and in good taste. Choose a price that is appropriate for the product and target market (see Chapter 7).

Finally, place the product so that the target market will think it is accessible. In other words a speech should be in a building or other location people can easily find. An inner-city hospital basement where parking is limited and a person's safety is at risk is a poor place for a nighttime speech. Another example might be for a consultant to be sure to have good telephone coverage. Business is sacrificed when the customer can't reach you with reasonable effort.

for their services it becomes necessary to determine what needs already exist and to fill those. A marketing plan then describes and organizes your plan of action.

How Do You Begin Market Research?

Without knowing it, you have probably already started your market research. Have you been watching to see if other nutritionists or weight loss programs are successful in your area? Have you discussed the possibility of starting a business with physicians, clinics, health clubs, other dietitians, clients, or any commercial businesses? If you have, then you have started to "test the waters."

It is highly recommended that you keep records of your contacts, plus their addresses, phone numbers, and other feedback (see Figure 4.1). Use the telephone book, Yellow Pages, professional mailing lists (usually sold for a fee), and what-

Figure 4.1   Portion of a Sample Market Survey

LOCAL PHYSICIANS
(G.P., Family, Internal, OB-GYN, Allergy, Ped., Endo., Cardio.)

1. Dr. Phil McCrady, 3402 Hampden   832-4218   G.P.

    Believes in nutrition care; receptionist (Gladys) gives out Lilly diet sheets;
    runner—prescribes walking for patients; will refer patients, especially for
    weight loss. GOOD CONTACT.

2. Dr. June McElwain, 34 Garden Center   427-6829   Family

    Believes in nutrition, but seldom refers patients out for it; has had some
    training; I will keep in contact. POTENTIAL.

3. Dr. Charles Jones, 8550 Zuni   429-8110   Internist

    Won't give appointment; secretary (Mary) states that he gives out all his own
    diets; St. Joseph Hospital dietitians state he is difficult—gives inconsistent
    care. DOUBTFUL.

4. Dr. Don Roberts, 155 Madison   832-8148   Endo.

    Wants to refer patients immediately; diabetic and overweight patients; good
    reputation; empathetic. GOOD.

5. Dr. Sheldon Wainwright, 453 Elmhurst   427-7171   Ob-Gyn

---

ever other sources you may have available to compile marketing lists. To evaluate
what the public will buy, keep an eye and an ear open to how your competitors
are doing, and what they offer for what fee. Look at the ads in the newspaper;
see what firms are trying to attract new business.

Whom Should You Include?

The private practice avenues you want to develop will determine the people and
businesses to contact or observe. However, there are at least five major target
markets; also other practitioners and competitors may be included in a survey.

   Public   The public at large can be studied by observing trends in the media
and advertising. Also, it can be reached through talking to people at clubs and
community, church, school, and professional organizations.

   Local physicians   Contact especially those trained as general and family
practitioners, internists, OB-GYN, allergists, pediatricians, endocrinologists, and
cardiologists. If this list is too large in your locale, eliminate the specialties that
are unfamiliar to you or that you don't want to pursue or reduce the size of the
geographical area where you will solicit business.

Clinics (government or private)   Contact cardiac, WIC, HMO, PPO, emergency, or family practice clinics in retail centers, dental, and so on. Don't just assume that they want an employee on staff. You may be able to generate a part- or full-time consultant position.

Private agencies   Contact visiting nurse associations, home health, wellness, mental health, dialysis, day care, alcohol rehabilitation centers and so on. You may have to sell and document the value of having a consulting nutritionist on staff, if it is not required by law.

Corporate   Contact employee health centers, food manufacturers, public relations firms, fitness centers, sports teams, restaurants, grocery chains, kitchen equipment manufacturers, and so on. When you want to write to a corporate account, call first to find out specifically what department and person the inquiry should be addressed to.

Other private practitioners   Inquire whether there is an organized Consulting Nutritionist (ADA) group in the area or state. Ask what their individual specialties are and for any words of advice. If you want extensive advice on starting a private practice, offer to pay for their consulting time. Ask, do physicians regularly refer patients? Is the medical community open to new ideas?

Competition   There are weight loss programs, chiropractors, physicians, and Ph.D.s who specialize in nutrition, wellness programs with nutritionists, and so on. Don't be afraid to talk to people who are your competition—they may offer a lot of advice, pro and con. Be careful to evaluate the validity of the advice.

Survey Methods

There are two major ways that are feasible for a small business owner to evaluate the market. It should be mentioned that you can pay someone to conduct a market survey for you; although a marketing specialist may charge several thousand dollars to do it, it is still an alternative.

Personal Interviews   Appointments can be made with physicians, clinics, and businesses to solicit feedback. Many private practitioners have found that the most common interviews are held in hallways, over a cup of coffee, or for a few quick minutes in an office or over the phone. Try to interview the top person if you can, but don't be discouraged if you are routed to the head nurse or business assistant—they often make many of the decisions and referrals. Personal contact with individuals helps build trust and confidence in you and your services.

Ask open-ended questions and try to offer concrete suggestions on how your service would supplement or improve their business's or clinic's function. Ask physicians, who presently gives the nutrition instructions, and if patients comply well. Ask businesses if they would be interested in a luncheon speaker, nutrition coordinator, media representative for their products, or whatever would be appropriate to the company's needs.

If you are unable to get a positive response for scheduling an appointment, ask the person quick questions over the phone. Make sure that you record the person's name, any referral names they may mention, and pertinent comments about the conversation.

Mail Surveys Many consulting nutritionists try to solicit feedback about whether clinics, sports centers, or physicians are interested in their services through a mail survey. It usually consists of an introductory letter that requests a personal interview and may include a stamped postcard response (see Figures 4.2 and 4.3).

The response rate is extremely variable ranging from 30 percent in smaller

Figure 4.2   Sample Letter of Introduction

755 Hartford Avenue, Suite 101
Middletown, CT 06457
(203) 922-5565

February 1, 1987

Dr. Nathan Roberts
155 North Madison Street
Middletown, CT 06457

Dear Dr. Roberts:

Your name was given to me by Dr. James Bowen. He felt that you would be interested in hearing about the service I offer.

I am a consulting nutritionist expanding my private practice into the North Middletown area. I have specialized for the past seven years in working with patients with obesity and eating disorder problems. I offer group and individual consultations and long-term follow-up to help assure compliance. Copies of letters of reference from Dr. Bowen and several patients are enclosed.

I will call you this week. Perhaps we can schedule a luncheon appointment at your convenience in the near future.

I look forward to meeting you.

Sincerely,

Mary Jones, R.D.

encl.

Figure 4.3   Postcard Response Sample

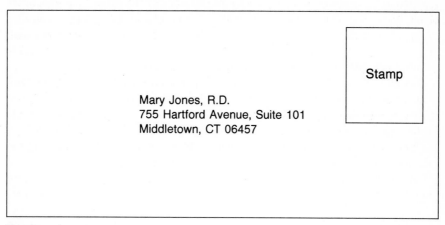

Stamp

Mary Jones, R.D.
755 Hartford Avenue, Suite 101
Middletown, CT 06457

Front

Dear *(Fill in name before sending)*:   Date

Do you presently offer nutrition counseling to your patients?

May I interest you in one or all of the following?

_____Personal interview

_____Brochure and calling cards

_____In-service nutrition training for your staff

Thank you for your time.

Sincerely,
Mary Jones, R.D.

Back

communities where the practitioner is known to about 2 percent in metropolitan areas. Such a low level of feedback makes the usefulness of this method doubtful in large metro areas. However, the fact that the response card was not returned does not mean that the letter wasn't read, or that the person had no interest in your services. You may receive feedback, but not in the time frame you established.

If you want to try this method, it is suggested that you call each target person's office to let them know that a letter and postcard will be coming in the mail, and that it would be of great benefit to you if the manager or physician did see it and took a few minutes to fill it out. Professional surveyors also suggest that a second phone call could be made to each office to thank them for sending back the card or to remind them to send it back. If you do not want to make the call yourself, have a friend or hire someone with a good phone voice to call for you.

U.S. Bulk Mail can be used to save money, when a practitioner plans to send out more than 200 copies (the required minimum) of a survey, booklet, order blank, and so on. If your time is too valuable to spend on this process, consider hiring a bulk mail service to do the mailing for you. Depending upon how much of the bulk mail process you decide to do for yourself, you could save nine cents or more per item when compared to first class postage.

Call your local post office to find the closest bulk mail terminal. The bulk mail center will sell you a bulk permit for $50 a year and give you the instructions, rubber bands, code seals and mail bags for the mailout. You will be responsible for having the bulk permit number stamped or printed on each item; for having all items separated by zip codes with rubber bands and seals; for prepaying the total mailing fee; and for delivering the mail to the bulk center. At the center you will need to weigh the mail and fill out destination slips and the mailing form (in duplicate so you have a copy). The process is not complicated, just time consuming.

From personal experience I found that as I became proficient at sending out bulk mailings, I also became terminally bored. I could not justify spending my professional or personal time doing the work, so I hired a secretarial service who in turn hired minimum wage labor to produce the mailout.

Get to Know the Area

Along with the above survey methods, start talking to people, business owners, and service organizations in the area you want to start your business and keep notes. Is the area growing? What is the mean income of residents in the area? Are there many hospitals or clinics that offer nutrition services to outpatients? Is rental space for an office readily available and affordable? Are there printers, typists, answering services, small local newspapers (to advertise in), and good professional advisors in the area?

MARKETING PLANS

Marketing plan components (1):

- Define product
- Define competition
- Identify and describe customer
- Identify and describe customer's needs
- Analyze market saturation and potential
- Analyze personal, professional, and support assets
- Set marketing goals

Marketing plans can be as detailed as you need (see Table 4.1). The main components are to identify the potential markets to go after, to list the competition, to identify, prioritize, and date the different tactics or tools you plan to use to reach that market, and finally, to estimate the costs. This plan should be

Table 4.1 SPORTS NUTRITION MARKETING PLAN

Service: Individual and group consultations, lectures, computer assessment, skinfolds

Goal: 15 hours/week at $40.00/hour net in 60 days.

	Strategies	Competition	Tools	Date	Cost
Sports Medicine Clinics					
Dr. Stanford's Clinic	*Sell idea that athletes will love it and it's individualized.	*Staff biases	*Call and letter	10/15	$45.00
Clinic for USFL Team	*Will augment present programs.	*St. Lukes Hospital Sports Medicine (nutritionist)	*Interviews	ASAP	Time, travel
Greenlief Sports Medical Center	*Will generate money.		*Proposal	As needed	$75.00 each
Alpine Sports Clinic	*Will give marketing edge in city to their program.	*Drs. Green and Brown (exercise physiologist gives info)	*Become speaker at sports conferences	ASAP	Varies, some income
Dallas Sports Center	*My reputation is known in the area—will be promotional plus.		*Contact local newspapers/media	ASAP	Varies
			*Develop booklet	12/85	$1,000.
			*Send articles to national magazine	1/86	Time, phone
Health Clubs					
Presidents'	*Will make them money by:	*Staff biases	*Call managers	10/15	Time
Racquet City	Programs presented	*No budget for it	*Interviews	ASAP	Time, travel
Spa Lady	Individual consults	*May want to pay as employee, not consultant	*Proposals	As needed	$75.00 each
Las Colinas	Attracting new members	*May want exclusive in the area	*"Brown bag" talks	ASAP	Time, travel
East Side Nautilus	*Gives new promotion tactic: Nutrition Wellness				
Sports Teams					

Source: Copyright, 1985 Kathy King Helm, R.D.

continually updated as it is used. It must be flexible enough to adapt to market changes.

Potential markets can be prioritized according to any criteria. Some potential markets will represent little challenge or excitement but will offer good steady income. Others can give your business a lot of exposure and notoriety (a sports fair or Governor's Council on Fitness), but little money. However, for public relations value they may still be worth putting at the top of the marketing list. Throughout their careers many successful practitioners say they continue to take high exposure-low paying jobs for the fun, public relations value, and to meet new people. Later, as your reputation grows, you can more realistically weigh the expected benefits against the amount of time and effort you must donate.

Good marketing ideas must be adequately financed and given time to produce. If an idea does not produce results or bring attention to your business, change it or try another.

Evaluating Your Results

After you have concluded your market survey you will know better than anyone else, including your professional advisors, which nutrition services will "sell" at what price to whom in the area. That is a wealth of knowledge and worth a lot. How much will sell is still only a guess, however. Your marketing advisor can help you prepare or review your marketing plan (see Chapter 6). The research can help substantiate loan requests, and plan your short and long term goals in the business plan (see Chapter 3).

This initial market survey is just the beginning of a continual awareness that you should develop for your business. The marketplace is always changing, and what sells today, may not next year. You should always be watchful of business trends, changes in the public buying habits, stories that make the news, and the economy, as well as feedback from your clients and physicians in forecasting market changes.

REFERENCES

1. Finn, Sue Calvert: Marketing presentation at the Alabama Dietetic Association, May 1985.
2. Leonard, Rodney E.: "Private Practice: On Our Own," *The Community Nutritionist,* Washington, D.C., July–August, 1982, 1:4.
3. King, Kathy: "Starting A Private Practice," Study Kit 3, The American Dietetic Association, 1982.
4. Marketing Manual, The American Dietetic Association, 1986.
5. Stevens, June: "The Coming Physician Surplus," Journal of American Dietetic Association, Chicago, IL, March, 1982.
6. Mancuso, Joseph: "What Business Are You Really In?" *Success,* New York, September, 1985.

chapter *5*

Legal Forms of Business Ownership

When starting your business, there are three basic business structures from which to choose. You can go into business as a sole proprietor, a partnership, or as a full or S Corporation (see Table 5.1).

The type of structure chosen is often vital to the success of a business. It can affect your ability to attract financial backing, what you pay in taxes, and the extent that your personal belongings are at risk if the business gets into trouble. The structure also affects the amount of control you will have in running the business and the amount of bookkeeping you must do. The more partners or investors you have, the more bookkeeping required (1, 2).

No business form is best for all purposes. A sole proprietorship offers freedom, but if a person needs money it may be useful to find a willing partner with the capital. At the same time, disagreement between partners on something so simple as how to spend the profit has undermined many new ventures. A corporation may require too much money and bookkeeping time to make it feasible for a very small operation. (See Figure 5.1.)

To organize your business in the most advantageous way, talk with a good small business lawyer at the outset. Because tax laws are in a state of flux, consult with a tax or accounting specialist. To help you and your advisors decide which form to use, it would be helpful for you to have made decisions about the ownership and financial support of your business. At least review the options and determine your resources.

To be recognized for tax purposes, whatever form you choose must be a genuine business—in other words, started and pursued in good faith to make a

Table 5.1   FORMS OF BUSINESS OWNERSHIP IN THE UNITED STATES 1980

	Proprietorships	Partnerships	Corporations	Total
Number of firms	12,702,000	1,380,000	2,711,000	16,793,000
% Total receipts	7.0	4.0	89.0	100.0
% Total firms	75.6	8.3	16.1	100.0

Source: Statistical Abstract of the United States, 1984

profit. This makes it different from a hobby or philanthropic work. Your work will be classed as a business if it produces a profit in any two out of five consecutive years, unless you can get an Internal Revenue Service ruling to the contrary. It is the Internal Revenue code, not local or state laws, that determines your federal tax and business status (1).

FEDERAL IDENTIFICATION NUMBER

To be registered as a business with the Internal Revenue Service, a Form SS-4 (see Figure 5.2, p. 56) should be submitted. This form requests a Federal Identification number and should be used when filing your taxes and when you are paid by a client, instead of your Social Security number. Local IRS offices can give you the form or your accountant will have it.

PERMITS, LICENSES, AND DBA TRADE NAME FORMS

In most localities, a person can do business under his own name without registering it with anyone. There are some places with local rules that require business permits, sales tax licenses, or various other documents that someone at City Hall and the County Court House can advise you about.

If you want to use a trade name or fictitious business name *other than your own,* an owner or partnership will probably need to register it at the county clerk's office or some similar place as a "fictitious" or Trade or DBA (Doing Business As) Name (see Figure 5.3, p. 57). This form lets people know that "Seattle Nutrition Consultants" is Jane Jones's business. This form may be necessary to obtain bank accounts in the business name or to legally bill clients in your county.

PROPRIETORSHIPS

If you plan a small, low risk private practice, and/or you do not own a lot of assets, a sole proprietorship may be your best bet. It means a one owner (or two spouses) operation. Although there are no studies to support it, this is probably the business form chosen most often by new private practitioners. The owner is responsible for all debts of the business, and he reaps all its profits. Other than for initial questions and occassional problems, a lawyer is seldom needed because a proprietorship really is without legal business organi-

Figure 5.1 Forms of Business Organization

(*Source:* Reprinted by permission of the U.S. Small Business Administration from *Starting and Managing a Small Business of Your Own.*)

WHAT FORM OF BUSINESS ORGANIZATION?

SOLE PROPRIETORSHIP

Advantages

1. Low start-up costs
2. Greatest freedom from regulation
3. Owner in direct control
4. Minimal working capital requirements
5. Tax advantage to small owner
6. All profits to owner

Disadvantages

1. Unlimited liability
2. Lack of continuity
3. Difficult to raise capital

PARTNERSHIP

Advantages

1. Ease of formation
2. Low start-up costs
3. Additional sources of venture capital
4. Broader management base
5. Possible tax advantage
6. Limited outside regulation

Disadvantages

1. Unlimited liability
2. Lack of continuity
3. Divided authority
4. Difficulty in raising additional capital
5. Hard to find suitable partners

CORPORATION (FULL)

Advantages

1. Limited liability
2. Specialized management
3. Ownership is transferable
4. Continuous existence
5. Legal entity
6. Possible tax advantages
7. Easier to raise capital

Disadvantages

1. Closely regulated
2. Most expensive form to organize
3. Charter restrictions
4. Extensive record keeping necessary
5. Double taxation

---

zation. It is the least involved of the business structures under the least government control (3).

Starting a Proprietorship

Anyone can start a proprietorship by simply stating that you are "open for business." Fill out a Form SS-4 to receive a Federal I.D. number. To legally

Figure 5.2 Application for Employer Identification Number
(*Source:* U.S. Department of the Treasury, Internal Revenue Service, 1983.)

Form SS-4
(Rev. 9-82)
Department of the Treasury
Internal Revenue Service

Application for Employer Identification Number
(For use by employers and others as explained in the Instructions.
Please read the instructions before completing this form.)
For Paperwork Reduction Act Notice, see page 2.

OMB No. 1545-0003 Expires 9-30-85

1 Name (True name and not trade name. If partnership, see page 4.)
2 Social security no., if sole proprietor
3 Ending month of accounting year
4 Trade name, if any, of business (if different from item 1)
5 General partner's name, if partnership; principal officer's name, if corporation; or grantor's name, if trust
6 Address of principal place of business (Number and street)
7 Mailing address, if different
8 City, State, and ZIP code
9 County of principal business location
10 Type of organization ☐ Individual ☐ Trust ☐ Partnership ☐ Other (specify) ☐ Governmental ☐ Nonprofit organization ☐ Corporation
11 Date you acquired or started this business (Mo., day, year)
12 Reason for applying ☐ Started new business ☐ Purchased going business ☐ Other (specify)
13 First date you paid or will pay wages for this business (Mo., day, year)
14 Nature of principal business activity (See instructions on page 4.)
15 Do you operate more than one place of business? ☐ Yes ☐ No
16 Peak number of employees expected in next 12 months (If none, enter "0") ► Nonagricultural | Agricultural | Household
17 If nature of business is manufacturing, state principal product and raw material used.
18 To whom do you sell most of your products or services? ☐ Business establishments (wholesale) ☐ General public (retail) ☐ Other (specify)
19 Have you ever applied for an identification number for this or any other business? ☐ Yes ☐ No
If "Yes," enter name and trade name. Also enter approx. date, city, and State where you applied and previous number if known. ►
Under penalties of perjury, I declare that I have examined this application, and to the best of my knowledge and belief it is true, correct, and complete.
Telephone number (include area code)
Signature and Title ► Date ►

Please leave blank ►	Geo.	Ind.	Class	Size	Reas. for appl.	Part I

conduct business in your area you may need a local license, permit, or Trade Name form filed. But otherwise, very little is required of you (1).

Taxes

At the end of the year your tax advisor can help you fill out and file the appropriate forms that briefly list your income and expenses and arrive at a net profit or loss. The IRS will look closely at your deductions, and whether it appears you are actively pursuing your business or just trying to write off your purchases and travel.

As a sole owner, your profits are only taxed once, as your personal income. The business profit is not taxed separately. A business loss can be deducted from any other income for that year. You will pay self-employment social security taxes. If you have employees, you will also pay payroll taxes, workman's compensation, unemployment tax, fringe benefits, and so on (1). A proprietor may invest in an IRA (Individual Retirement Account) and KEOGH (HR-10 Pension Benefit Plan) to help reduce his taxable income.

Advantages

Many practitioners choose the sole proprietor route in business because they like to have as much control as possible and have the option of making all the decisions. There are no partners or stockholders trying to lobby you, usurp your

Figure 5.3 Sample Trade Name Affidavit

(*Source:* Bradford Publishing, Golden, Colorado.)

Recorded at ___8 1 0'9 0'5 0 6 M.,___

Reception No.___

1981 MAY -4 PM 1: 48

Recorder.

County of Jefferson State of Co

STATE OF COLORADO,

County of **Jefferson** } ss.

KATHY L. KING ___ of the

County of **Jefferson**, in the State of

Colorado, being first duly sworn, upon oath deposes and says that

PRIVATE PRACTICE SEMINARS

is the name under which a business or trade is being carried on at **P.O. Box 5267**

GOLDEN, CO. 80401

in the ___ County of **Jefferson**, and State of Colorado.

The full first names and surnames and addresses of all persons who are represented by the

said name of **PRIVATE PRACTICE SEMINARS** are as follows:

KATHY L. KING

P.O. BOX 5267

GOLDEN, CO 80401

The affiant is (one of the persons) (the person)*carrying on said business or trade under the

above name.

Kathy L. King

Subscribed and sworn to before me, this **30**th day of **april**, 19__

My commission expires **april 22, 1985**

Witness my hand and official seal.

Jim L. Codman

Notary Public.

*Strike as applicable

NOTE—The foregoing Affidavit must be filed in the county in which any person, partnership or association of persons does business or carries on a trade in the State of Colorado under any other name than the personal name of its constituent members. The Affidavit is to be refiled for any change, whether by withdrawal, additional, or otherwise, of the parties represented by the name. Unless filed, suits for collection of debts may not be prosecuted and failure will warrant a misdemeanor charge which upon conviction carries a fine of not less than $10.00, nor more than $300.00. C.R.S. 7-71-101 (1973) et seq.

No. 298. TRADE NAME AFFIDAVIT. Rev. 79— Bradford Publishing, 15165 West 44th Avenue, Golden, Colorado 80401 — (303) 278-0644 — 8-80 power, or change the quality of service. If you do not like the way the secretarial service answers the phone or how your lawyer works with you—you make a change. This way of doing business can be very efficient and fast, with only one person making the final decisions.

A sole proprietorship can offer a business owner the opportunity to have the freedom to act out his dreams or wishes with only the obvious limitations of time, effort, and money. At least no person is in the position of changing your company name or the way you counsel patients unless you allow him to.

Many consulting nutritionists choose this type of business structure or an S Corporation because it is less cumbersome and less expensive to manage. Lawsuits can be minimized by being very careful and clear about all business agreements and by having them in writing. If a practitioner plans to have a business that publishes controversial exposés, pursues large contracts with other businesses, or in other ways handles large sums of money, or if he personally owns many assets, for peace of mind, another type of structure that limits the owner's liability may be more in order.

Disadvantages

The most obvious disadvantage to a sole proprietorship is the unlimited liability the owner must assume. An owner is personally liable for all the business' debts, its obligations, and suits against it. Your house, car, savings, and other possessions may be claimed by people who have won a suit against you. Additionally, your business assets are potentially at risk if you have personal debts that are unpaid. Malpractice insurance will cover you in case of a lawsuit against your professional abilities, but not for your business ventures, financial responsibilities, and unpaid bills.

Another disadvantage that many sole proprietors, especially women, experience is lack of credit. Credit is difficult to attract, both personal, from lack of assets, and business, due to lack of track record and business experience. Limited credit makes it hard when an owner needs extra money to expand into a new office, publish a booklet, or cover the cash flow when a big creditor does not pay on time (1).

A sole proprietorship's success is very dependent upon the abilities, energy, and output of the owner. We are not all good at all business functions, so we must be willing to delegate. Also, if the owner gets sick or has personal problems that affect his work, the business usually suffers. Should the owner die, the enthusiasm and knowledge of conducting the enterprise usually goes with him.

PARTNERSHIPS

Two or more people may begin private practice as partners. The advantage of this type of arrangement is that one partner may compleme:.t the talents or resources of another.

Often money, a broader base of expertise, or influential personal contacts is the ingredient needed. A partner may be a well-known person who will attract business. Legally, a partnership is a group of persons having a common business interest, each doing something to make the business succeed (2). However, because of internal problems, our mobile society, and changing partner priorities, the average partnership only lasts 18 months to 2 years (3).

Partners must get along well. They should be clearly able to do better as a team than they could separately. Partnerships take special understanding and a definite amount of patience. The biggest hurdles to work out are differences in value systems and expectations, lack of delineation of roles (partners step into each other's territory), and unequal contributions of start-up money (the major contributor may expect final say on all decisions) (2).

Successful partners often attribute their working relationships to the fact that they had talked about exactly how the business would run and what would be done "in case this happens" before the partnership was formed. Also, they had to accept that in many instances the "good of the business" had to prevail over their own opinions.

A partnership agreement should always be put in writing with the aid of your lawyer. The agreement should describe the proposed business in detail, and state the business name. It should tell (1,2,3):

- What each partner's initial investment will be, either in money or in other valuable consideration
- The percentage ownership of each partner, and how profits and losses will be divided
- How much time each partner will give to the business
- Who can sign the checks or if two signatures are required
- Who can sign contracts, incur liabilities, and sell assets
- What each partner's functions, duties, and powers are
- How the business will be managed
- What happens if a partner wants to get out
- How a new partner can be admitted
- Who will arbitrate if partners disagree
- How the partnership can be dissolved
- How the value of any partner's interest will be computed
- What happens when a partner dies, divorces, goes bankrupt, or becomes unable to function
- The size and nature of key person insurance policies to be carried

Financially, a partnership may be able to get bank loans more easily than a sole owner. Many times this is true just because the assets of two people instead of one are used to secure the loan.

The partnership must file a year-end tax return, but it does not pay taxes. The return is for information only, identifying each partner and showing her or his income and deductions from the partnership. The profit (or loss) is divided among the owners using preagreed-upon percentages. Each partner must attach a copy of the partnership's tax return to his or her personal one.

Partnership Pitfalls (1,2)

1. To be recognized as a partner for tax purposes, a person must actually contribute either money, time, reputation, or something else of value. A joint venture merely to share an office or other expenses is not a partnership to the IRS.
2. Conversely, people may sometimes be liable as partners even though no partnership agreement was drawn up.
3. Bookkeeping for a partnership can become complicated if the partners own different percentages or draw unequally for expenses.
4. Partnership income is taxed to each partner each year, even when the partnership decides to retain the profit for future expansion. Taxes may be owed on money that is never actually received.
5. A partnership is only as stable as its weakest member. Usually it dissolves if a partner dies or withdraws, becomes insane or incompetent, or goes bankrupt.
6. *The riskiest drawback is that every partner can be held liable for what the other partners do.* This means that one partner binds the other when she or he signs a contract or check. If an accident is caused by one partner, all can be sued. And if one partner is dishonest, all may be prosecuted.

Partnership Buy-Sell Agreement (2)

In case a partner wants to leave the business, a preagreed-upon Buy-Sell Agreement could help make the dissolution easier. The agreement should include the following points:

- A formula to determine the value of the business at the time of a sellout, taking into account initial contributions by each partner, assets, debts, and goodwill generated since the business start up.
- Terms governing the sale—for example, monthly payments over a 5-year period at 12 percent interest.
- Provisions in the event of death of a partner to protect the survivors against the estate of the deceased. To cope with the added expense of one less person running the business, partners should consider carrying insurance on each other.
- An agreement should be made up front before it ever becomes necessary to determine how deadlocked negotiations can be resolved—probably through arbitration.

Limited Partnerships

If a limited partnership is formed, the "limited partners" will have no personal liability for business indebtedness or the acts of their partners. To have a limited partnership there must be at least one "general" partner who is legally responsible for all business indebtedness and the acts of all general partners. A primary drawback to using a limited partnership, depending upon how you look at it, is the requirement that limited partners cannot play an active role in the management of the business or the partnership affairs. Limited partnerships are used

most often when the partners want to have some of the advantages of a corporation (limited liability) but pay income taxes as a partnership (1).

CORPORATIONS

A corporation is a legal form of business granted by states. A corporation can
be created from a new business or an already existing one (a sole proprietorship
or partnership). The corporate structure is the second most common business
form in America, but incorporated businesses generate over 88 percent of total
profits (see Table 5.1).

A corporation is a legal entity separate from its owners with its own property, debts, and responsibilities. Even though shareholders may own the corporate stock, they do not owe the bills. As a shareholder, your personal property
is not at risk for your business debts (1).

State laws differ on the specifics of a corporation, but generally a corporation is formed by filing articles of incorporation along with paying a fee to the
Secretary of State of any state in the United States (see Figures 5.4 and 5.5). The
records are checked to make sure that no one else is using your proposed business
name, and the forms are checked for completeness. If all is well, you will automatically be sent a charter (see Figure 5.6, p. 65).

The new corporation then issues *shares* of its total issue of *stock* (3). In a
closely held corporation only the owner(s), family, and friends own shares. No
shares are sold to others so that control of the business is maintained. Selling
shares is one way to generate capital to run the business, but because it dilutes
control and can complicate business as you grow, many advisors recommend
trying to borrow the money first. People who buy your stock take a chance that
the corporation will be successful; they do not have to be paid back if it is a failure.

The corporation name must include one of the three following words:
"Inc.," "Corp.," or "Ltd." It is required so that others will know they are doing
business with a corporation (1).

It is important that a business owner seek legal advice when planning to
incorporate. It is possible to incorporate your business yourself. However, if you
are sued or audited and the appropriate records and forms have not been filed
or filled out, it could be far more costly to remedy. Fees charged by lawyers to
incorporate a business can vary from $400 to $3500; check around to find the best
fee for service. The more you know about incorporation, the more you can do
for yourself; seek out information.

Some of the advantages of a closely held corporation (1,3):

- Owners risk only the money they put into their corporation. It can go
  broke, and the owners can stay solvent.
- The corporation generally has greater borrowing power than other business structures.
- A shareholder can transfer his part ownership to someone else instantly
  by selling it, giving, or bequeathing his stock certificates.
- Corporate federal income tax rates are below the top brackets for individuals.

Figure 5.4   Sample Articles of Incorporation (Colorado)

ARTICLES OF INCORPORATION
OF
DIET CONTROL, INC.

The undersigned natural persons, each more than twenty-one years of age, hereby establish a corporation pursuant to the statutes of Colorado and adopt the following articles of incorporation:

FIRST: The name of this corporation shall be Diet Control, Inc.

SECOND: This corporation shall have perpetual existence.

THIRD: The business and purpose of the corporation is to engage in and carry on the general business of nutrition consultation, public speaking, publishing and menu development. In furtherance of the foregoing purposes the corporation shall have and may exercise all of the rights, powers and privileges now or hereafter conferred upon corporations organized under the laws of Colorado. In addition, it may do everything necessary, suitable and lawful for the accomplishment of any of its corporate purposes.

FOURTH: 1. The aggregate number of shares which the corporation shall have to issue is 50,000 shares of common stock, each having no par value.

2. Each shareholder of record shall have one vote for each share of stock standing in his name on the books of the corporation and entitled to vote, except that in the election of directors he shall have the right to vote such number of shares for as many persons as there are directors to be elected. Cumulative voting shall not be allowed in the election of directors or for any other purposes.

3. At all meetings of shareholders, a majority of the shares entitled to vote at such meeting, represented in person or by proxy, shall constitute a quorum.

4. All shareholders of the corporation shall have preemptive right to subscribe for any additional shares of stock, or for other securities of any class, or for rights, warrants or options to purchase stock or for script, or for securities of any kind convertible into stock or carrying stock purchase warrants or privileges.

5. The Board of Directors may from time to time distribute to the shareholders out of its assets, in cash or property, subject to the limitations contained in the statutes of Colorado.

FIFTH: Three Directors shall constitute the initial Board, their names and addresses being as follows:
              a. Jane Smith   8403 Bryant, Westminster, CO 80030
              b. Reed Jones   1414 Grant, Denver, CO 80218
              c. John Doe   2034 Sage Circle, Golden, CO 80401
Thereafter, the number of Directors constituting the Board of Directors shall be not less than the minimum number of Directors permitted by the statutes of Colorado, nor more than five, the exact number thereof to be fixed from time to time by the By-Laws of the Corporation. Directors need not be shareholders of the corporation.

Figure 5.4 *(Continued)*

SIXTH: The address of the initial registered office of the corporation is 8403 Bryant, Westminster, Adams County, Colorado 80030. The name of its initial registered agent at such address is Jane Smith. The corporation may conduct part or all of its business in any other part of Colorado, of the United States or of the world. It may hold, purchase, mortgage, lease and convey real and personal property in any of such places.

SEVENTH: The following provisions are inserted for the management of the business and for the conduct of the affairs of the corporation, and the same are in furtherance of and not in limitation or exclusion of the powers conferred by law.

1. *Contracts with directors, etc.* No contract or other transaction of the corporation with any other person, firm or corporation, or in which this corporation is interested, shall be affected or invalidated by (a) the fact that any one or more of the directors or officers of this corporation is interested in or is a director or officer of another corporation; or (b) the fact that any director or officer, individually or jointly with others, may be party to or may be interested in any such contract or transaction.

2. *Indemnification of directors, etc.* The corporation shall indemnify any and all persons who may serve or who have served at any time as directors or officers, and their respective heirs, administrators, successors and assigns, against any and all expenses, including amounts paid upon judgments, counsel fees, and amounts paid in settlement (before or after suit is commenced), actually and necessarily incurred by such persons in connection with the defense or settlement of any claim, action, suit or proceeding in which they, or any of them, are made parties by reason of being directors or officers, except in relation to matters as to which they shall be adjudged in any action, suit or proceeding to be liable for their own negligence or misconduct in the performance of their duties.

3. *Negation of equitable interests in shares or rights.* The corporation shall be entitled to treat the registered holder of any shares of the corporation as the owner thereof for all purposes, including all rights deriving from such shares, and shall not be bound to recognize any equitable or other claim to, or interest in, such shares or rights deriving from such shares, on the part of any other person, including but without limiting the generality hereof, a purchaser, assignee or transferee of such shares or rights deriving from such shares, until such becomes the registered holder of such shares, including: to receive notice of shareholder meetings; to vote; to examine a list of the shareholders; to be paid dividends; or to own, enjoy and exercise any other property or rights deriving from such shares against the corporation.

EIGHTH: The name and address of each incorporator is:
      a. Jane Smith   8403 Bryant, Westminster, CO 80030
      b. Reed Jones   1414 Grant, Denver, CO 80218
      c. John Doe   2034 Sage Circle, Golden, CO 80401

Executed this 25th day of September, 1987.

Figure 5.5 Sample Articles of Incorporation

(*Source:* State of Colorado.)

SS Form DI (Rev. 1/86)

FOR OFFICE USE ONLY

MAIL TO:
Colorado Secretary of State
Corporations Office
1560 Broadway, Suite 200
Denver, CO 80202
(303) 866-2361

TOTAL OF FEES: $11.00
MUST BE TYPEWRITTEN (BLACK)
SUBMIT ORIGINAL AND ONE COPY

ARTICLES OF INCORPORATION

I/We the undersigned natural person(s) of the age of eighteen years or more, acting as incorporator(s) of a corporation under the Colorado Corporation Code, adopt the following Articles of Incorporation for such corporation:

FIRST: The name of the corporation is _____

SECOND: The period of duration if other than perpetual: _____

THIRD: The purpose or purposes for which the corporation is organized if other than Any Legal and Lawful Purpose Pursuant to the Colorado Corporation Code. _____
_____

FOURTH: The aggregate number of shares which the corporation shall have the authority to issue is
_____ and the par value of each share shall be _____
(dollar amount or "no par value")

FIFTH: Cumulative voting shares of stock is _____ authorized.
(not)

SIXTH: Provisions limiting or denying to shareholders the preemptive right to acquire additional or treasury shares of the corporation, if any, are:

SEVENTH: The address of the initial registered office of the corporation is _____
_____
(Address must include Building number, Street (or rural route number), Town or City, County and ZIP CODE.)

and the name of its initial registered agent at such address is _____

EIGHTH: Address of the place of business: _____
_____
(If different from registered office)

NINTH: The number of directors constituting the initial board of directors of the corporation is _____, and the names and addresses of the persons who are to serve as directors until the first annual meeting of shareholders or until their successors are elected and shall qualify are:

The number of directors of a corporation shall be not less than three; except that there need be only as many directors as there are, or initially will be, shareholders in the event that the outstanding shares are, or initially will be, held of record by fewer than three shareholders.

NAME	ADDRESS (include zip code)

TENTH: The name and address of each incorporator is:

NAME	ADDRESS (include zip code)

Signed _____

Signed _____

Signed _____
Incorporators

DC-28-1602a-85

Figure 5.6　Certificate of Incorporation
(*Source:* State of Colorado.)

DC-1
(Rev. 12-75)

STATE OF COLORADO

DEPARTMENT OF
STATE

PROFIT
CERTIFICATE OF
INCORPORATION

I, MARY ESTILL BUCHANAN,

Secretary of State of the State of Colorado, hereby certify that pursuant to the provisions of the Colorado Corporation Act, Articles of Incorporation were delivered to this office, found to conform to law, and filed in this office.

Accordingly the undersigned, by virtue of the authority vested in me by law, hereby issues this Certificate of Incorporation of

------------------------SPORTS SCIENCE ASSOCIATES, INC.------------------------
(A COLORADO CORPORATION)

Dated this------Twenty-Second-*day of*-------July------, *A. D. 19* 76.

Mary Estill Buchanan
SECRETARY OF STATE

- A corporate executive can deduct many expenses from his gross income that he probably could not deduct as a sole proprietor, for example, the costs of health insurance can be deducted as legitimate business expenses if the insurance is offered to all employees.
- If an executive or any employee lives on company premises "for the convenience of the corporation," he need not pay anything for it, as well as company-supplied food, and so on.

- Fringe benefits can be better in terms of pension plans, profit sharing and stock purchase plans.

Corporate Disadvantages (1,3)

- Incorporation is more costly—both to begin and maintain (added bookkeeping, records, and fees).
- Corporate income is taxed twice—first on its profits, then shareholders pay tax on the distributed dividends.
- Owners cannot write off the loss from their personal income if the corporation loses money.
- Many banks and businesses will not accept a corporate signature without a personal guarantee by one or more of the executives.
- An executive's salary must be "reasonable" in IRS's eyes, or it may be disallowed as a business expense.
- Shareholders may sue a director if his incompetence or misdeeds causes the corporation to lose money.
- Some states tax corporations more heavily.
- If corporate stock is offered to the general public, the corporations must conform to the complicated rules of the Securities and Exchange Commission (SEC).

S Corporation Election

If a business has fewer than 35 shareholders and meets other specifications, an "S Corporation" offered by the federal government for small businesses should be considered (see Figures 5.7 and 5.8). It offers the same limitation on liability as a "full" corporation, but like the sole proprietorship and partnership, the business itself pays no income tax. All profits or losses become part of the individual's personal income tax responsibility. Benefits are also slightly different than a full corporation, so talk to your attorney and accountant about the pros and cons for you. Many private practitioners have been advised to choose this business form for the above reasons.

Final Words on Corporations

Dietitians, as members of the health care professions, are being advised more and more to think seriously about some form of incorporation for their businesses because of the interest in suing health care professionals. If a practitioner chooses this route, it is important to emphasize that all business and contracts should be done in the corporate name, using its Federal Identification Number instead of her or his own Social Security Number to establish that it is the corporation doing the work.

CONCLUSION

It is not necessary to become overly concerned about areas of business that are completely unfamiliar to you. There are many resources and advisors to offer

Figure 5.7   Form 2553, Used for Electing S Corporation Status

(*Source:* U.S. Department of the Treasury, Internal Revenue Service, 1983.)

Form **2553** (Rev. May 1983) Department of the Treasury Internal Revenue Service	**Election by a Small Business Corporation** (Under section 1362 of the Internal Revenue Code) ► For Paperwork Reduction Act Notice, see page 1 of instructions. ► See separate instructions.	OMB No. 1545-0146

Note: *This election to be treated as an "S corporation" can be approved only if all the tests in Instruction B are met.*

Part I

Name of corporation (see instructions)	Employer Identification number (see instructions)	Principal business activity and principal product or service (see instructions)
Number and street		Election is to be effective for tax year beginning (month, day, year)
City or town, State and ZIP code		Number of shares issued and outstanding (see instructions)
Is the corporation the outgrowth or continuation of any form of predecessor? . . . . . ☐ Yes ☐ No If "Yes," state name of predecessor, type of organization, and period of its existence ►		Date and place of incorporation

A If this election takes effect for the first tax year the corporation exists, enter the earliest of the following: (1) date the corporation first had shareholders, (2) date the corporation first had assets, or (3) date the corporation began doing business. ►

B Selected tax year: Annual return will be filed for tax year ending (month and day) ►
See Instructions before entering your tax year. If the tax year ends any date other than December 31, you must complete Part II or Part IV on back. You may want to complete Part III to make a back-up request.

C Name of each shareholder, person having a community property interest in the corporation's stock, and each tenant in common, joint tenant, and tenant by the entirety. (A husband and wife (and their estates) are counted as one shareholder in determining the number of shareholders without regard to the manner in which the stock is owned.)	D Shareholders' Consent Statement. We the undersigned shareholders, consent to the corporation's election to be treated as an "S corporation" under section 1362(a). *(Shareholders sign and date below.)	E Stock owned		F Social security number (employer identification number for estate or trust)	G Tax year ends (Month and day)
		Number of shares	Dates acquired		

*For this election to be valid, the consent of each shareholder, person having a community property interest in the corporation's stock, and each tenant in common, joint tenant, and tenant by the entirety must either appear above or be attached to this form. (See instructions for column D, if continuation sheet or a separate consent statement is needed.)

Under penalties of perjury, I declare that I have examined this election, including accompanying schedules, and statements, and to the best of my knowledge and belief it is true, correct, and complete.

Signature and
Title of Officer ►   Date ►

See Parts II, III, and IV on back.

---

help. You will know more with every discussion and decision you make. Rest assured also, once a decision has been made on the business structure, it can be changed if it needs to be with some additional effort and money. Nothing is forever "cast in stone."

Figure 5.8   Instructions for Completing Form 2553

(*Source:* U.S. Department of the Treasury, Internal Revenue Service, 1983.)

Department of the Treasury
Internal Revenue Service

Instructions for Form 2553

(Revised May 1983)

Election by a Small Business Corporation

(*Section references are to the Internal Revenue Code, unless otherwise specified.*)

Paperwork Reduction Act Notice.—We ask for this information to carry out the Internal Revenue laws of the United States. We need it to ensure that you are complying with these laws and to allow us to figure and collect the right amount of tax. You are required to give us this information.

A. Purpose.—To elect to be treated as an "S Corporation," a corporation must file Form 2553. The election permits the income of the S corporation to be taxed to the shareholders of the corporation except as provided in Subchapter S and section 58(d). (See section 1363.)

B. Who May Elect.—Your corporation may make the election only if it meets the following tests:

1. It is a domestic corporation.
2. It has no more than 35 shareholders. A husband and wife (and their estates) are treated as one shareholder for this requirement. All other persons are treated as separate shareholders.
3. It has only individuals, estates, or certain trusts as shareholders.
4. It has no nonresident alien shareholders.
5. It has only one class of stock. See sections 1361(c)(4) and (5) for additional details.
6. It is not an ineligible corporation as defined in section 1361(b)(2). See section 6(c) of Public Law 97–354 for additional details.
7. It has a calendar tax year or other permitted tax year as explained in Instruction G.
8. Each shareholder consents as explained in the instructions for Column D.

See sections 1361, 1362 and 1378 for additional information on the above tests.

C. Where to File.—File this election with the Internal Revenue Service Center where the corporation will file Form 1120S, U.S. Income Tax Return For An S Corporation. You should keep a copy for the corporation's files.

If the corporation's principal business, office or agency is located in	Use the following Internal Revenue Service Center address
New Jersey, New York City and counties of Nassau, Rockland, Suffolk, and Westchester	Holtsville, NY 00501
New York (all other counties), Connecticut, Maine, Massachusetts, New Hampshire, Rhode Island, Vermont	Andover, MA 05501
Alabama, Florida, Georgia, Mississippi, South Carolina	Atlanta, GA 31101
Michigan, Ohio	Cincinnati, OH 45999
Arkansas, Kansas, Louisiana, New Mexico, Oklahoma, Texas	Austin, TX 73301
Alaska, Arizona, Colorado, Idaho, Minnesota, Montana, Nebraska, Nevada, North Dakota, Oregon, South Dakota, Utah, Washington, Wyoming	Ogden, UT 84201
Illinois, Iowa, Missouri, Wisconsin	Kansas City, MO 64999
California, Hawaii	Fresno, CA 93888
Indiana, Kentucky, North Carolina, Tennessee, Virginia, West Virginia	Memphis, TN 37501
Delaware, District of Columbia, Maryland, Pennsylvania	Philadelphia, PA 19255

D. When to Make the Election.—Complete Form 2553 and file it either: (1) at any time during that portion of the first tax year the election is to take effect which occurs before the 16th day of the third month of that tax year (or at any time during that year, if that year does not extend beyond the period described above) or (2) in the tax year before the first tax year it is to take effect. An election made by a small business corporation after the 15th day of the third month but before the end of the tax year is treated as made for the next year. For example, if a calendar tax year corporation makes the election in April 1983, it is effective for the corporation's 1984 calendar tax year.

For purposes of this election, a newly formed corporation's tax year starts when it has shareholders, acquires assets, or begins doing business, whichever happens first.

E. Acceptance or Non-acceptance of Election.—IRS will notify you if your election is accepted and when it will take effect. Until then, do not file Form 1120S. If you are now required to file Form 1120, U.S. Corporation Income Tax Return, continue filing it until your election takes effect. You will also be notified if your election is not accepted.

F. End of Election.—Once the election is made, it stays in effect for all years until it is terminated. During the 5 years after the election has been terminated, the corporation can make another election on Form 2553 only if the Commissioner consents.

See section 1362(g). However, the 5-year waiting period does not apply to terminations made under Subchapter S rules in effect for tax years beginning before January 1, 1983. See sections 1362(d), (e), and (f) for rules regarding termination of election.

G. Permitted Tax Year.—Section 1378 provides that no corporation may make an election to be an S corporation for any tax year unless the corporation has a permitted tax year. A permitted tax year is a tax year ending December 31 or any other tax year for which the corporation establishes a business purpose to the satisfaction of IRS. The tax year requirement applies to any election made after October 19, 1982. See section 1378(c) for additional requirements when a 50 percent shift in ownership occurs in an existing S corporation.

H. Investment Credit Property.—Although the corporation has elected to be an S corporation under section 1362, the tax imposed by section 47 in the case of early disposition of investment credit property will be imposed on the corporation for credits allowed for tax years for which the corporation was not an S corporation. The election will not be treated as a disposition of the property by the corporation. See section 1371(d).

Specific Instructions

Part I.—Part I must be completed by all corporations.

Name and Address of Corporation.—If the corporation's mailing address is the same as someone else's, such as a shareholder's, please enter this person's name below the corporation's name.

Employer Identification Number.—If you have applied for an employer identification number (EIN) but have not received it, enter "applied for." If the corporation does not have an EIN, you should apply for one on Form SS–4, Application for Employer Identification Number, available from most IRS or Social Security Administration offices. Send Form SS–4 to the IRS Service Center where Form 1120S will be filed.

Principal Business Activity and Principal Product or Service.—Use the Codes for Principal Business Activity contained in the Instructions for Form 1120S. Your principal business activity is the one that accounts for the largest percentage of total receipts. Total receipts are gross sales and gross receipts, plus all other income.

Also state the principal product or service. For example, if the principal business activity is "Grain mill products," the principal product or service may be "cereal preparation."

Number of Shares Issued and Outstanding.—Enter only one figure. This figure will be the number of shares of stock that have been issued to shareholders and have not been reacquired by the corporation. This is the number of shares all shareholders own, as reported in column E, Part I.

REFERENCES

1. Lowry, Albert: *How To Become Financially Successful by Owning Your Own Business,* Simon and Schuster, New York 1981.
2. Shyne, Devin: "In Business: From Friendship to Partnership," *Working Woman,* August 1983, pp. 48–49.
3. Curtin, Richard T.: *Running Your Own Show,* New American Library, New York, 1982.

chapter 6

Developing Your Business Management Team
Olga Satterwhite, R.D.

Now that your practice is developed on paper, you need to evaluate who will make up your team of professional advisors. You could go it alone, but it is advised to at least initially contact professional help for the start up of your venture. A team of professional advisors should include a lawyer, accountant, banker, business or public relations consultant, and an insurance agent. By using a group of consultants you will gain the benefit of each profession's expertise as well as different perspectives on the same issues. These advisors will evaluate your business liability, marketability, set up or advise you on bookkeeping systems, determine business structure, make you aware of potential problem areas, and assist in dealing with state and federal regulations concerning the practice.

LOCATING ADVISORS

When seeking good professional guidance obtain several different names of highly recommended specialists. Ask for referrals from your friends, other small business owners, the Small Business Administration, physicians who have started their own practices, other dietitians, and local professional groups. Look especially for professional consultants who have experience setting up and working with *small* businesses—you will save yourself from a lot of headaches and grief if you are specific in what you are looking for. Remember too that *you* interview the consultant. They work for you, so do not be intimidated and feel you must hire the first person you talk with. Consider the following questions as guidelines when discussing a business consultant's services and her or his suitability for your practice:

1. What is the consultant's experience in your area of business—a divorce lawyer or large corporate banker or accountant will probably not fit your needs.
2. What specific services does the consultant propose for your practice?
3. Approximately how much will you be charged? If it will be on an hourly basis, obtain an estimate of how many hours the consultant feels your practice will take. Will phone calls be charged? Although fees are important, be aware that bargain rates sometimes only get you bargain services.
4. Does the professional advisor have the time to take on your practice? Will you get both adequate advice and reasonable turn-around times on contracted work?

The better you know the needs of your practice and the more work you can do for yourself, the less you will have to pay someone else. Before you commit yourself to a specific consultant, ask yourself: Was I comfortable with him or her? Did she or he seem interested in me and my practice? Keep records of all correspondence with a contract consultant. Follow up any telephone conversations with a letter reiterating any points you feel uneasy about or that you feel were important. Keep a copy of the letter for yourself. Do not assume anything about an agreement—ask! Do not be afraid to change to another consultant and transfer your records if you are unhappy with the work you receive.

It is never wise to use family and professional friends as anything but personal advisors because it is so hard to fire them when a job is not being done to your satisfaction. Well-qualified strangers always make the best business advisors.

It is important to know how to use each consultant's expertise to your best advantage. Talking with other business owners and professionals will help supplement the research and reading you must do before going into private practice.

ATTORNEY

When choosing your attorney, you should look for someone whom you can trust and can work with and whose fees you consider reasonable. Trust is believing that the attorney can do the job, is competent, and cares about helping you (1).

The legal fee you will be paying is important. Often the lowest hourly rate is not always the lowest total bill, especially if the attorney is not familiar with the legal problems of your type of business. An attorney may spend a lot of time at your expense learning what to do. Legal services are the last of the "cottage industries," meaning that each item is custom made (1). There is a great deal of discretion involved as an attorney does his or her job, so take the time to find a good one.

On matters such as suing or countersuing it is highly suggested that you obtain a second (independent) decision before pursuing it. Make sure that you agree with the language and possible consequences of any legal action before you let your lawyer take action in your name. You will have to live with the results.

Legal advice incorporated at the beginning of your practice can prevent misguided decisions that could affect your business for years to come. A lawyer will help you understand state and federal regulations and licenses that you will need to decipher. An attorney can help with copyrights for materials and assist with trademarking your practice's logo. He or she will write and/or look over *all* contracts or letters of agreement that you must sign in setting up the practice. Most importantly, a lawyer will help you decide on and develop the appropriate structure for your practice—sole proprietorship, partnership, or corporation. Attorney fees range from $50 per hour in smaller communities up to $150 per hour or more for specialized work, and they usually charge for phone calls.

ACCOUNTANT

Accountants are divided into two groups: those who are Certified Public Accountants (CPAs) and those who are not certified. Certification is awarded by the state of residence and verifies that the recipient has completed a two-year apprenticeship under a CPA and has passed a series of difficult tests in the areas of auditing, accounting, accounting theory, and business law. CPAs are accountants with an assured high level of skill; however, other accountants may be highly qualified, but not certified.

As you look for an accountant, ask other business people whom they use. Your best source of information is a satisfied customer.

Your accountant should provide tax advantage information to you to help structure the practice to your best advantage. He or she can recommend your salary level or commission based on projected cash flow, with an eye to all possible tax savings. Your financial advisor should keep you aware of all the legitimate tax deductions due you, such as mileage, equipment expenses, furnishings, materials, insurance, and so on. She or he will be valuable in helping choose a bookkeeping or record system that will fit your needs. If the system is set up correctly and simply, you should be able to do the bookkeeping yourself, aided by year-end income tax assistance. Often an accountant will prepare financial reports that are invaluable tools in determining future business strategy, marketing and tax analysis, or for obtaining financial backing. Some accountants also give advice on how a business should be operated—called management services.

The hourly fee for an accountant or CPA usually ranges from $30 to $125 per hour or more. Always ask for an estimate of time and fee before the work is begun. Inform your financial advisor of any time limitations you have and request that the work be completed by that date. Again, beware of "bargains," such as new people on staff for "special" rates—they may take twice as long to complete the work, *and* you may have to pay the full price for a supervisor to look over the work. Most importantly, the person may not have any business experience, and an accountant should be a valuable resource in this area.

BANKER

Spend time becoming acquainted with your area banks and the services they offer. Even if you do not intend to borrow working capital from a bank, your business accounts will make you a welcome customer. Get to know a bank officer. A friendly banker is more important than which bank you use. Discuss your plans for your practice with him. An experienced banker can give you a wealth of valuable business information not only on financial matters, interest rates, and so on, but on trends in the community. Try to use the same personnel when doing your banking and speak up if you are always directed to new inexperienced ones. Banking personnel never charge for their services and can be one of your best resources when starting out.

BUSINESS CONSULTANT

A business consultant can advise you on major business decisions such as locale, image development, fees, marketing, new market areas, and so on. Good, affordable consultants for small businesses are hard to find, but well worth the research time. Their fees range from $40 per hour on up.

Very good *free* services available in your area are the SCORE (Service Corps of Retired Executives) and ACE (Active Corps Executives) programs of the Small Business Administration. These two programs will work to match you with a retired or active business person who will be able to answer your business questions. These people have been at the starting point where you are now and their knowledge and experience can be one of your most valued resources. Many local banks, local Chambers of Commerce, YMCA or YWCAs, universities, and evening high schools offer new business classes or seminars to help the beginning business owner.

PUBLIC RELATIONS

Seeking out a public relations expert can help you let the world know you have arrived. The services they provide can include logo development, business card and brochure design, market research, and advertising savvy. Many private practitioners have stated that their business image was so greatly improved by having a public relations firm develop outstanding promotion materials that the expert's fee was worth every cent. As the nutrition practice becomes more sophisticated, public imaging will, no doubt, be more important. Hiring a public relations firm is expensive, so be careful and specific in your negotiations on prices and services. To assure that you like what is produced, ask to be involved in all stages of development.

If you want to do your own marketing and feel confident that you can generate the art work and/or wording, look into using the *free* advertising/sales consultants offered by the ad departments of all newspapers, magazines, radio, and television stations. Not only can they assist with simple layout suggestions, but can advise you on the best time to run your ad, e.g., morning spots on radio or Sunday newspapers, and so on. Use the experts to help sell your knowledge in nutrition.

FINAL WORD

The wise use of professional advisors will in the long run save you from lost time, wasted energy, and misdirected capital. Their combined expertise will enable you

Table 6.1   BUSINESS MANAGEMENT TEAM

Consultant	Assistance
Attorney	Form of business structure Partnership agreements Licenses Contracts and letters of agreement Office leases Copyrights, trademarks, patents Zoning ordinances Lawsuits
Accountant or CPA	Financial statements Audits Cash flow projections Tax deductions Income tax records and reports Bookkeeping systems Investment analysis Management services (sometimes available)
Banker	Loan/venture capital Credit information IRA and Keogh accounts Business checking and savings accounts Community trends
Business Consultant	Locate office Image development Networking and contacts Setting fees Marketing and promotion Business agreements Setting priorities Management
Public Relations	Logo design Develop business cards and brochure Market research Promotion ideas Advertising layouts Media contacts Image development

to enter into your practice confident that your organization will run at its optimum. (See Table 6.1.)

REFERENCE

1. Curtin, Richard: *Running Your Own Show,* New American Library, New York, 1982.

chapter 7

Money, Fees, and Bookkeeping

Jan Thayer, R.D., and Kathy King Helm, R.D.

The *bottom line* in business—the measure of success—is to make money. A business that does not make money is either a hobby or one that has a limited lifespan. Entrepreneurs soon appreciate the importance that generating a profit, not just income, means to the success of their businesses.

Components of the process to generate good cash flow and a profit include sufficient capital investment up-front to start the business, quality service at a fair price, good collection of revenue, timely payment of bills, and appropriate record-keeping for yourself, the IRS, and the lender. Managing money and keeping records should not be difficult tasks, especially since accountants and Certified Public Accountants (CPAs) are available to help you set up the system or do it for you. The challenge is to know what needs to be done.

Before anyone will be able to help you secure a loan or set up your books, she or he will need to know what you plan to do. The information generated in the business concept and plan will be beneficial, as well as knowing the type of business structure you will use and an estimation of your start-up costs (see Chapter 9).

INITIAL INVESTMENT

Good financing offers peace of mind, the option of changing your mind, and freedom to create without survival being in peril. When asked, successful private practitioners estimate that years ago they invested $5,000 to $20,000 or more their first year in business (1). With the large quantity of sophisticated competition today, plus inflation, the start-up money may have to be two to five times what was needed ten years ago.

Practitioners with well-equipped, well-staffed offices in their own rented space pay the higher fees. They *may* also realize success much faster because of the stability, quality of service, and image that they portray. Investing more money into a business will not necessarily make it more successful. However, if the business is managed and promoted well and the owner makes intelligent and timely decisions, an adequately financed venture has a better chance of becoming a lucrative business faster.

Smaller investments are made by practitioners who either have more time than money and/or those who want to keep the risk and investment low. This is best accomplished initially by sharing office space in a physician's office or clinic or health club and using the staff and services already available in return for a small fee. Care must be taken while in this situation to develop a separate, successful identity as a consultant.

SOURCES OF FINANCING

One of the first realities to face in business is establishing a money commitment. Business and financial experts usually encourage new business owners to try to use someone else's money to finance their venture if possible instead of exhausting personal assets. The main reason for this is so that financial strength is better maintained in case a follow-up loan is needed later, or so that the owner can contribute later during financial emergencies or expansion projects. There are several options for obtaining money, depending upon your assets, business expertise, or connections.

Lending Institutions

Lending institutions are in business to make money by loaning money for an interest fee. Loaning money involves taking a risk that the new business will be successful, and the owner is honest and reliable. Your job would be to convince the loan officer that you are committed, sincere, and qualified to establish this business. Seldom will a new business without any assets for collateral be given a loan, but the owner may be able to obtain one on a signature or by securing it with personal assets. It is also possible to place your money in a lending institution account and borrow against it. The interest you pay is tax deductible and you will still own the original money.

Commercial Banks

Commercial banks are the most common lending institutions. They offer a wide variety of services beside checking and savings accounts. Basic financial counseling and credit analysis are often offered at no cost to regular customers. Most commercial banks are prepared to make short, intermediate-term and long-term loans. You may be asked to put personal property, Certificates of Deposit, savings, or other assets of value up as collateral. In some cases where you have established credit, you may be asked only to sign for the loan. When assets are used to secure a loan, they presumably are not to be sold, spent, or used without approval by the lending institution. Read your loan agreement carefully.

Industrial Banks

Industrial banks usually give loans by offering second mortgages on real property (home, building, or land). The interest rates are usually higher than those asked at commercial banks. Not all mortgage loans or states allow second mortgages on homes so be sure to check. Also, look to see if they ask for a substantial prepayment penalty.

Finance Companies

Finance companies offer credit on a variety of different types of inventory, equipment, and personal assets, but the rates, especially on short-term loans are usually much higher. Companies may charge 30 to 40 percent interest per year.

Savings and Loan Associations or Savings Banks

Savings and loan associations or savings banks usually offer long-term loans on real estate, for example, on land, buildings, and homes. For the practitioner considering purchasing a condo office or other office complex, this may fit your needs.

The Small Business Administration (SBA)

The SBA of the United States Government is another resource alternative for a new or established business loan. The law stipulates that SBA loans can be made only to businesses that are unable to get funds from banks or other private sources. This is usually because the personal assets or type of business will not qualify for a regular loan, not because the person is a poor risk. A commercial bank, however, will usually make the loan, but it is guaranteed by the SBA up to as much as 90 percent of the total loan. Especially with new businesses, the SBA may ask that the owner contribute 15 to 50 percent of the initial investment to start the business before a loan is granted. Occasionally, the SBA will make the loan itself, but this is rare. It is also important to note that only one-quarter of the total 30,000 or so loans that the SBA makes or guarantees each year goes to new businesses, so competition is tough. Interest rates on an SBA loan are attractive because they are lower than banks usually offer. As attitudes change in the federal government SBA money becomes more or less available.

The SBA requires extensive information about you and your business venture. An accountant or CPA can be hired to put the proposal together for you or to guide you in assembling and filling out the documentation required. When pursuing this type of loan be sure to allow plenty of time because the process may take many months before approval or rejection is announced.

Outside Investors/Venture Capital

Outside investors, friends, or relatives may have venture capital that they would like to invest in your company. Most financial and business advisors state that they consider the ideal situation is when a loan is made without the owner having to give up any control of the business. Also, be aware that business and friendships or relatives do not always mix, and it may *not* be a wise choice of funds. Discuss what you can offer in the way of return on investment, limited or silent partnerships, or percentage of ownership with your professional advisors. Consult with your lawyer about drawing up any legal agreements.

LOAN PACKAGE

The loan package is the finalized presentation compiled to secure a loan from a bank, investor, venture capitalist, SBA, or a combination of these sources (2). It succinctly presents your basic idea through the business concept and plan. In a nutshell it explains who you are, your financial status, and how the money will be used and repaid.

It is generally believed that having an accountant or CPA provide a review of the figures presented substantially improves the chances for getting a loan. A review is less involved and less expensive than an audit and only as accurate as the figures used, yet it often satisfies bankers because it offers some limited assurance about the reliability of the financial information (2).

Typically, bankers will request or appreciate having the following (2,3):

    I. A business concept and plan with its market analysis (see Chapter 3)
   II. Personal history of each owner (resume, business experience, letters of reference, etc.)
  III. Company information: copies of contracts you already have signed, lease agreements, insurance carried, etc.
  IV. Personal balance sheet and your personal income tax returns for the past three years (see Figure 7.1, p. 81)
   V. If already in business:
     A. Company balance sheet and tax returns
     B. Company profit and loss statement (see Figure 7.2, p. 82)
     C. Aging of accounts receivable and payable as of current date
  VI. Business cash flow projections for at least one year (see Figure 7.3, p. 83)
 VII. Amount of loan requested
VIII. Purpose of loan
  IX. Source of repayment
   X. Duration of loan
  XI. Collateral to be offered to secure the loan (official appraisals of assets may also be supplied, especially when their market value is not easily determined)

Q & A

Buying An Ongoing Private Practice

A local private practitioner is moving and wants to sell her practice. How do we determine what it is worth, and are there alternatives to paying a lump sum up front?

Determining the value of a service-type business whose success is closely associated with the personality of the owner is not easy. The following factors should be considered (1):

Profitability You are concerned about the future profit potential of the business. Start by analyzing balance sheets and profit and loss statements of the present owner for the past five years or however long the practice has existed. If these forms are not available, ask for copies of the income tax forms. Are the profits satisfactory? Have profits continued to grow? Ask the seller to prepare a projected statement of profit and loss for the next 12 months and compare it to your own estimations.

Tangible assets The most common are inventories, typewriter, furniture, and teaching materials. Make sure that they are in working order, and that they are not outdated. Consider whether the items are something you can use. If the asking values seem too high, call around to obtain estimates of similar equipment from dealers of new or secondhand items.

Goodwill This is the dollar amount that the owner is asking for the favorable public and physician attitudes toward her or his going concern. You should be realistic in determining how much you should pay for goodwill. Since it is payment for favorable public attitude, you should make some effort to check this attitude. A way of judging the value of this intangible asset is to estimate how much more income you will receive through buying the going business than by starting a new one. How much of the business will stay and how much will be lost because of the present owner leaving?

Liabilities You should be sure that there are no outstanding debts or liens on the assets. The seller should pay off all accumulated debts before an agreement is signed.

Business worth After you have researched the above variables there is still the question of worth. This is determined through negotiation and bargaining. Are you sure that physicians and contracts will use your services? Do you have any verbal or letters of agreements (with contract accounts) to that effect? Have you carefully evaluated the lease agreement, zoning, the growing competition, and other possible factors that may affect your business? Will the seller train the buyer in running the business or offer any other intangible services?

Some business owners have sold out only to start a new business in competition with the buyer. Consider placing limitations upon the seller's right to compete with you for a specific period of time and within a specified area.

As a safeguard against costly errors, legal advice should be obtained before any agreement is made. Items typically covered in a contract selling a small business are (1):

1. A description of what is being sold
2. The purchase price
3. The method of payment
4. A statement of how adjustments will be handled at closing (prepaid insurance, rent, inventory remaining, etc.)
5. Buyer's assumption of contracts and liabilities
6. Seller's warranties (against false statements and inaccurate financial data)
7. Seller's obligation and assumption of risk pending closing
8. Covenant of seller not to compete
9. Time, place, and procedures of closing

The seller and buyer must comply with the bulk sales law of the state in which the transaction takes place. The purpose of such a law is to make certain the seller does not sell out, pocket the proceeds, and disappear, leaving creditors unpaid. The seller must furnish a sworn list of her or his creditors and you, as the buyer, must give notice to the creditors of the pending sale. Otherwise, the seller's creditors may be able to claim the personal property which you purchased.

Payment   There are several ways that practitioners have negotiated the payment for a practice. One is, of course, a lump sum of money up front. Another way is time payments with either a balloon note at the end of three to five years, or money up front followed by regular payments for several years. Another option is to pay an up-front amount followed by a percentage of the gross income for a period of one to five years.

When the buyer and seller cannot seem to agree on the worth of the goodwill for sale, the option that several have used is the last one—up-front money followed by a percentage. As the seller, it would be advisable to also train the buyer on how to run the business and market so that sales do not drop appreciably, if this method is chosen.

Reference

1. "Starting and Managing a Small Business of Your Own," U.S. Small Business Administration, 4th edition, U.S. Government Printing Office, Washington, D.C., 1982.

Before beginning to prepare all of these documents, ask your individual loan agent what forms he or she needs. Many business consultants suggest that the loan package be typed and bound in an attractive folder or notebook (3).

Numerous options exist on loans so work with your loan officer and financial counselor to choose one that fits your needs. Practitioners have found that loans that are termed "line of credit" are very helpful for peace of mind and yet do not usually cost anything if the money is not needed. Loans may also be set up so that only interest payments are made every three to six months the first year.

Once a loan has been awarded, the bank may request that quarterly, semiannual, or yearly status reports be submitted, and occasionally, if all payments are made on time, nothing may be needed.

A "no" answer should not be seen as a total defeat. Ask the banker to be specific on what else is needed and be prepared to go back several times to achieve your desired results or until an agreement will not work out.

MANAGING MONEY

Whether you decide to incorporate your business or not, when your business begins to make money, it has a life of its own. The money that is generated must be accounted for. Records on incoming revenue must match bank deposits into the business bank account. All business expenses, plus the owner's salary or consultant fee, are then paid by check from that account. Personal expenses for groceries or the house note should only be paid out of funds appropriately transferred to the owner's personal account.

Large amounts of business money should not be left in a noninterest-bearing checking account when it will not be used immediately. A savings, money market, or other interest account should be used even for just a few weeks to generate interest.

When petty cash is needed for the office, a business check should be written for that purpose and cashed. Cash taken in as payment from clients should be recorded as income and deposited, not pocketed or used.

Cash Flow

Cash flow is just what the name states, the flow of money through the business. Cash flow is concerned with how much money is coming in regularly as compared

Figure 7.1   Sample Balance Sheet

BALANCE SHEET

Assets

Cash in checking account $_____

Cash in savings account   _____

Credit union savings account   _____

Life insurance cash value   _____

House fair market value   _____

Car   _____

Furniture and personal effects   _____

Other   _____

                                     _____

   Total assets $_____

Liabilities

Department store account balance $_____

Balance on car loan   _____

Home mortgage   _____

Other   _____

                                     _____

   Total liabilities $_____

Net worth
(Assets minus liabilities) $_____

___

to that needed to pay current bills. It could be compared to not having more monthly bills to pay than your paychecks can cover.

As a new business owner it should be assumed that it may take six months or more before enough money will come in to cover all expenses. When planning

Figure 7.2   Sample Profit and Loss Statement

PROFIT AND LOSS STATEMENT

Income
Nutrition counseling $ _____

Public speaking   _____

Nursing home consultation   _____

Book royalties   _____

Other   _____

    Total income
    (To date, monthly, yearly) $ _____

Losses (or Expenses)
Rent $ _____

Utilities   _____

Telephone and answering service   _____

Equipment   _____

Salaries or consultant fees   _____

Insurance   _____

Auto   _____

Benefits   _____

Supplies   _____

Other   _____

    Total expenses $ _____

    Net income $ _____

Other reductions
Taxes $ _____

Depreciation   _____

Other noncash reduction   _____

    Adjusted net income $ _____

Figure 7.3　Sample Cash Flow Planning Form

CASH FLOW IN

	Jan.	**Feb.**	**Etc.**
1. Beginning cash balance			
2. (Income sources)			
3.			
4.			
5.			
6.			
7.			
8.			
Total cash available			

CASH FLOW OUT

Operating Expenses

1.
2.
3.
4.
5.
6.
7.
8.

Capital Expense

1. Loan payments
2. Income tax and Social Security

Total cash required

Cash available less cash required

Money to be borrowed
(if negative total)

Debit payments (if positive)

Ending cash balance

Operating loan balance
(at end of period)

---

for working capital in your start-up costs, allow enough to keep cash flowing and bills being paid. Limited cash flow is not only frustrating, but if it becomes serious, more money (working capital) may have to be borrowed or supplied by the owner, or the business may have to close.

Suggestions for improving cash flow include:

- Request all payments at the time of the visit.
- Improve collection efforts on outstanding accounts, especially the larger ones.
- Keep low purchased inventories of teaching materials, printed diets, and promotion tools.
- Avoid making new purchases that will increase the business overhead and either deplete savings or create additional time payments.
- Deposit temporary excess funds in a savings account or money market fund to draw interest.
- Evaluate, for your own situation, when to take cash discounts if offered and pay a bill quickly to save money, or when to delay paying bills until the end of the payment period to conserve cash outflow.

FEES AND COLLECTION

Valuing Your Time

An important element of managing money is knowing the value of your time and effort. Too often we spend countless hours doing $8 per hour secretarial work when we should be doing management work like writing ads, making public appearances, or negotiating contracts. If you have something more important that you could be doing, don't sit around doing work that can be easily delegated.

Establishing Fees

It is illegal (price-fixing) for us to discuss what charges you could ask for your services. It is also illegal for you to call around your area to ask the going rates of other health professionals. We can, however, discuss ways that you can determine for yourself what you need to charge. The factors to evaluate when you establish fees for any work you perform are:

- How much expertise and experience does the work require?
- How difficult or demanding is the job?
- How much total time will the job, paperwork and follow-up take?
- How much direct overhead cost (handouts, teaching materials, travel expense, hiring another consultant to help, secretarial time, computer use, etc.) and indirect overhead (to maintain office, telephone, insurance, etc.) will be expensed to this job?
- What will the market bear, so that you don't price yourself out of it?

After you have considered all of the variables in establishing fees, charge whatever you want since it's your business and your decision. Business advisors vary in their recommendations, but most feel you are doing well if you can *net* 40–60 percent of the asked fee to cover your salary, taxes, and Social Security.

Fees are a curious item. If you charge a small fee, sometimes, not always, patients, physicians, and clients think that you are not as good as the competition. If you charge a fee that your reputation, years of experience, or expertise can't support, no one will pay it. Arriving at "correct" fees for different types of jobs is more a process of negotiation and learning from past experience. As a private practitioner becomes known for quality work and a good reputation, new business will come his or her way. The fee will become less important because people are willing to pay for what they feel is the best.

Diet instruction fees should be consistent so that patients feel that they are charged fairly. Practitioners do not agree on whether offering flexible fees to certain clients produces the desired results, but it is an option. Patients should be told what the fees are when the appointment is first scheduled. Also they should be told that the payment is requested at the time of the visit—even if insurance coverage is available. This gives patients the opportunity to back out or plan ahead to have their checkbook or cash along. Telling them in advance makes bill collection easier.

There is no standardized way of charging for nutrition consultations. Some practitioners charge by the hour, but charge a minimum fee for very short appointments. They give their patients an estimate when asked how much the fees are. Other practitioners charge by the visit and then try to keep the appointment within a certain time range.

Several practitioners have programs where the initial diet consultation takes three to eight or more visits. Printed diets are given out only after much education and assessment has taken place. The program commitment is made very clear in the beginning. The fees are either charged as they go, payments are heavily weighed up front, or they are paid in cash or by credit card up front.

Following this same way of thinking, many practitioners automatically include several follow-up visits in the fees charged to patients. It is commonly agreed that a one-visit instruction *rarely* changes behavior. Patients aren't always aware of that and will not always attend follow-up visits unless their importance is stressed.

Group classes for weight loss, gourmet, "natural," or diabetic cooking are very popular with the public. For the practitioner group classes represent challenge, a creative outlet, and the possibility of making more income per hour because of reaching more people at a time. Here are two hints that may be helpful to a practitioner thinking about doing group classes: First, preregister attendees instead of letting them show up at the door, so that you can cancel if attendance will be poor or adjust your room and handouts if a large number plan to come. Second, collect the fee for ongoing classes at the first session, or when preregistering so that attendance will be better and your budget more stable.

Public speaking or speaking to professional groups can be very satisfying and fun. It should also be financially rewarding. Organizers often work harder to have a better audience turnout when they are excited about the speaker and there is a fee to cover. Occasionally, there will be times when you choose to give a free talk, but at that time let the organizers know that you are waiving the normal fee. If the organization is nonprofit, ask for a receipt from the organization, for tax purposes, showing that you donated your speaking fee.

When you first begin public speaking, you may not be familiar with what organizations are willing to pay. The best way to find out is to ask the person who calls to set up an engagement. They know what their fee boundaries are, and most local people are very willing to share and negotiate with you. If the fee is low, try asking for more; also ask that your travel and handout costs be covered. Also make sure that you can pass out your calling cards.

As you become an established and sought-after speaker or an author of some note, your fees can reflect this. Travel and accommodations will be included for out-of-town travel. However, although the fees will be much higher, when you consider the travel time to distant speeches and any lost income while away from the business, the actual net income may be modest. Speakers often look on the opportunity as one to grow professionally, to travel and meet new people, and to sell books or whatever.

Consulting to business usually comes after years of specialized training or experience in the field.   However, young practitioners with expertise in nutrition assessment, sports nutrition, wellness, and other new emerging areas are also being asked to consult at this time.

If you are stumped on how much to ask for a consultant job, ask the client to make an offer. At least then you would know the ballpark they are in, and you can then negotiate if it is too low. Clients are often hesitant about mentioning a fee first, in case you would have been willing to work for much less. So, if you must set the fee yourself, use your best calculations on what it will cost you to do the job, estimate your hours and needed profit, and then estimate more hours to do the job by approximately one-fourth to one-third. Most often the problem is not that we set our fee too low, but that we underestimate how long a job will take and we barely break even. Coming in under budget is always acceptable, if it happens. More negotiating suggestions are found in Chapter 15.

Credit Cards

A number of consulting nutritionists offer the use of credit cards to their clients as a means of payment. Many patients like this convenience and the fact that they can then delay their payments. Credit cards help attract patients who would have delayed coming due to lack of ready cash. People who conduct group classes have found that there is less resistance to the up-front fee when credit cards can be used.

A representative from your local bank can explain the service to you. Forms and a printer are available, usually for a small fee. The credit card forms are deposited into your bank account just like other checks, except for one item: a service charge is charged to you on every patient who uses this service. The company charges usually vary between 5 to 12 percent per bill. You can increase your fee slightly to cover the service charge cost but that would mean that all patients are subsidizing the credit card users. Some other types of businesses have tried to offer discounts for cash or extra fees for using credit and they have found a mixed response. Actually, the increase in business may offset the added service charge so that no fee increase would be necessary.

Q & A

Charging Commercial Clients

I was recently asked to write the script for a video on wellness nutrition for a health club chain. They will offer the video for sale and lease to its members. I want to do it, but I want to be compensated fairly. I don't have any idea what to ask for. Can you give me some ideas?

Let's start with the overall considerations:

- You can always negotiate with the club to arrive at the final agreement. What you want to avoid is coming in too low so you don't make money or coming in so high that you sour the client on using your services. A well-thought-out beginning asking price with room to negotiate is what you are looking for.
- Professional advisors will tell you that *most* people assume that you will charge commercial accounts differently than if you were charging for services given to an individual who uses the information personally.

The factors to consider in pricing your services are:

- The popularity and recognition factor of your name and reputation.
- How the product will be used and the profit potential for the client.
- Your best estimate plus a cushion on the number of hours and other resources this project will cost you.
- Consider asking for a royalty for as long as the video script is in use. Ask for editorial or revision rights to up date the script as needed or yearly. And finally, if the club wants to state that you are a staff member or consultant, ask for a retainer fee and have a letter of agreement on your rights and liability limitations. Talk to your professional advisors concerning your protection, proposal, fees, and before signing anything.
- Have your agreement on fees, expected outcomes, review process, project aborting, etc. down in writing *before* you start writing the script.
- Ask for a nonrefundable portion of your fee up front to cover some expenses in case the project plans change.

Collecting Fees

The older your accounts receivable grow, the more stale they become. In a service business such as nutrition counseling, since no inventory is lost, no write-off can be taken for bad debts (except for actual expenses such as teaching materials, computer printouts, etc.). Therefore, new practitioners must realize that the money must be collected or else the diet appointment did not have financial value.

A written contract or letter of agreement for a completed consultant job is very good proof that the other party should pay you, but you may have to retain a lawyer and go to court to get the money. You will be able to deduct your actual expenses for the job and the cost to recover the money. But the actual cost of time, aggravation, and legal fees may mean you are only breaking even or less. Timely collection of funds should be a business priority.

Precautionary action can often keep an entrepreneur from having to bill in the first place. Many times the purpose of establishing credit policies and setting credit limits is not so much to assure collection of accounts, but to set limits on the risk of loss. Patients should be asked to pay at the time of the visit. If they know that their insurance company will cover your charges, ask that you be paid and give them a paid, itemized receipt (see Figure 7.4 and examples in Chapter 8).

Contracts or letters of agreement can be written so that ongoing bills can be submitted monthly and paid in two weeks. Another option is to break the total expense for a project into thirds, for example, and have one portion paid when the proposal is given final approval, another halfway through the project, and one at the end.

Figure 7.4   Sample Receipt or Statement

DATE: _____

JANE JONES   LICENSE No. R392300
REGISTERED DIETITIAN

PATIENT'S NAME: _____

ADDRESS: _____

_____

DIAGNOSIS: Diabetes, hypertension

SERVICE: Initial nutrition evaluation
and consultation as ordered by
Dr. Glen Murphy

(1 hour) $ _____

PAID

If billing becomes necessary, here are some hints. Date statements as of the last day of the preceding month rather than the first day of the current month. The customer will be inclined to pay sooner since the statement appears to be a month older.

Quickly identify delinquent accounts and speed up the collection process by a more vigorous follow-up. Delinquent accounts of over two months should receive a pleasant, tactful phone call from either you or someone representing your business, requesting that a payment be mailed by a deadline date. If no payment is received or a partial payment is not followed shortly by the balance, a second tactful call should be made, requesting immediate payment before the account is turned over to collection.

Collection agencies state that small medical bills are one of the hardest types of bills to collect on. They state that any account over six months old, and often only two to three months, is usually uncollectable. Most agencies charge 50 percent of the bill as their fee if they collect it, and few will touch an account with under $100 outstanding.

Credit is costly if you can't collect. As an example, you provide $100 worth of services to a patient, and your profit margin is 25 percent. If the patient never pays, you will have to collect $400 worth of fees just to recover the uncollected $100 (4). When you consider how much you have invested in your business, you can easily appreciate why business people do not tolerate delinquent accounts.

BOOKKEEPING

Accounting keeps track of money you earn and spend, what you own and owe: your worth. Your income equals revenue minus expenses and is recorded on an income (profit and loss) statement (see Figure 7.2). Your assets are capital worth minus liabilities and are recorded on the balance sheet (see Figure 7.1) (5).

A good bookkeeping system is necessary to record all of your financial transactions, but it should be simple enough for you to use yourself. The larger and more complex the business is the more comprehensive, but not necessarily the more complicated, the bookkeeping system must be. The information generated will help you know your financial position, evaluate success, and pinpoint problems. These records can also help you make comparisons from year to year and help make more accurate projections for the future.

A good accountant or CPA will be able to help you choose the system that is most appropriate for your business. Office supply stores have a variety of simple bookkeeping record systems. One of the most popular is the Dome book entitled "Simplified Monthly Bookkeeping Record" (6). More elaborate "pegboard" systems are available from accounting supply companies. Pegboard systems use carbonless paper to make recording a patient bill receipt, bank deposit, appointment card, and patient ledger card a one-step process. This system can be imprinted with the business name, address, and phone. And it is becoming more reasonable in cost as competition between companies increases. This system is commonly seen in physicians' offices and clinics.

Budget

In his book *Private Practice,* Jack D. McCue, M.D., states that "fewer than 2 percent of (medical) practices have a budget" (5). If a survey were conducted of nutrition private practitioners, those using a budget would no doubt be as small. Agreeing on a budget forces you to examine projected expenses and agree on the gross income, hours of work, and charges necessary to generate the projected net income. A monthly check of your records allows you to examine the actual figures and make adjustments if necessary.

Cash versus Accrual Accounting

The IRS will ask that you indicate which form of accounting you use in your bookkeeping—cash or accrual. Cash accounting is when you record income as you receive it and expenses as you pay them. Accrual accounting takes place when income is recorded as it is earned, not necessarily when it is received, and expenses are recorded when they are incurred, not when they are paid. Accrual accounting is usually used in businesses that have large inventories where flexibility of figures and dates may be beneficial. Financial consultants usually suggest that service businesses such as private nutrition practices use cash accounting because it is simple and easy to use.

Recordkeeping

The following list shows the typical progression of recordkeeping for a physician-referred clinical patient visit.

1. Appointment is recorded for patient's visit.
2. Medical diagnosis or written or verbal diet order is obtained from referring physician along with pertinent chemical scores.
3. Initial interview sheet, assessment history, and food analysis, etc., is filled out.
4. Written information/handouts are given to patient.
5. As the patient gets ready to leave, an itemized bill is given to him or her and payment is requested.
6. The payment is recorded.
7. The bill is marked paid.
8. An appointment card is given to the patient if there is to be another visit and an entry in the appointment book is made.
9. The payment is listed on the bank deposit slip.
10. A follow-up communique is sent to the referring physician.
11. The patient's interview sheet or folder is filed.

If a payment is not made, the unpaid statement is given to the patient, and a ledger note is made. Patients are requested to send back the payment as soon as possible. Some practitioners even put the statement in an addressed, stamped envelope to make the process easier.

Daily, all income (checks, credit card receipts, and cash) is recorded on the business bank deposit slip. The total income is listed in the accounting records under daily receipts. All bills should be listed as they are paid under expenses. The date, check number, amount, and deduction code if you use one should be listed also (see Figure 7.5).

Monthly, all income and expenses should be tallied and totals to date brought forward (see Figure 7.6). You should also know how much money is uncollected in accounts receivable and how old each account is. Bills may be sent out biweekly or monthly.

You may choose to do your own bookkeeping, hire an experienced accountant or CPA to just do your reports and taxes, or simply deliver all your figures regularly to your accountant. If you carry a heavy client load, you may not have the time or energy to complete your financial analysis as often as you should. As computers become more commonplace in dietitians' offices, their use in financial recordkeeping and assessment has become a tool of great value. Whatever the mode you choose for bookkeeping, never lose sight of the fact that, as the owner, you will ultimately be held responsible for the accuracy of the reporting system and its figures.

Record Retention

Files need to be kept on your business for important documents and records of business transactions. There isn't total agreement among experts as to the actual length of time to hold records, so check with your own advisors.

Suggested record retention schedule:

Permanent

- Audit reports of accountants, financial statements
- Capital stock and bond records
- Cash books and charts of accounts
- Cancelled checks for important payments
- Contracts and leases still in effect
- Correspondence (legal and important matters)
- Deeds, mortgages, bills of sale, appraisals
- Insurance records, claims, policies, etc.
- Patient files
- Corporate minute books of meetings
- Tax returns and worksheets
- Trademark registrations and copyright certificates

Figure 7.5   Sample Income and Expense Record

DATE								
Income				Expenses				
Day	Name	Check No.	Amount	Day	Name	Check No.	Account No.	Amount

Figure 7.6 Sample Monthly Bookkeeping Record

(*Source:* Nicholas Picchione, *Simplified Monthly Bookkeeping Record,* Warwick, R.I.: Dome Publishing Co., 1983. Reprinted by permission of the publisher.)

MONTH OF *March* 19

TOTAL RECEIPTS FROM BUSINESS OR PROFESSION			EXPENDITURES				
DAY		AMOUNT	ACCT. NO.	ACCOUNT	TOTAL THIS MONTH	TOTAL UP TO LAST MONTH	TOTAL TO DATE
1		221 60		**DEDUCTIBLE**			
2		187 93	1	MDSE.-MATERIALS	5,704 47	12,087 12	17,791 59
3		201 69	2	ACCOUNTING	50 -	100 -	150 -
4		400 82	3	ADVERTISING	27 50	140 80	168 30
5		571 57	4	AUTO EXPENSE	59 34	134 15	193 49
6		901 42	5	CARTONS. ETC.			
7		0	6	CONTRIBUTIONS		20 -	20 -
8		112 71	7	DELIVERY EXP.	96 33	316 05	412 38
9		65 22	8	ELECTRICITY	27 12	54 48	81 60
10		104 61	9	ENTERTAINMENT	9 58	66 62	76 20
11		130 34	10	FREIGHT & EXP.	62 85	173 67	236 52
12		423 68	11	HEAT	42 84	136 16	179 -
13		666 44	12	INSURANCE	40 -	136 32	176 32
14		0	13	INTEREST	10 17	22 23	32 40
15		124 10	14	LAUNDRY			
16		65 12	15	LEGAL EXPENSE		100 -	100 -
17		95 76	16	LICENSES			
18		176 33	17	MISC. EXP.	35 50	105 06	140 56
19		374 75	18	OFFICE EXP.	60 24	162 15	222 39
20		690 40	19	POSTAGE	18 -	45 61	63 61
21		0	20	RENT	150 -	300 -	450 -
22		204 97	21	REPAIRS	16 50	16 43	32 93
23		162 02	22	TAX—SALES	80 61	140 67	221 28
24		182 24	23	TAX — SOC. SEC.	27 70	55 40	83 10
25		263 53	24	TAX — STATE U. I.		26 03	26 03
26		505 18	25	TAX — OTHER		58 06	58 06
27		920 09	26	SELLING EXP.		25 -	25 -
28		0	27	SUPPLIES	11 80	58 17	69 97
29		210 14	28	TELEPHONE	38 67	104 54	143 21
30		150 21	29	TRADE DUES, ETC.		20 -	20 -
31		163 48	30	TRAVELING EXP.	50 -		50 -
TOTAL THIS MONTH		8,276 35	31	WAGES & COMM.	834 58	1,769 16	2,603 74
TOTAL UP TO LAST MONTH		18,052 71	32	WATER			
			33				
TOTAL TO DATE		26,329 06	34				
			35				
				SUB-TOTAL	7,453 80	16,373 88	23,827 68
				NON-DEDUCTIBLE			
			51	NOTES PAYABLE			
			52	FEDERAL INC. TAX		200 -	200 -
			53	LOANS PAYABLE	150 -	300 -	450 -
			54	LOANS RECEIV.			
			55	PERSONAL	400 -	900 -	1,300 -
			56	FIXED ASSETS			
			57				
				TOTAL THIS MONTH	8,003 80		
				TOT. UP TO LAST MO.		17,773 88	
				TOTAL TO DATE			25,777 68

MEMO

```
   8,276.35
 - 7,453.80
   ─────────
     822.55
```

Profit this month

```
   26,329.06
 - 23,827.68
   ──────────
    2,501.38
```

Profit to date

COPYRIGHT DOME ENTERPRISES

Seven years

- Accident reports and claims
- Accounts payable and receivable ledgers
- Cancelled business checks (see permanent listing)
- Contracts and leases (expired)
- Invoices
- Payroll records
- Purchase orders and sales records

Three years

- Correspondence (general)
- Employee applications and personnel records (terminated)
- Insurance policies (expired)

One year

- Bank reconciliations
- Correspondence (routine)

TAXES

Filing income tax and Social Security tax forms is made easier by working closely with an advisor to learn: forms to file and how to fill them out, dates to file, and tips to minimize over- or underpayment. Even if your accountant or CPA fills out the forms, you should be familiar with what they are doing (see Figure 7.7).

Who Must File

Any single person who grossed more than $3,300 or a surviving spouse who grossed more then $4,400, or a married couple who grossed more than $5,400 must file a tax return (6). Partnerships must file returns and state specifically the items of their gross income and deductions. Corporations must file and pay taxes on any profit. S Corporations do not pay taxes, but have their profit or loss reflected on the shareholders' tax returns.

Deductions

Practitioners are usually allowed to deduct the following expenses (6):

- Cost of supplies, postage, teaching materials, etc.
- Rent paid for office rooms
- Cost of fuel, water, lights
- Advertising and promotion
- Telephone, answering service
- Hire of office assistants and subcontractors
- Dues to professional societies (social clubs, usually excluded)
- Cost of operating an automobile for business
- Furniture, instruments, equipment, business computer, etc.
- Books, newsletters, journals   *(List continues on p. 95.)*

Figure 7.7   Sample Tax Calendar

(*Source:* Nicholas Picchione, *Simplified Monthly Bookkeeping Record,*
Warwick, R.I.: Dome Publishing Co., 1983. Reprinted by permission of the
publisher.)

(Dates and information may change without notice.)

Jan. 1 Form W-4. Employee status determination date.

     15 Amended declaration return of estimated tax may be filed.

     15 Final payment of estimated tax by individuals and corporations who
have previously made declarations.

     31 Employer furnishes each employee Form W-2, showing amount of taxes
withheld during prior year.

     31 Form 941. Quarterly return by employer of taxes withheld during
preceding quarter plus employer and employee Social Security taxes.

     31 Quarterly return by employer of state unemployment taxes.

     31 Form 940. Annual return by employer of Federal unemployment taxes.

Feb. 28 Forms 1096 and 1099. Annual information of dividends, salaries, and
other payments.

     28 Form W-3. Reconciliation of withholding taxes.

Mar. 15 Form 1120. Corporation income tax return due for those on
calendar-year basis.

Apr. 15 Form 1040. Individual income tax return for prior calendar year. (Note:
Individuals may file this form on January 31 and thus avoid filing
amended estimate.)

     15 Final income tax return of taxpayer who died in prior year.

     15 Form 1065. Partnership return due for those on calendar year basis.

     15 Form 1040 ES. Important: Declaration return and payment of
one-quarter of current year's estimated tax due.

     15 Form 503. Depository form and payment of corporate estimate due.

     30 Form 941. Quarterly return by employer of taxes withheld during
preceding quarter plus employer and employee Social Security taxes.

     30 Quarterly return by employer of state unemployment taxes.

June 15 Payment due of one-quarter of current year's estimated tax.

     15 Form 1040 ES. Amended declaration return may be filed.

     15 Form 503. Depository form and payment of corporate estimate due.

July 31 Form 941. Quarterly return by employer of taxes withheld during
preceding quarter plus employer and employee Social Security taxes.

     31 Quarterly return by employer of state unemployment taxes.

Sept.15 Payment due of one-quarter of current year's estimated tax.

     15 Form 1040 ES. Amended declaration return may be filed.

     15 Form 503. Depository form and payment of corporate estimate due.

Figure 7.7 *(Continued)*

Oct. 31   Form 941. Quarterly return by employer of taxes withheld during preceding quarter plus employer and employee Social Security taxes.

    31   Quarterly return by employer of state unemployment taxes.

- Expenses incurred in attending business conventions
- Job hunting expense, if not looking for first job or a position in an unrelated field

Any additional types of deductions should be discussed with your tax advisor.

Personal, living, or family expenses are not deductible. These would be items such as:

- Withdrawals of money by owner
- Insurance paid on a dwelling house
- Life insurance premiums (except key person insurance for business owners)
- Payments made for house rent, food, clothing (except uniforms), servants, upkeep of pleasure auto, etc.

Loans

Since money borrowed is not considered taxable income, neither is the repayment of the loan considered an allowable deduction. Interest paid can be deducted.

Retirement Plans

IRA, KEOUGH (HR-10 Pension benefit plan), and profit sharing plans are forms of retirement plans. These plans allow an entrepreneur to invest in tax deductible accounts that accrue interest tax free until retirement. Each option has its advantages and limitations. Before choosing the program(s) you will use, talk to your banker, accountant, lawyer, and also to financial institutions that offer new twists to the traditional programs.

WAYS TO IMPROVE YOUR BUSINESS

Regardless of the type of business you have and what you sell, there are common problems shared by most businesses. There are also common business practices that may improve a business:

- Use a budget and become involved in the regular evaluation of your business output and financial status.
- Keep accounting systems relevant and effective—reevaluate regularly.

- Take calculated, well-thought-out risks.
- Use prosperous periods to reduce your firm's debts and strengthen its finances.

Many businesses and financial consultants encourage new business owners to use their first year in business to become established in the marketplace while keeping overhead minimized. The second year should be used for gaining stability and becoming financially secure. The third year and on could be used for expansion and calculated risks. To be rewarded with longevity, a business must first have a stable income generated from clientele support.

REFERENCES

1. Leonard, Rodney E.: "Private Practice: On Your Own," *The Community Nutritionist,* Washington, D.C., July–August, 1982.
2. Curtin, Richard T.: *Running Your Own Show,* New American Library, New York, 1982.
3. Wexler, Hildegarde: *A Businesswoman's Guide to Working with Professional Advisors,* Mid States Bank, Denver, CO, 1980.
4. "How To Collect Accounts Receivable" in *Business Perspectives,* United Bank of Denver, December, 1979.
5. McCue, Jack D.: *Private Practice,* The Collamore Press, Lexington, MA, 1982.
6. Picchione, Nicholas: *Simplified Monthly Bookkeeping Record,* Dome Pub., Warwick, RI, 1983.

chapter *8*

Third Party Reimbursement

When someone other than the patient pays your fee for nutrition counseling, that is called third party payment. That "other" party is usually an insurance company or government program. At this time independent private practitioners report only inconsistent and sporadic coverage of their fees by third party payers, but it is improving.

As insurance coverage for nutrition services becomes a reality, it is hoped that more people in need of nutrition counseling will seek it out. We know that good nutritional care can make a big difference in the maintenance of good health. Unfortunately, third party programs, both public and private, have been slow to recognize the contributions registered dietitians can offer their beneficiaries. They have been particularly hesitant to cover nutrition services offered by an independent practitioner outside of the standard institutional setting or physician's office.

COVERAGE CRITERIA

The major criteria that insurers use in deciding whether to offer coverage of a new service is whether the public is already willing to pay for it and whether there are requests for coverage for it—as in dental insurance coverage. In other words there must be public demand not just professional pressure. As new insurance policies are negotiated, nutrition counseling could be an added "perk" offered by employers or a new coverage item used by insurance companies to attract new business. However, if there are no private practitioners in the area to make the public or the companies aware of the valued services, no changes are likely to be made. Most insurance policies are written for specific businesses or regions; very few are national. Therefore, changes will probably have to be initiated on a more local or state-wide basis. And it should not be assumed that because a company offers coverage in one state or region, it will automatically offer it somewhere else.

Another major criteria insurance companies use in determining what services to cover is whether the service provides cost-benefits. Will it save health care costs in the long run for the patient to see a dietitian? Are the services vital and effective? Surveys are being conducted at this time by practitioners and organizations to help substantiate the cost-benefits of nutrition counseling, but each of us can develop statistics in our own setting.

Most states do not require that dietitians be licensed, therefore they are not legally recognized as the sole or best providers of nutrition counseling. This may keep some providers from offering coverage on nutrition counseling.

THIRD PARTY PROGRAMS

The major programs that provide medical health insurance, as discussed by The Bennett Group/Health Services report to The American Dietetic Association entitled "Noninstitutional Third-Party Reimbursement For Nutrition Services" are private commercial companies, Blue Cross/Blue Shield, Medicare, Medicaid (1). It is important to know the major differences between these programs so that efforts to solicit coverage are more specific and thus productive. Other systems of payment are also emerging on the medical scene that will be important to our careers and future livelihoods: Health Maintenance Organizations (HMOs), Preferred Provider Organizations (PPOs), and prospective payment systems using Diagnose Related Groups (DRGs).

Private Commercial Companies

Private insurance companies are autonomous of one another, and have the ability to offer their customers whatever benefits they see fit. Private practitioners report that by far the best chance of reimbursement of their services is by private insurers. Reimbursement is usually tied to whether the patient is referred by a physician and whether the nutritional services are medically necessary and appropriate for the diagnosis. Suggestions to improve the chances of fee coverage will be listed later in this chapter.

Blue Cross/Blue Shield (BC/BS)

According to The Bennett Group report,

> Blue Cross and Blue Shield were started back in the late 1930s by hospitals and doctors, respectively, to assure payment of their own bills. Both organizations (which have officially merged as of July 1, 1982) were set up as nonprofit service entities. BC/BS has traditionally offered very complete coverage for lower premiums than other private health insurers. This was partially due to their

nonprofit status. . . . From an organizational standpoint, BC/BS is quite insistent that each plan has autonomy to decide what benefits to offer as part of their various packages. While they often emulate other plans, most particularly the federal Medicare program for which they are a claims processor in many states, policy is set at the individual plan level (1).

Independent private practitioners report that some of their patients have been reimbursed for nutrition consultation under Blue Cross/Blue Shield Major Medical policies. Blue Cross/Blue Shield offices will usually offer independent practitioners the opportunity to submit supporting evidence as to the dietitian's qualifications, an explanation of the services rendered, plus time and cost information to their medical review board for consideration of coverage. Provider numbers like those given to physicians are necessary to bill the company directly. For now an itemized nutrition bill can be attached to the common insurance form, and it will sometimes be covered. At this time nutritionists do not qualify for provider numbers.

Medicare

It is well known that Medicare will reimburse an institution based on reasonable cost for dietary services, but federal rules do not permit coverage of noninstitutional nutritional services. Nonetheless, some practitioners report that several of their patients have received reimbursement for nutrition services under Medicare Part B—Supplemental Insurance.

Medicare has two segments: Part A where care is given as an inpatient at a hospital, at a nursing home, or by home health care, and Part B, which is a voluntary supplemental program that covers services that complement Part A.

Medicare is a federally run program and it was established to cover the *acute* medical costs for persons over 65 years of age, disabled Americans, and patients with End Stage Renal Disease. Medicare was not intended to cover the cost of preventive health care—which is the usual category for nutritional counseling. Legally, it would take an amendment to the Medicare program to include preventive health care services.

Medicaid

Medicaid (Title XIX) is a program of medical assistance, funded jointly by the federal government and the individual states. The beneficiary populations are state residents who are medically and/or financially needy and are also aged, blind, disabled, or a member of families with dependent children. Medicaid, like Medicare, is administered by the Health Care Financing Administration, part of the Department of Health and Human Services in Baltimore, Maryland. Medicaid, however, is primarily a state program with the state determining who is eligible, exactly what the benefits are (within Federal guidelines), the scope of the care, who can provide the services, and how much the state will reimburse the accepted providers. Medicaid coverage of dietetic services is a state-by-state phenomenon.

HMOs and PPOs

HMOs and PPOs are prevention-oriented health care providers. They make money by keeping their insured members healthy. They may offer programming for free or at low cost on weight control, smoking cessation, alcohol control, and stress management. The insurance premium may also include a yearly physical, exercise classes, prescriptions, or office visits at low or no cost.

These two programs differ from each other in at least one important manner. HMOs hire their own staffs to work at their clinics and members come to see them there. PPOs contract with medical staffs who ordinarily remain in their own offices and members go to the office for care. In practice, insurers may use some of both systems.

Dietitians may be hired as employees or consultants to HMOs. PPOs may add you to their list of covered providers (sometimes you may have to pay to be on the list) or hire you. Hospitals may also be on a PPOs list and may offer nutrition services in the outpatient clinic, food service, home health rehabilitation, corporate wellness or fitness areas. You could be hired as an employee or consultant to the hospital programs.

Billing for HMO or PPO members takes place in many different ways depending upon the individual program. The members may have to pay up front and then be reimbursed, or you may be asked to bill the company. Whatever the method, make sure it is clear before instructing insured members.

Prospective Payment System with DRGs

The prospective payment system uses the Diagnose Related Groups to estimate the cost associated with having a certain medical problem. This system is being used by the government to stop the rampant overspending for government paid hospitals bills. If the system proves successful, it may be adopted by private insurers. The philosophy may be adapted to cover all reimbursable medical fees. Although it is too early to guess all the ramifications of this payment system, it is certainly worth watching closely.

BILLING SUGGESTIONS

Consultants suggest that, for purposes of cash flow and effective fee collection, nutrition consultants ask for payment of their fees at the time of the visit. It is then the responsibility of the patient to make sure the forms are filled out correctly and sent in to the insurance company. If less than the entire fee is reimbursed, the patient, not the consultant, absorbs the difference. Claims should be sent to insurers even when it is known that funding is probably not available. This may help create an increased awareness of the nutrition services and would check whether the rules are being interpreted differently.

GROUNDWORK FOR PAYMENT SYSTEM

The seven major steps to implementation of a Nutrition Services Payment System in any dietetic setting are (2):

1. Establish a rationale and plan for implementation.
2. Review the Uniform Nomenclature and select the terms that are appropriate for the services provided in the practice setting.
3. Establish a fee-for-service system.
4. Process charges and bill patients/clients or third party payers.
5. Monitor payment and reimbursement.
6. Document services rendered and the value of services.
7. Educate users—market nutrition services.

Terminology

Prerequisite to obtaining third party coverage, it is imperative that practitioners document their work, its cost, and its benefits to the public. To compare services and outcomes and to keep more accurate statistical information, we must speak the same language. To that end the American Dietetic Association organized a task force that developed a "Nutrition Services Payment System" manual (2).

Establishing Legal Professional Identity

It is important that dietitians establish a professional identity for themselves not only in the eyes of the public but also on a legal basis. Using the initials "R.D." or words "Registered Dietitian" after your name is protected under trademark law for dietitians who are registered by the Commission on Dietetic Registration of The American Dietetic Association. But, in states without entitlement or licensure anyone can call him- or herself a dietitian or nutritionist and not have any legal problem. To obtain third party reimbursement for nutrition counseling, insurers state they will eventually demand that there be some control over who can call themselves a qualified nutrition counselor and what they will be qualified to do. It is curious to note that chiropractors and naturopaths in California can legally be reimbursed for nutrition consultations, but not dietitians because they are not licensed.

Standards of Practice

The American Dietetic Association has had members working very hard for several years to determine the standards that would be considered good dietetic care and service. These standards are agreed upon and published. They will become the basis for evaluation of ethical, quality dietetic practice.

Reimbursement   To help improve the patients' chances of obtaining reimbursement, the following suggestions are given:

1. Have the referring physician write the request for a diet instruction down on a prescription pad (see Figure 8.1). Include this order along with the

Figure 8.1   Sample Prescription/Referral Form
(*Source:* Reprinted by permission of The American Dietetic Association.)

```
(name)    Jane Doe, R.D.
(address) 4110 22nd Street, Suite 213
          Dallas, Texas
(phone)   863-4111

Nutrition counseling referral


patient's name_____   phone _____

address_____   date of birth _____

diagnoses  _____

_____

other medical conditions _____

_____

medications  _____

relevant lab data  _____

_____

_____

nutrition prescription_____

_____

exercise restrictions _____

_____


                              _____
                              physician's signature

                              _____
                              date
```

completed insurance form and the nutritionist's bill to the insurance company. The chances are poor if a client is self-referred.

2. On the nutritionist's bill, state the medical reason(s) for the nutrition consultation, being careful *not* to list weight loss as the primary diagnosis, if possible. Insurance companies must be afraid that they will have to cover the expense of every dieter in the nation, if they once start. The bill should also indicate the referring physician, date, and the type of visit (initial or revisit) or the amount of time spent. (See superbill Figure 8.2 and sample bill Figures 7.4 and 8.3.)

Figure 8.2   **Sample of a Superbill**
(*Source:* Reprinted by permission of The American Dietetic Association.)

---

patient's name: _____   date: _____

place of service: ____hospital ____office ____extended care ____home

diagnosis_____

referring physician   _____

service description	fee		service description	fee
Consultation, with initial history of current life-style, habits of nutrition, environment, exercise, and stress	_____		Hospital visit and re-assessment	_____
			Follow-up evaluation	_____
Comprehensive consultation with complex disease and diagnostic nutrition assessment	_____		Office visit —brief	_____
			Follow-up evaluation	_____
Consultation and re-assessment of nutrition status and disease management	_____		Initial screening with limited assessment	_____
			Structured health management program (group)	_____
Screening assessment to rule out malnutrition	_____		Crisis intervention/ emergency phone consultation	_____
Nutrient intake analysis—comprehensive	_____		Special reports	_____
			Educational materials	_____
Nutrient intake analysis—limited	_____		Telephone conference	_____
Behavioral/ psychosocial counseling	_____		Home visit	_____
Patient-related team conference	_____		Dispensing pharmaceutical products, administration of supplies and equipment	_____
Prescription and formulation of enteral nutrition product	_____		Follow-up evaluation	_____
Preparation and/or dispensing of proprietary supplements and defined formula diets	_____		Activities of daily living	_____
			Miscellaneous, unlisted nutrition service	

today's charges _____

previous balance _____

Jane P. Doe, R.D./L.D.
00001   total charges _____
Board of Dietetic Examiners
12 Main Street, Suite 567   _____
Houston, Texas 77204   dietitian's signature

                                  _____
                                     registration number

Figure 8.3   Sample Itemized Bill
(*Source:* Reprinted by permission of The American Dietetic Association.)

name: _____   mailing address: _____

_____

_____

client's name: _____   referring physician: _____

diagnosis: _____

_____

_____

date first consulted for this condition: _____

date of service	service rendered	code	charges

additional information: _____

_____

_____   _____
        date   dietitian's signature

                                         _____
                                         registration number

3. Proper terminology on the nutritionist's bill is also very important. It is suggested that you do not use the words "diet" because it connotes weight loss diet or "nutrition education" because it conveys a luxury not medically based.

4. Insurance companies want to have a physician's provider code number on an insurance claim. The referring physician's provider code is used appropriately only when nutrition counseling takes place in the physician's office. However, some private practitioners have found that their patients have been reimbursed when the dietitian was obviously a separate service at a different locale, but the insurance form (with the prescription note and nutritionist's bill) had been signed by the physician's office.

5. Consultants should make a special effort to document improvement in patients' health not only in subjective terms, but also in lab values, skinfolds, and other anthropometric, physiologic, or cardiac values. Documentation of results may prove very beneficial in future negotiations on the need for third party coverage and the contribution of nutrition consultation.

MARKETING

As a private practitioner desiring third party coverage of your services for your clients, you are encouraged to contact your local insurance headquarter offices

Figure 8.4 Sample Statement of Cost Benefit
(*Source:* Reprinted by permission of The American Dietetic Association.)

TO   : Third-Party Payers
SUBJECT: Coverage of Nutrition Counseling Services

This information statement is provided for your company to clarify the listed services for nutrition, the qualifications and role of the registered dietitian practitioner, and the rationale for referral by the attending physician.

Reimbursement for treatment and health maintenance can prevent and control unnecessary and inflated medical costs to your company. Nutrition intervention is a vital component of primary treatment in medical and health care. Individuals are frequently referred to the registered dietitian for nutrition assessment, counseling, and management.

The referring physician realizes the cost benefit of nutrition management by the practitioner trained in this specialty, the registered dietitian. As a skilled professional, the registered dietitian has been trained extensively in accredited universities and medical centers on implementation of nutrition prescriptions. The R.D. practitioner has also had extensive training in educational and psychological techniques for effective patient/client compliance.

From the cost-benefit perspective, a visit to a registered dietitian for nutrition counseling, tailored to the individual's eating habits, life style, and nutrient needs, is much less expensive in the long term than recurrent office visits or hospitalization due to poor control, compliance, and disease management. These poor results are evidenced when inflexible, preprinted diet sheets and vague or no advice are the primary mode of corrective, maintenance, and preventive nutrition counseling.

---

to see what steps they would suggest. You may also contact state agencies that govern workmen's compensation and Medicare programs. Ideally, we would like to see provider numbers be given to consulting nutritionists, so ask about the possibility. Some private practitioners have offered academic information, resumes, nutrition services definitions, plus their approximate cost and time

Figure 8.5   Sample Correspondence with an Insurance Company
(*Source:* Reprinted by permission of The American Dietetic Association.)

DATE : March 10, 1983

TO   : Aetna Life Insurance Company

FROM: Jane P. Doe, R.D.
        Consulting Nutritionist

RE   : Susan Murray
        #175-16083-0007029

I am treating Susan Murray for malnutrition, ICD Code No. 263.9. Relative to the denial of coverage, because I was not recognized as a "physician" provider under the plan definition, please be advised that this patient was referred to me by my associate, Dr. John Smith, for care.

A registered dietitian is a recognized health care provider in the state of California, listed under the Business and Professions Code, Chapter 501. This was established by legislation, SB 213, in 1982. I am enclosing a cost-benefit statement, indicating that my services are provided upon referral by a physician for those consultations requiring the expertise and skill of a registered dietitian. Please note that no other health care provider is specifically trained as a nutrition counselor.

As an associate in a physician practice, I work with physicians to provide the skills and nutrition intervention necessary for patient care that is beyond the scope of medical practice.

Although in the past the physician or her or his nurse handed out a diet sheet, it has been recognized that this was not quality care nor did it facilitate results. On the other hand, recent cost-benefit studies have indicated that the nutrition counselor, namely the registered dietitian, produces results.

In my negotiations with the National Life Insurance Company, it was specifically indicated that with a diagnosis and referral by a physician, consideration would be given to the services of a registered dietitian. Realizing that this is a new aspect perhaps to your policy coverage, I would appreciate further review of this case, as this is a physician-referred order.

Thank you for your consideration in this regard.

Enclosures (3)

---

allotments and patients' outcomes as supporting evidence of the quality and validity of their care. Letters may also be written to third party payers to introduce your services or to defend patients' requests for coverage (see Figures 8.4 and 8.5, pp. 105 and 106).

CONCLUSION

On the negative side of third party payment, if patients delay payment and expect you to fill out their insurance forms, it could mean added problems and financial burdens for the practitioner. Also, as has happened in other medical professions when third party coverage arrived, it did not guarantee better patient care, and it supported a few incompetent professionals who took advantage of the program.

As a positive result of third party payment, it will surely mean more patient referrals to consulting nutritionists and longer follow up. This should result in better and more comprehensive nutritional care of clients. More dietitians will be able to begin or better maintain their own businesses. Also, it will mean more recognition of the dietitian and dietetic profession.

REFERENCES

1. The Bennett Group/Health Services report to The American Dietetic Association: "Noninstitutional Third-Party Reimbursement For Nutrition Services," 1983.
2. *Nutrition Services Payment System,* The American Dietetic Association, 1984.

chapter *9*

Start-up Costs

The cost of starting a private practice can vary greatly depending on the region of the country and the tastes of the practitioner. Some feel that if they are going to start a business, they are going to do it right. Others try to see how little they can spend to make the venture fly. Both can be successful, but both have also failed.

Investing a large sum each month in overhead to cover prime office space, extensive advertising, a secretary's salary, and new furnishings can create a successful stable image right from the start, which should logically attract more business—eventually. Eventually is the important word. There is a point where adding more money to create a good business will not necessarily bring in more clientele faster. However, an equally bad error can be made by not investing enough to give clients the feeling that you will be there next week.

Before trying to guess how much you are willing to spend on this venture, first decide what kind of office, furnishings, services, staffing, and marketing you would ideally like to have. Then estimate the cost to see if you can afford it. Compromises may have to be made. It may be that the office must be shared with another professional to cut the rental fee, the computer diet analyses and photocopying sent out, or a typing service called in as needed.

As mentioned earlier, most business consultants encourage new business owners to buy only the essentials, look for affordable quality, and keep the overhead low, especially the first year. The second year, increase the profit and savings and ordinarily, wait until the third year to expand and invest in more expensive ventures. The years involved are not as important as the business and financial growth that should logically take place first.

It is a well-known fact in business that the more metropolitan the area and the more ideal the rental space, the higher the cost, unless the area is overbuilt. This is especially true on the East and West coasts as compared to rural America. Competition for office space and higher service fees drive up costs that you must pay to run your business. Fees that a consultant charges can reflect these higher costs. The figures that follow are just rough estimates of the costs involved. Call around in your local area to get more accurate figures (see Figure 9.1).

IMPORTANCE OF WORKING CAPITAL

Up-front money will be invested to buy or rent the essentials to start your business, for example, office space, printed materials, calling cards, scale, calipers, insurance, telephone, answering service, furniture, and so on. The money that maintains these essentials and your salary is the working capital. Therefore, when estimating your expenses, recognize that there are two categories: up-front money to open the doors and maintenance money (working capital) to sustain the business. When planning a business, these two categories do not include the money being generated by clients.

The working capital should be readily available, but it does not have to be in your checking account. It could be a prearranged line of credit from your bank that isn't used unless it is needed—or any one of a number of other choices mentioned in Chapter 7. As a reminder, for your peace of mind, arrange to have six months' working capital available.

OFFICE SPACE

Choosing the correct office space, along with good marketing, may determine your ultimate success in business more than your nutritional expertise. Your office space can be instrumental in conveying stability, credibility, and success to patients and clients—or just the opposite.

Novices to business often do not know what kind of office space to look for. Some choose office space that costs very little, but unfortunately, they often get the quality they paid for. Others sign leases for beautiful space that destines them to work just to pay the rent. Some practitioners have found that sharing office space with a physician or even renting space in the same building as an influential or controversial physician may keep other physicians from referring patients. Knowing that some practitioners work successfully out of their homes, others try it, but have dismal luck. Most of these problems may be avoided with a little research and objective evaluation.

Rental Office Space

The ideal office location is convenient, accessible, and presents a good image. Clients will become more tolerant of inconveniences such as limited or paid parking, no elevator service, and little or no waiting room space as your reputa-

Figure 9.1   Sample Start-up Cost Estimates

Working Capital
Have six months' capital available before starting.

Lease
Deposit: Damage and last month's rent?
Monthly rent: $6 to $30+/square foot/year.
Nameplates: $5 to $150 (be sure to check).
Parking: Is staff parking included in rent? Is cost high?

Utilities
Deposit: Amount varies.

Telephone
Deposit: Amount varies, but may run from $100 to over $400.
Installation: $60 to $800; you may have to buy a phone system.
Monthly rate: $15 to $65+ per line.
Yellow Pages listing: One line is free; everything else is extra.
White Pages listing: Listing is free, but boldface is extra.
Long-distance service: $5 to $10/month, plus phone bill.

Services
Answering service: $25 to $80/month.
Answering machine: $150 to $300, depending on features.
Call Forwarding: $2+/month.
Call Waiting: $5 or less/month.
Accountant fees: $30 to $125.00+/hour.
Attorney fees: $50 to $150+/hour.
Temporary secretarial service: $8 to $24.00/hour.
Typing service: $7 to $24/hour.
Receptionist-secretary: Salary varies, but the best are expensive.
Cleaning service: Cost varies.

Insurance
Office liability and fire: $50 to $125.00+/year.
Malpractice: About $50/year when working part-time; $140 to $180/year when
            working full-time; costs reflect size of nutritional staff.
Disability: $15 to $40.00/month.
Health: Amount varies.
Life: Amount varies.

Office Supplies
Announcements: $25 to $40 per 100.
Business cards: $20 to $65 per 1000.
Letterheads: $10 to $30 per 100 (next 100s are less).
Envelopes: $10 to $30 per 100 (next 100s are less).
Brochure: Varies greatly; get several quotes. Ranges from 15 to 35 cents per
            brochure plus typesetting.
Logo: Artist fees vary greatly.
Bookkeeping system: $40 to $650 to establish.
Copying and printing: Price around; prices vary greatly.

Figure 9.1 *(Continued)*

Postage and miscellaneous: Keep supplies in modest amounts.
Handouts and teaching materials: Keep in modest supply.

Equipment and Furniture
Medical scale: $300+.
Typewriter: $250+.
Copier: $50+/month to rent or $1500+ to buy.
Calipers: $175 to $450.
Computer and software: $1500 to $6000 to buy; may also be leased, or send
           food lists out for analysis.
Impedance analysis machine: $200/month on lease or $6000 with computer
           purchased.
Furnishings and carpet: Amount varies greatly.

Advertising
Amount varies greatly.

Incorporation
$400 to $3500+.

---

tion grows. However, these problems possibly could be avoided by anticipating them and seeking a better location.

It may take several years before your business will attract clients from very far away. Practitioners suggest that offices be located near prospective clientele. Market research should help identify that area of town.

If you choose office space in a medical complex instead of an office building, you may find that you will attract more business. Fewer patients may get "lost" between being referred and actually scheduling a nutrition consultation.

Although "store-front" businesses in shopping malls or corner retail centers can do very well, private practitioners are not known for choosing these locations —yet. As emergency medical centers and daytime outpatient services become more prevalent in retail areas, maybe dietitians will opt to be there too.

There is one final point on a rental location: before signing a lease closely evaluate your neighbors, surrounding businesses, and the landlord. If you are signing a long-term lease, it is important to know if the area is going downhill, if neighboring renters are disruptive, or if the landlord maintains the property well.

Seeing Patients at Your Home

Before starting a private practice out of your own home, realize that the home environment can be a blessing or a big mistake. The home setting should be as professional as any private office. That means no family interruptions or phone calls during patient interviews and a comfortable yet clean and uncluttered setting. If the home does not have an appropriate waiting area, it may be necessary to allow more time between patient appointments.

A positive benefit of working out of one's home is that patients and clients seem to relax more quickly. This facilitates the consulting sessions or interviews. Also, it is convenient, requires no travel, and overhead is reduced; therefore profit per hour can be higher.

On the negative side of using the home: it may be an intrusion into the family's privacy, patients or physicians may be hesitant to use your services, and the dietitian may feel tied to the work setting. Some dietitians report they do not work out of their homes because they are concerned that their business images would not appear as established and successful. It is inconvenient when the practitioner's residence is in a large apartment or condominium complex and difficult to find.

If a den or other room is used exclusively for seeing patients or as your office, a percentage of the square footage and a portion of the related expenses or a rental fee may be a business tax deduction. A multipurpose room such as a living room or den with the family TV cannot be used as a deduction. Consult with your financial advisor on your specific situation.

Zoning laws for your neighborhood should be checked before starting to see patients at your home. The laws were written to protect the neighborhood quality of life from any undue disruption, excessive traffic, or commercialism. Practitioners who already work quietly out of their homes and have only one or two patients per hour have not found that zoning was a problem. If it becomes one, it may be possible to obtain a zoning variance for your business. Unless the zoning is correct for a business at home, an outside sign is usually not permitted.

Home Visits

Private practitioners in both rural and affluent areas have had success seeing patients in their own homes. Patients enjoy the convenience and are willing to pay extra, if they can afford it.

For the practitioner home visits are not an efficient use of time, if they pull him away from the office where other patients could be seen. If, however, the practitioner works at home and does home visits instead of renting an office, the savings could make it a good option.

Travel time, gas, and other related costs must be figured to help determine home visit fees. Some practitioners charge their patients a flat rate, while others charge according to the total time involved.

As the surplus of physicians grows and home visits become more common-place, or when insurance coverage more readily applies to home rehabilitation, this option may be very viable and popular.

Office Layout

If you can afford it, it is always a nice touch to have a receptionist or secretary —even one shared in common with other offices—to greet patients as they arrive. Patients expect to have a place to sit down and wait and a more private place for the diet consultation. Except for group meetings and large families, there will seldom be times when the waiting room will need more than four chairs and your office more than two for patients.

Most practitioners decorate their offices to fit their own tastes, not as a medical clinic. Patients seem more at ease with warmer surroundings and the break from what is traditional.

To establish credibility immediately, practitioners' certificates, diplomas, and awards should be framed and displayed in their offices. Patients do notice and read these items.

Office Safety

For the sake of safety, it is advisable to have an office fire extinguisher, flashlight, and smoke alarm. A diagram of the exits should be attached to the back of the main door. The furniture and decorations in the waiting room and your office should not be obviously dangerous or fragile. Any steps should be well marked and lighted.

When clients are being seen in the evenings it is best to ask group members to leave together or to call the building security person to make sure the client or you get into your cars without problems. When you are working before or after normal business hours (when few people are around), care should be taken to keep the office door locked. This precaution also applies whenever working out of your home—do not just let people walk into an unlocked house. With a little care, potentially negative situations may be avoided.

OFFICE AGREEMENTS

Rental or Lease

The following guidelines may be helpful to you when renting space:

- Do not accept the stated rental fee at face value. Virtually all rents are negotiable.
- Be on the lookout for especially attractive bargains caused by the economy or overbuilding. Many property owners are strapped for cash and are willing to make attractive offers.
- Look for ways to operate with a minimum amount of space. Should the firm be successful, chances are good you will be able to find additional space when it is needed.
- Practitioners seeking to serve a large market area should consider renting two smaller offices at different locations (one close to downtown and one in the suburbs) rather than one large one. This can double the firm's exposure and convenience to clients without doubling the cost of doing business, if it is planned well.
- Be aware that many leases have additions that boost the space costs well above the base price per square foot. Maintenance or management fees may not have limitations on escalation. Compute these costs into the amount of the lease.

- In negotiating for consulting space, be sure to mention that your business will not need special plumbing, extra electrical outlets or lavatory facilities—this will mean less expense and fewer problems for the building owner and rental could begin sooner.
- Be sure to ask what the rental fee includes, such as, shared waiting room, receptionist, utilities, insurance, carpeting, and so on. Discuss who will own any shelving, carpeting, or other additions you may pay for in your office—usually the landlord takes ownership unless some other arrangement was agreed upon.
- Will any months of free rent be offered to you as an enticement to rent?
- Check to see that the lease allows you to sublease your space in case the need arises.
- Most leases run a minimum of one to five years, but occasionally special concessions can be made for new or small businesses. Realize that the shorter the term of the lease, probably the sooner the rent will go up.
- Have a lawyer review the terms of the lease.

The major advantages of having a rental space of your own are that you can control its use, you can decorate it to your tastes, materials and records are readily available, and a business phone can be permanently installed. All of these elements help contribute to a more smoothly run operation and the appearance of order and prosperity. In a food management or similar practice, the office locale can be more flexible, especially when clients seldom come to the office.

Before moving into rented space it may be necessary to pay not only the first month's rent, but also the last month's rent and a sizable damage deposit. In all it may amount to three or more times the monthly rent! Ask your financial advisor about local state laws governing the money held by the landlord and your rights to interest, early payback, and so on.

Rental fees are quoted in two basic ways: a monthly rate, such as $350 per month, or as cost per square foot. The cost per square foot is usually for one year unless indicated otherwise. It may range from $6 per square foot in some locales to $30 or more in others. To figure your rent first determine the total number of square feet to be rented then multiply that figure times the cost per square foot to arrive at the total cost per year; divide by 12 months to arrive at your monthly rent (see Figure 9.2).

Coleasing

Coleasing takes place when two partners or other people agree to rent an office jointly. This is often an advantage when the square footage is too large for one and it is useful to share the cost. If the office space is only large enough for one person at a time, the days are alternated.

It is not advisable to colease with another nutritionist, unless you are partners and working for the same goals. Otherwise, trying to advertise two businesses selling the same service under the same telephone number and handling "walk-in" patients without intruding on each other's territory could prove too troublesome.

Figure 9.2 Figuring Rental Square Footage

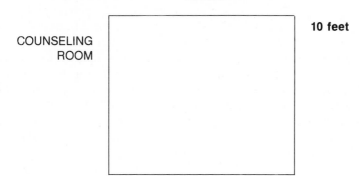

Full Time Use

12 feet $\times$ 10 feet = 120 square feet
120 square feet $\times$ \$10/square foot rent/year = \$1200 rent/year
\$1200 $\div$ 12 months = \$100/month rental fee

Subleasing Part-Time Use

Office used: 2 days/week $\times$ 4 weeks/month = 8 days/month
Percentage of month used: 8 $\div$ 20 working days = 40%
40% $\times$ \$100 rent/month = \$40/month rent (plus any other expenses or fees for other services)

It is again extremely important that you choose a coleasee well, and that a lawyer review the lease agreement. The agreement may hold you both responsible for damage or theft that your coleasee or his clients inflict. It may also leave you with the full responsibility if the other person moves or leaves and does not fulfill the entire lease agreement. Read the agreement carefully, change terms as necessary, have your lawyer review and make additions, and then submit it back to the landlord.

Sharing Office Space or Subleasing

Sharing office space is an alternative for those who want all of the amenities of a nice office and locale, but at less expense. In addition to the office, the telephone and answering service, copy machine and receptionist/secretary may also be shared. Again, all agreements should be in writing and reviewed by a lawyer.

An office may be subleased from another professional such as a speech therapist or psychologist who only needs the office several days per week or who has too much space for his or her business. The office rent and expenses can be split according to the percentage of the week each uses the office or for whatever amount you agree upon. Be sure to negotiate and get the best deal for yourself as you would with any landlord.

Office space can also be shared with a physician or clinic. Several different options are possible in this instance (see Chapter 16). The private practitioner could remain independent and do his own billing, marketing, printing of materials, and scheduling of own appointments while subleasing or renting space. Another option would be to give a percentage of the consultant fee in return for the use of the office and its amenities. A third option is to negotiate a retainer fee where you would always be available to see patients for the physician or clinic during a designated time in return for your receiving a specified fee—this is a good option when your services are sought after but the patient load is variable. A final option that some practitioners are still able to find is office space offered for free so that nutrition services are more accessible to the patient.

As you negotiate rent with a physician or clinic, consultants warn that doctors sometimes tend to overestimate the number of persons you will see. Agree on a fee that you can afford, not one that is based on ultimate expectations.

Close association with other professionals can provide numerous benefits. Several very successful practitioners report that much of their success when they first started in business came from having one or more "mentor" physicians who promoted them. Some of the physicians sublet space to the dietitians, but others just did it out of friendship and respect for the practitioner and aid to the patients.

Depending upon your individual situation, some important questions need to be discussed with the physician: Will you be able to see other doctors' patients at the office? Who will schedule patient appointments, pull and file charts, and bill patients? Can you use the copy machine? Who will market you and how? Remember the more services you request the more you may have to spend. Write down all agreements and have a signed copy for each party. A simple letter of agreement will work. A termination clause is advisable. When a contract is coming up for renewal, you should start negotiating at least a month in advance to allow both parties a chance to work out differences.

Parking

In some locations parking space is at a premium, especially in downtown or medical center areas. If a parking lot is owned by your building, are spaces included for the leasee? Can they be added when negotiating the lease?

Name Plates and Floor Directories

Most office buildings have some kind of directory outside the building, in the main lobby, or on each floor, in addition to door name plates. Seldom will a landlord of a medical building allow you to print your own—they like them standardized. This again could be a lease option to negotiate. Don't assume anything; one practitioner had to pay up to $26 per line for four partners on six floors.

Utilities

When utilities are not included in the lease, the utility companies can give you an estimate of your monthly bill. For electricity they will need to know the number of watts of each light and how many hours per week it will be used, in addition to the estimated usage of other equipment such as air conditioning, a typewriter, or computer. For gas heating, the square footage of your office can be used in determining an estimate. A money deposit or a letter of credit may be necessary to obtain new service.

Telephone

The recent and ongoing changes after the break up of AT&T will necessitate that each practitioner check on the best telephone coverage available locally. To survive a business must have good telephone service and coverage.

A business phone system costs approximately $60–$800 to install. Converting an existing private line at home to a business one is usually only a fraction of that cost, however, your business phone would then be at home. More telephone considerations are discussed in Chapter 18. If you have never had a business line, the telephone company may ask for a deposit—call for an estimate. The monthly fee for the telephone line will range from approximately $15–$65 per line.

Other services that you may consider for your phone are call waiting, call forwarding, and a limited service line. Call waiting will allow you to accept a second incoming call while keeping the first call on the line. Call forwarding allows you to transfer your incoming phone calls to another phone number where you or your answering service can answer it. Limited service lines are not available everywhere, but the line allows a limited number of outgoing calls to be made each month for a reduced rate. Calls above the limit are charged extra; in-coming calls are not counted. The rates and availability of these services vary—call your local company for more information.

Whenever you pay for a telephone line, business or personal, you will be given a listing in the white pages for free; bold print is extra. To have a Yellow Pages listing, you must have a business line. One listing under the most appropriate heading (probably "Dietitian" or "Nutritionist") will be given to you. Additional listings, bold print, extra lines, logo, a large ad, and so on will cost extra and will be billed monthly or however you arrange. (See ad samples in Figure 17.9.) If you share office space with someone who already has a business phone, for an added fee you can have your name added to that line. It will then be in directory information and in the Yellow Pages.

Answering Service

When you begin your business, the phone should be answered during normal business hours, Monday through Friday. An answering service or recording machine can give you coverage when you are away from the phone.

An answering service that receives your call through call forwarding and does not answer with your company name is the most inexpensive while giving a personal touch. Prices range from approximately $25 per month for the previously mentioned service to $40–$80 per month for private lines answered with your company name.

A telephone answering machine with a remote call device can also give you coverage. The public is becoming more familiar with talking to a machine. If the message is clear, creative, and of good quality, callers will use it. Answering machines range in cost from $150–$300.

SERVICES

Accountant or CPA

Fees for accountants or Certified Public Accountants range from $30 per hour to $125 per hour or more. Some accounting firms will teach you how to set up your books so that you can keep your own books; the firms then do tax returns. Others will take care of the books monthly for a flat rate and complete the tax return for free or a nominal fee. The more work you do yourself, the more reasonable the cost.

Secretary/Receptionist

There is little doubt that a private practitioner would enjoy using the services of a secretary/receptionist, however, there are ways to have the duties covered without having the full cost of an employee. According to surveys conducted by popular women's magazines, a good secretary is usually paid as much as a good dietitian with years of experience. Some alternatives are to hire someone part-time for several mornings per week, send out your typing, set up your office so that you can handle it yourself, use a temporary secretarial service at peak times, or find office space where a secretary's services are included. Most typing services charge from $7–$24 per hour. Temporary secretarial services charge approximately $8–$24 per hour with a minimum number of hours.

INSURANCE

Malpractice

At this time we know of two companies that offer dietitians' malpractice insurance: Bill Beatty Co. (through ADA), and St. Paul. An insurance broker will help you get a quote from St. Paul. On the average the cost is $50 per year when working part-time and approximately $140 per year when in private practice full-time for $200,000/$500,000 coverage. Prices go on up for larger amounts of coverage.

Office Liability and Furnishings

When a practitioner opens an office people will visit, there is always the risk that someone will get hurt on the premises. In rental space the landlord usually carries liability coverage, but often on a limited basis. When sharing space at a physician's office or clinic, good liability coverage may already be available to you under their policy—check. When working out of your home, home insurance companies ask that they be notified so that coverage can be increased. Insurance for office contents in case of fire, theft, or other loss is easily acquired along with the liability coverage. The fee for good liability and furnishings' insurance ranges from $50–$125 or more per year, depending upon the value covered.

Disability

Disability insurance will provide a certain level of limited income while you are ill. The most expensive coverage begins after only 15 days of illness and lasts for 2 years on up to life; depending upon several variables, the price may range from $30–$40 per month for $800–$1300 income per month. To reduce the cost, disability payments could begin after 30 or 60 days of illness and last for only 1 year. This policy will range from approximately $15–$25 per month for $800–$1300 per month disability income. The premium and disability coverage are dependent upon your age, health, and present income. Unfortunately, self-employed individuals have a more difficult time qualifying for this type of insurance according to several companies. Check with several insurance companies to see what they have to offer and compare costs and coverage.

Health

Health insurance is a necessity with today's health care costs. One hospital stay for one week or more could wipe out an uninsured person's savings. To help reduce the cost of a policy, try to join under a spouse's policy, contact local HMOs or PPOs, or join a group policy (through The American Dietetic Association, executive clubs, rural cooperatives, small business owners, local chambers of commerce, or those offered by local insurance brokers). In some cases if you have two or more employees in your business, you can qualify as a group. Another way to keep premium payments lower is to choose major medical coverage instead of a comprehensive top-of-the-line policy. You would have to pay the first $500 or so of a bill but then coverage may be 80 to 100 percent after that. Prices and coverage vary so greatly that you will need to take the time to get several quotes.

Life

Life insurance to pay off your loans and debts, as well as to help support your family in case of your death, is an important consideration. Term life insurance is usually the least expensive for the amount of coverage if you are younger and in good health. A 35-year-old practitioner may pay between $150 to $200 per year for $100,000 coverage. However, as the person grows older, the yearly premiums may increase quickly. Variations of whole life policies are readily available today. This type of policy is more expensive from the beginning, but eventually can act as a savings account to be borrowed against. This type of policy has a definite total price; therefore, premiums do not continue indefinitely as with term insurance.

OFFICE SUPPLIES

Business Cards

Before ordering cards make sure that your address and phone number will be more than temporary. Several practitioners have had cards printed with either the phone or address missing and had the information calligraphied in later. Allow two to three weeks to have cards printed. Because of the cost savings, most businesses order 500 or 1000 cards at a time. Cost for printing ranges from about $20–$65 per 1000 cards, depending upon the layout, paper, ink, embossing, and number of different colors of ink. For the first run there may also be a typesetting and layout fee.

Letterheads

Paper that is standard stock can be printed easily when more is needed. When the letterhead is on special paper, it can be more economical and time efficient to order the paper by the ream and keep it on hand yourself. Take it to be printed as you need it. If the letterhead printing or ink is special, it is more economical to print a larger amount because of the one-time fees to change ink colors, emboss, imprint, and so on. Letterheads range from about $10/100 sheets to more than $30/100 sheets for special paper and printing. Each additional 100 sheets is usually printed for a lower cost.

An economical way to send out a large mailing or form letter is to type the letter on one of your letterheads and have it reproduced on good paper (logo, your name and address, letter, and all). The date, heading, and your signature can be added whenever you use the letter.

To have a professional looking letter it is important that the color of paper you choose has correction tape or liquid to match. Plain paper should be purchased to match the letterhead for additional pages of a letter. Business letters are usually sent on 8½″ × 11″ paper, but notes can be any size with the appropriate size envelopes.

Envelopes

Envelopes are used quickly and are usually purchased in amounts of 500 or more at a time. The prices range from $10–$30/100 with each additional 100 costing less. Legal size is traditionally used in business.

Brochures

Good quality brochures are an asset to a business; typesetting is highly recommended. To save money the brochure could be a self-mailer, but for times when the best image is required, use an envelope. The cost of printing a simple brochure on colored paper on both sides with black ink is approximately $15–$35/100, folding included. Typesetting will vary between $15–$40/page. Before printing your brochure have several people read it and offer suggestions. Some pharmaceutical companies have offered to print brochures for private practitioners as a professional service. If you are interested in this service check with your local representatives.

Bookkeeping System

A beginning bookkeeping system with an appointment book, cash ledger, receipts, file folders, and yearly ledger can be purchased for under $40. Your accountant or CPA may request that you purchase a definite kind of system, but most are reasonable.

As the business grows and becomes more complex, it may be necessary to look into purchasing a "peg board system" so popular in medical offices. This is the system that uses carbonless paper to make writing a receipt, ledger entry, and next appointment a one-step process. This system is readily available commercially through companies listed under "Bookkeeping Systems" in the Yellow Pages or from an office supply business. This system retails for approximately $350–$650 to start and just the cost of the personalized forms from then on.

Diets and Handouts

The most important aspect about printed materials given to a client is to keep them simple, clear, and impressive. Also, don't load the patient down with every free booklet available on a subject—pick the best ones, free or not. One sheet of white paper printed on one side costs between $4–$9/100 sheets; colored paper is more. Diets that are not needed regularly can be photocopied when needed.

EQUIPMENT AND FURNISHINGS

Medical Scale

If a scale is used, a good balance beam medical scale is suggested. A waist-high balance beam is not suggested because it is awkward for very heavy patients to stand on the scale without touching the beam. Spring scales are not always accurate. A good scale retails for about $300 and up; used ones are less.

Skinfold Calipers

For consultants who work with weight loss, sports nutrition, or nutrition assessment, calipers are a must. They range in price from approximately $3.50 for the plastic ones to $175–$250 for the metal ones to $450 for the computerized ones.

Impedance Method of Body Composition Measurement

As an alternative to the skinfold method of measurement the RJL Impedance machine may be leased or purchased. The accuracy of this method is comparable to skinfolds and underwater weighing for most individuals (there are some exceptions), but like those methods is only as accurate as the technician's skill and control of the testing variables. This system is portable and easy to use. Considering the high price, a practitioner would invest in this product because clients are intrigued by it. Handled correctly and promoted well, it should open new doors and attract more business.

The entire system with the small computer retails for $6,000. Without the computer (if you already have access to an IBM or Apple) the price is $4,000. The system can be leased for 3 or 5 years for prices ranging from $110–$150/month without the computer to $160–$240/month with the computer. The longer the lease the higher the final price, but the monthly fee is lower.

Typewriter

If you decide to buy a typewriter, look for one that can also print diets and handout materials. It is suggested that it be pica-size type so that elderly patients can easily read it, not script style, and have the ability to use "film," not just cloth ribbon, for clearer printing. The cost for a good typewriter will begin at approximately $250 and go on up to $2,000 or more for the top of the line.

Computer

A computer, its components, and software can be a tax deduction if it is used for business. Businesses are springing up that rent computer or word processor time —you just supply the software. Computers and software packages range from $1,500–$6,000 on up. Systems may also be leased monthly for a minimum number of months.

Copier

When the volume warrants it, consider leasing or buying a photocopier. Many practitioners state that having a plain paper copier that can print their letterhead and reproduce office forms, bills, bulk mailings, instruction materials, and so on is a necessity. At the start of a business it may be more economical to share a copier or find a convenient quick copy store. Leases can range from $50–$100 per month. Used copiers may be available for reasonable prices also.

Office Furniture

Prices will vary with personal taste. Make the setting comfortable for yourself and the client. For dietitians who will be seeing very large patients, buy sturdy chairs without armrests or with a wide area between armrests, and not so soft so that standing up becomes embarrassing.

Carpet and Interior Improvements

It is assumed that any "permanent" improvements that you or your landlord pays for, such as carpeting, secretary's window, shelving, and so on are the property of the landlord when you move unless you have made another agreement (have it in writing). If you don't want to pay for carpeting you can't take with you, buy an area rug. Free-standing shelving can be purchased. Costs of changes to walls, doors, and windows can be negotiated. Keep receipts for all purchases and check with your accountant or CPA concerning deductions, depreciation, and using items from home.

MARKETING

Announcements

Announcements to mark the opening of your office will cost approximately $25–$40/100, including a one-time typesetting fee. Pharmaceutical companies again occasionally pay for printing announcements for new medical/nutrition practices.

Advertising

Business consultants suggest that at least 15 percent of your budget be allocated to cover the cost of the first year's kick-off campaign in marketing, such as newspaper ads, business lunches, brochures, direct mail letters, and so on. Also allow 5–10 percent or more of each additional year's budget for on-going marketing.

LEGAL

If you decide to incorporate your business before opening your doors, it will cost between $400–$3500. Licenses to open a business in your local city, county or state will range from none needed to an estimate of $15–$150. As mentioned earlier, a lawyer may charge $50–$150 per hour, plus more for phone calls.

MISCELLANEOUS

Although we like to feel that we have anticipated all of the applicable expenses, we of course haven't. Memberships and subscriptions may need to be budgeted. A dependable car may have to be purchased. A "cushion" needs to be planned to cover petty cash expenses and unexpected larger expenses.

Good preplanning makes the evolution of a business an anticipated pleasure instead of a crisis management seminar (see Figure 9.3).

Figure 9.3   Anticipated Costs Worksheet

	Start-up	Cost/Month	Total/Year
Working Capital		_____	_____
Office Lease	_____	_____	_____
Deposit	_____		_____
Last month's rent	_____		_____
Parking	_____	_____	_____
Nameplates	_____		_____
Utilities (gas, electricity, water)	_____	_____	_____
Deposit	_____		_____
Telephone (monthly rate)	_____	_____	_____
Deposit	_____		_____
Installation	_____	_____	_____
Call Waiting	_____	_____	_____
Call Forwarding	_____	_____	_____
Yellow Pages Listing	_____	_____	_____
White Pages (extra fees)	_____	_____	_____
Other _____	_____	_____	_____
Answering Service or Recorder	_____	_____	_____
Attorney Fees	_____	_____	_____
Accountant or CPA	_____	_____	_____
Secretary-Receptionist	_____	_____	_____
Typing Service	_____	_____	_____
Janitorial Service	_____	_____	_____
Other _____	_____	_____	_____

Figure 9.3 *(Continued)*

	Start-up	Cost/Month	Total/Year
Insurance			
Malpractice	_____	_____	_____
Office liability and furnishings	_____	_____	_____
Disability	_____	_____	_____
Health	_____	_____	_____
Life	_____	_____	_____
Other _____	_____	_____	_____
Office Supplies			
Business cards	_____	_____	_____
Letterheads	_____	_____	_____
Envelopes	_____	_____	_____
Brochures	_____	_____	_____
Bookkeeping system	_____	_____	_____
Diets (printing, research, etc.)	_____	_____	_____
Handouts, educational materials	_____	_____	_____
Other _____	_____	_____	_____
Equipment and Furnishings			
Medical scale	_____	_____	_____
Typewriter	_____	_____	_____
Copier	_____	_____	_____
Skinfold calipers	_____	_____	_____
Computer	_____	_____	_____
Software	_____	_____	_____

Figure 9.3 *(Continued)*

	Start-up	Cost/Month	Total/Year
Impedance machine	___	___	___
Furniture	___	___	___
Carpet	___	___	___
Office improvements	___	___	___
Other ___	___	___	___
Marketing			
Announcements	___		___
Advertising (on-going)	___	___	___
Kickoff	___		___
Other ___	___	___	___
Legal			
Incorporation	___	___	___
Licenses	___	___	___
Other ___	___	___	___
Miscellaneous			
Memberships	___	___	___
Subscriptions	___	___	___
Car care	___	___	___
Petty cash	___	___	___
Other ___	___	___	___
Totals	___	___	___

three

MANAGING YOUR BUSINESS

chapter 10

Computers in Nutrition Practice

Cecelia Helton, M.A., R.D.

Computers are not new to the field of dietetics, however, many of us are just learning to appreciate the myriad of functions they can perform. Computers are categorized as fast, but dumb, pieces of equipment—they can process words and data quickly, but they are totally dependent upon input from the outside for them to function. The output that computers produce is only as accurate as the information that is fed into them. Therefore, the persons who use computers largely determine how well computers work.

WHAT CAN A COMPUTER DO FOR A PRACTITIONER?

Before investing in the expense of computer equipment (hardware), the program instructions (software), and training to learn how to use the system, decide what you want the computer to do. Too many small business owners buy a computer because they think they must need one. But, they have no idea (other than for bookkeeping and nutritional analysis) what to do with it. What an expensive and limited investment!

Nutrient Analysis

Nutrient analysis of recipes, menus, and food intakes is probably the most familiar computer function to dietitians. Before the use of the computer, it was so time consuming to analyze foods for nutrient levels that it was not done with any regularity, except perhaps in research settings.

Q & A

Computer Replacing a Dietitian

I see so many weight loss and wellness programs run by laymen and nurses who feel they can do nutrition counseling because they can nutritionally analyze a person's diet. Am I overreacting or am I being replaced by a floppy disk?

I always tell dietitians that if they can be replaced by a floppy disk, they are not doing dietitian-level work. I tell potential consultant accounts that the nutritional analysis of a person's diet is an easy way to arrive at "ball park" estimates of the days analyzed. But the interpretation and application of the results, along with the motivational counseling, behavior change training, medical score interpretation, and individualized nutritional care are really what a trained nutritionist has to offer.

We have got to market ourselves and perform to standards that are above the competition.—Kathy King Helm, R.D.

Today many practitioners offer nutrient analysis to institutional settings such as jails, nursing homes, and hospitals. Nutrient analysis is used to help write menus, to document the nutritional value of the foods offered, and to calculate the nutritional value of food eaten by any one resident. The computer can also calculate food orders, cost analysis per vendor or menu item, inventory control, employee scheduling and paperwork, and of course many other bookkeeping functions.

Many private practitioners also use nutrient analyses while working with individual patients, corporate clients, or athletes and sports teams. Clients are impressed and fascinated with computer printouts that show "scientifically" how nutritious their diets are. The truth, of course, is that the results are only ball park figures. The foods analyzed may not have been representative of the client's normal eating patterns. The amounts and ingredients of foods may even be 30 percent or more wrong because of the guesswork involved in a layman's food diary or recall. And, finally, the database used to analyze the foods may not be complete enough, so entire foods are left out of the calculations, or their ingredients are estimated. To help avoid these pitfalls as much as possible, a practitioner should instruct the client on how to measure foods (ideally by weight). A week's record could be recorded with three representative days chosen for analysis. And care should be taken to find analysis software that has an accurate and adequate database.

In April, 1983, dietetic students, enrolled in my community nutrition class at Idaho State University, used the Nutrichec computer program at a health fair to provide on-the-spot nutritional analyses for interested consumers. On the first day of "Health Fair 83" we had one student operate the computer and a second student assist with pamphlet distribution and answering questions from the participants. The lines at our center were so long we decided to add another computer on the second day of the fair. Our lines didn't seem to get any shorter; we were just able to serve more people—approximately 200 throughout the two-day period. Since this was our first experience with dietary analysis for the public, the students discovered that there was a high level of interest in foods and nutrition among the lay population. In today's technological society, I am certain that the presence of the microcomputer at our center was an effective means for attracting attention.

Teaching

Teaching nutrition to patients or clients can be carried out on a computer. Topics such as energy balance for weight control, sports nutrition, and menu planning, as well as diabetic or other clinical diet guidelines or behavior change lessons could be programmed onto software in a self-instruction format.

A computer may also be used for evaluating the effectiveness of your nutrition counseling sessions. By pre- and posttesting a patient in a nonthreatening environment, the patient and you will be able to tell whether the patient and his family understood the most important points. The posttest will also act as a summary.

Nutrition Histories

Nutrition histories, fitness, and lifestyle computer questionnaires can be developed or purchased for use by the patient or to be input into the computer by the practitioner from a written form filled out by the patient. The questionnaire results can be used to motivate the patient by showing specific areas for needed improvement, or where he is doing well.

Patient and Client Records

Records of all sorts can be "filed" on computer software. In fact, unless you feel you must have a folder to hold the patient's pertinent information, there is no reason not to put all information on software (with a backup copy). When a patient arrives for an appointment, you could retrieve his record on the screen. Chemical scores, medical diagnosis, nutritional history, assessment, care plan, appointment summaries, and financial records can all be listed. The information can be used from the screen or printed as needed. After the appointment is over, the practitioner can update the payment record and input changes in status (chemical scores, percent body fat, habits, attitude, etc.) and future goals, including the date of the next appointment. Each patient can be assigned a patient number or his last name can act as the file code. The practitioner could also recall files by diagnosis name or code, referring physician's name, or whatever.

Other types of clients, such as wellness programs, restaurants, consultant contracts, and so on, and their key people can be listed. Reminders for appointments, reports, and marketing can be keyed in. Follow-up letters, proposals, and reports can be typed into the computer using word processing software, and as many copies as needed can be printed in minutes—each one originally typed.

Researching Literature and Reports

Researching is another function that can be carried out on a computer. Through use of a modem and the appropriate software, through your telephone you can access information in much larger databases at libraries, government offices, and banks. Companies in the business of placing journal reports, medical literature, media articles, stock reports, and so on, on databases for sale to subscribers can also be accessed for a fee. When practitioners want to write an article or book on a subject or appear on the media, they can have the most recent information at their disposal.

Word Processing

Word processing capabilities of a computer are well known. Articles, menus, reports, letters, individualized diets, and other written items can be typed, viewed on the screen, corrected or changed, and then printed. If the item is stored on software, it can be recalled and reused or corrected as needed. Bulk mailings can be typed to look like originals and individually headed. By preprogramming nutrition care plans onto software, a practitioner can individualize or adjust a plan for each patient and then print it for a personalized presentation.

Business Management

Business management of a private practice is possible through use of software with financial spreadsheets and accounting capabilities. Detailed records can be prepared more regularly and compared with past incomes, expenses, and forecasts. Bookkeeping records could be sent by telephone to your accountant for auditing and tax preparation.

SELECTING A COMPUTER SYSTEM

The most crucial question to ask yourself when thinking about purchasing a computer system is, "How do I plan to use the computer in my private practice?" Your response to this question is the key to the type of software you'll need. Currently, not all software is applicable to all computer systems, so it is important to match appropriate software to the right computer. Quality software is essential in obtaining the maximum use from your computer and investment.

Guidelines for Evaluating Software

The first step in evaluating software is to become aware of available programs that appear suitable for your needs. Keep in mind that new programs are being developed daily, and some are definitely better than others. Since it is difficult to thoroughly evaluate software from a written description, before buying obtain a copy of the desired software and run the program on an appropriate computer system. As you run through the program, ask yourself the following questions:

1. What is the objective of this program? Is it what I want?
2. Are the instructions clear?
3. Is the format appropriate and interesting?
4. Is the content accurate?
5. Does the program output provide useful information that is easy to understand?
6. Is the cost of the program worth it?

Since most types of software or its stored information can be destroyed by various elements, such as air pollutants, spilled liquids, magnets, heat, bending, power failures caused by severe weather conditions, and so on, it is legal to make a copy for your own use. A copy can also be made if it is necessary to use the program more effectively (1). Computer software is usually protected through a copyright by its owner.

Selecting Hardware

When selecting your computer, deal with a local, reputable company who is willing to provide good service, training, and maintenance. Talk to other people who own and use the machine you want to buy and ask how happy they are with it. Find out as much as you can about the operation and reputation of the equipment that is compatible with the software you want. Many books, magazines, and professional articles compare and review the major brands of computers. The choice is a matter of your own personal preference. For further reference, the article by Downs (2) describes twelve desk top models of microcomputers. Information relating to price, auxiliary equipment, and capabilities is discussed in the article.

The basic equipment included in a computer system is:

1. Keyboard (similar to typewriter keyboard)
2. Monitor (screen or CRT—cathode ray tube)
3. CPU—central processing unit (the brains of the computer)
4. Printer (to turn information into "hard copy")

Many salespeople also suggest purchase of a surge protector device to keep power changes from erasing data or programs.

Monitors differ in appearance, type face, and size. Some display information using white letters on a black background and others called monochrome use bright green print on a dark green background. Monitors with the capability of using a wide range of colors are also available. Characters can be in upper case only or both lower and upper case. Some features enhance the display of information, which is important since eye strain and fatigue are common complaints of computer users.

The CPU is the working brains of the computer. Always find out the number of "K's" (size of a computer memory) available before buying. One "K" is equivalent to 1000 bytes or characters of information storage. It is important to remember that your CPU must have a "K" that is equal to or greater than the software program you wish to use.

Printers vary with respect to:

1. Number of characters printed per second
2. Number of characters per horizontal inch (that is usually between 10 to 12 and comparable to pica/elite type on the typewriter)
3. Number of lines per vertical inch
4. Number of lines printed per minute
5. Type of print (dot matrix or fully formed characters—letter quality)

A printout from a printer with fully formed characters appears like a "typewritten copy." This does not mean that printers with fully formed characters are always superior to dot matrix printers. There is a wide range of print quality, so you need to decide which is most appropriate for your needs. Again, be certain that the printer you purchase is compatible with your other hardware and corresponding software.

By the time auxiliary equipment, print paper, and floppy disks are added, the purchase price is significant. Selection of the *right* equipment and software is prudent.

BASIC COMPUTER USE

Computer operation is very simple once you have familiarized yourself with the language and equipment. Computer programs may be stored on a variety of media. For microcomputers (small personal computers), programs are frequently stored on floppy diskettes. A diskette resembles a 5 1/4-inch phonograph record that contains the computer program. This diskette is inserted into a disk drive in the CPU. When the computer is turned on, it is able to "read" the information present on the diskette and display it on the monitor.

In order to use a computer you have to be able to enter information. This first step is the *input phase*. Information is entered into the computer by means of the keyboard. The typed information is then displayed on the monitor.

The second step is the *processing phase*. During this phase the computer (CPU) performs the instructions or commands on the program.

The last phase of computer operation is *output*. Processed data or words are displayed on the monitor or printed. A hard copy is output in a permanent form (printed on paper).

COMPUTER ADVANTAGES

Computers require time and commitment to work well but the effort is worth it. The major advantage that computers provide to the practitioner is a greater volume of quality business output. In today's market, computers can help give an edge to the practitioner who wants to offer more information and service than his competitors.

REFERENCES

1. "Computer Savvy. Copying Software: Legal or Not?" *Forecast of Home Economics,* April 1983, pp. 14–25.
2. Downs, J.: "Computers at Home," *The Community Nutritionist,* January–February 1983, 2:24.

BIBLIOGRAPHY

Ahl, D.H.: "Buying a Printer," *Creative Computing,* pp. 12–29, March, 1983.
Brown, J.E., L.W. Hoover, and J.K. Cross.: "Shopping for computers." *The Community Nutritionist,* 1:18–21, May–June, 1982.
Coffey, M.: "Form Fiddling," *Creative Computing,* pp. 50–53, September, 1982.
Kimmel, S.: "Better Nutrition Bite by Byte," *Creative Computing,* pp. 78–88.
Leventhal, L.A., and I. Stafford: *Why Do You Need a Personal Computer?* John Wiley and Sons, 1981.
McLellan, M.R.: "An Introduction to Microcomputers: What They Are and How They Operate," *Food Technology,* 35:79–83, October, 1981.
Spaeth, M.: "Do You Really Need a Computer?" *Family Weekly,* p. 25, May 22, 1983.
Willard, R.: "Computers in Dietetics," *Dietetic Currents,* May–June, 1982. Volume 9(3).
Youngwirth, J.: "The Evolution of Computers in Dietetics: A Review," *Journal of the American Dietetic Association* 82(1): 62–67, January, 1983.

RESOURCES FOR FURTHER INFORMATION

1. The Minnesota Educational Computing Consortium *(MECC)* will send a free (upon request) publication and programs price list. Although you may think this is specifically for educators, think again; dietitians are in the teaching business.
   Minnesota Educational Computing Consortium
   2520 Broadway Drive
   St. Paul, Minnesota 55113
   (612) 638-0627
2. *Creative Computing* is a magazine designed for inexperienced computer users who do not have a technical background in computer science. This monthly magazine frequently reviews various types of software. This is also a good way to keep up with the latest developments in the field.
   Creative Computing
   P.O. Box 789-M
   Morristown, New Jersey 07960
3. *Computer stores* will provide you with a source for a demonstration system, supplies, disks, paper and so on. These stores generally carry proven product lines and are a

source for local service and information. *Manufacturers brochures* are also available through these stores. A collection of these pamphlets allows you to compare and contrast computer systems at your own pace and time.

4. *Computer clubs* offer an opportunity for you to meet with people who share similar interests. You are able to learn about computer systems and programs from current users. Through these individuals you may obtain information about the reputation of local computer stores.

5. Don't forget about your city and university *libraries.* You may be able to read the monthly issue of *Creative Computing* without purchasing a subscription. Some libraries might have a computer learning facility open to the public. This would provide an opportunity for hands-on experience with the computer.

6. Industry or university sponsored *classes* offer a more structured learning environment with assistance from qualified personnel. An excellent opportunity to learn everything from "turning on the machine" to "basic programming."

7. The American Dietetic Association is publishing an annotated bibliography of nutrition software.

chapter 11

Creating a Good Business Image

Every new business and its owner will eventually develop an image in the mind of the public. The important thing is that the image be a good one. Having a positive, successful image is what many large corporations, politicians, and movie stars spend untold amounts of money to achieve. They know that their image will usually determine success—whether their products sell, they get a vote, or remain a star (1).

Consultant nutritionists report that as their professional images grow to look successful, their businesses attract new clientele with a minimum of effort. Good images make patients, physicians, and business people want to use their services. Everyone likes to feel that their nutritionist, as well as physician and dentist, is the best, the most sought after, the most qualified and successful.

INTRODUCTION

When creating an image the first thing that comes to mind is physical appearance. In addition to this are who we are and what we stand for, plus tactfulness, stability, credibility, and the appearance of success.

Successful private practitioners have a variety of professional approaches including those that range from very conservative in dress and manner and traditional in instructing patients to those that have flashy appearances and seek out unconventional nutrition information. As long as the person's practice is ethical and meets the clients' needs, it is *not* necessary for everyone's approach to be the same. Creativity and uniqueness in the development of a business will help create an image that is distinctive from its competition. One image is only better than another if the practitioner feels more comfortable with it, or if it is more successful in reaching more people and producing more income.

WHO WE ARE AND WHAT WE STAND FOR

Choose your battles carefully. Others' opinions of us are greatly influenced by what we choose to defend, by our honesty and how we fight our battles. It is important that we have opinions, and that they are well thought out and researched. Do not appear to be a person who lacks loyalty and changes opinions to please whoever is ahead. Defend your arguments with facts and fairly listen to other points of view. Also, be willing to accept a majority vote or new evidence that substantiates another point of view. Become known for your honesty, integrity and fairness.

APPEARANCE AND FIRST IMPRESSIONS

"You only get one chance to make a first impression." (Anon.)

Because of stiff competition and the fast-paced nature of this society a person seldom has the opportunity to make up for a poor first impression. A well-qualified dietitian may never get the chance to show what he knows because he did not "first get his foot in the door."

Having a good appearance increases the chances that a consultant's creative ideas will be heard. A counselor's effectiveness on the job is also influenced by appearance. Part of whether a patient or his family respond to counseling is dependent upon their first impression of the counselor, and whether credibility has been established.

Although it may seem vain and foolish to put too much emphasis on outward appearance, it is equally fool hardy to put too little value on it. A story about an East coast student illustrates the importance the public places on overall appearance and clothing. A student was dressed in two different ways on two different days and then went to ask people for money in a New York City subway. He used the same words both days, "I've lost my wallet; can I borrow 30¢ to get home?" The first day the student had a day's growth of beard and was dressed slovenly in old clothes. The second day he was clean shaven and dressed in a three-piece suit. The difference in the amount of money he collected was astounding—about $19 the first day and over $300 the second day! The public responded to how he took care of himself, dressed, and the status or power it implied.

To show examples of how dress and appearance influence feelings about someone, think how you would feel when:

1. A very close relative of yours is in the hospital and while you are visiting, a young medical person comes into the room. The fellow is wearing a white jacket with a stethoscope around his neck. He is also wearing a loud-colored paisley tie. Do you wonder whether he is really the physician in charge or just a student? Do you question his seriousness?

2. You are at an investment conference and two men speak about how to invest. One is dressed in a sports jacket and loafers and the other has on an expensive suit. Both speak equally well and have similar grooming. Do you have a tendency to feel that the one in the suit is more successful?

Historically, and even in recent surveys, a dietitian has been thought of as an inflexible, heavy woman in the hospital kitchen, dressed in white with a hair net on. Private practitioners are regularly reminded of this image when they are told, "But you don't look like a dietitian."

In his books on dressing for success for men and women, John Molloy states that to achieve a powerful, successful appearance the person should be clean cut and more traditional than fashionable or trendy (2,3). When power is necessary in business, the goal is to look stable and successful. His research has found that it is easiest to do that by wearing dark colored suits (skirted suits for women) with classic blouses or shirts, plain shoes, leather briefcases, expensive watches, and gold Cross pens: no double knits. Melodie Chenevert in *Special Techniques in Assertiveness Training for Women in Health Professions* states, "Where do John Molloy's suggestions leave you and me? Hundreds of thousands of us have been wearing white or pastel double knits with orthopedic shoes along with Timex watches and carrying Bic pens. Nothing about us non-verbally communicates success or power" (4).

Reaction to John Molloy's suggestions has taken an interesting turn in the last few years, especially in the way women dress. So many people followed his suggestions that they looked cloned. They lost their individuality! In fact, Karen Vartan, R.D., a former vice-president at Ritt and Ritt employment agency, says that one of her best prospects was not hired for a position because she showed up for her final interview in a "John Molloy outfit." The employer felt that if she couldn't think for herself, they didn't need her. Evidently, it is considered most appropriate to dress attractively but with a little individual flair.

Dietitians and nutritionists who now work in business have found that what they wear and their appearance have a lot to do with their effectiveness, especially while negotiating. Jean Yancey, a small business advisor in Denver, has stated that, "If you are rich and eccentric, you can forget about dress mores, but if not, you have to 'play the game' like the rest of us."

A private practitioner should strive to be a good example of the nutrition and health professions and "practice what he preaches," that is, have normal weight, eat well, and have a healthy appearance. Carolyn Worthington, a Registered Dietitian who has specialized in recruiting dietitians for many years, states that, "Nothing diminishes a candidate's job prospects more than being very overweight. The overweight dietitian destroys her or his credibility with clients and medical staffs." Just as a cardiologist who smokes or a preacher who swears loses credibility in the eyes of some of his or her clients and associates, extreme obesity and poor health habits can create a credibility problem for a nutritionist.

Other aspects that contribute to a good physical image and appearance are good posture, direct eye contact while speaking, a firm handshake, and body language that is confident and positive, not filled with nervous movement. Speak-

ing in a clear, bold manner and making sure that the statements are well thought
out also contribute to good image.

TACTFULNESS AND MANNER

Along with physical appearance, people notice and respond to a professional's
tactfulness and manner. The old adage holds true, "He was right, but he lost the
argument because of the way he handled it." People in business find that they are
not only selling a commodity or service, but also themselves to the client, their
families, and professional peers.

Business people have the task of finding the happy medium between being
aggressive and knowing when to be passive and pull back. They must learn when
to make a point and when to let another person's point of view dominate. Novices
tend to experience greater swings and react in one extreme manner or the other.
Experience and self-confidence help develop a more self-assured, moderate attitude and approach. This transition is difficult for most. Until recently women
have never been encouraged to be assertive. Consultant nutritionists have definitely experienced this confusion coming from meeker hospital roles into trying
to distinguish themselves as businesspersons. Time and experience in the field
prove to be the best teachers.

The "Rule of 250," developed by a sales promotion seminar leader, briefly
states that every person we meet has a sphere of influence with other people, such
as employer, family, professional peers, neighbors, and so on, that may affect as
many as 250 other people. That means that a tactless comment or a bad encounter
or a very positive experience can have influence on a potentially large number of
people. A businessperson's image in the eyes of the public is greatly affected by
the small day-to-day dealings and the manner in which they are handled.

Some suggestions that could improve tactfulness with your patients, clients,
referring physicians, leasing agents, professional counselors, etc., include:

1. Be very cautious about what is said when you feel that you have been
   attacked. Becoming defensive and "striking back" is *not* the best response. Instead try to relax and state something like, "I am sorry you
   feel that way" or "I don't feel that that was necessary to say."
2. Be brief and direct in your word choices and speak in a slow, nonemotional tone. Conduct your business directly with the individuals involved
   and do not leave long messages with spouses or secretaries. Secondhand
   messages have a way of being misinterpreted.
3. When people ask, "Are you worth that much money?" consultants can
   answer by saying, "I certainly am; let me explain what I can do for you."
4. If a physician states that he or she only charges $25 for a visit, why do
   you charge $45, a good answer is, "That's true, but the difference may
   be in how long we spend with the patient. I spend 45 minutes to one hour
   with a patient for that fee."
5. If a counselor recognizes that a patient is not responding to the counseling and probably has no intention of doing so, it is not out of line to
   suggest that, "We evidently do not respond well to each other, and I feel

that perhaps another counselor could help you more. Would you like for me to refer you to someone else?"

6. If a professional advisor (lawyer, accountant, etc.) has not performed your work well, talk directly with the individual and state, "I am not happy with what I see of your work. Are you interested in my business, and if so, what can you do to take care of this situation?" or "Your work is not the quality that I expected and I am disappointed. Some of it is not what we discussed. I would like you to reevaluate the charges on the bill you sent me."

STABILITY AND CREDIBILITY

In his book *Winning Images,* Robert Shook states, "People need to know that their relationships with you are durable. Everyone realizes that flash-in-the-pan types cannot be counted on, and such an image scares people away" (1).

People tend to equate stability and credibility with honesty, quality, and permanence. Banks and large corporations build large offices to symbolize their stability. Retail outlets have inventories and stores to create their images. A service type of business such as nutrition counseling is, by its nature, intangible, therefore, its need to look stable and credible is even greater. Most beginning practitioners will not be in a financial position to afford an expensive office in the best location, so other means to look stable, prosperous, and honest must be found.

Using high-quality business cards and brochures, as well as handout materials, gives the appearance of professionalism and can engender a sense of trust in others. Offering personalized instruction and development of high-quality programs gives a business and its owners credibility. Completing projects by the deadline and within the projected budget builds a good reputation. Doing something when you say you are going to do it sounds simple, but it is a rare individual or company that actually follows this principle.

Keeping appointments and arriving on time is important and is appreciated. Clients and patients also expect to come and meet with a consultant nutritionist at or near the appointment time. Physicians who are notoriously late in seeing their patients are finding that patients will not accept this discourtesy as they used to.

Shook states (1):

Second chances are seldom given today to professionals who do not perform as promised. Many people whose talents border on genius achieve only mediocre results in their careers because they lack the necessary follow-through and persistence to actually perform well. In business less-gifted people continually outperform highly educated and gifted persons because they provide consistently good service.

To enjoy a long and rewarding career, a nutrition consultant should provide outstanding work and good, timely information. The clients should feel that they receive full value of the services rendered.

SUCCESS BREEDS SUCCESS

People like to deal with successful people because being successful *must* mean they are good at what they do. When given a choice, people want to deal with the best. To create an image of success do outstanding work and become successful. The performance and reputation of a professional will attract the public and bring in business referrals as time passes.

When starting a new business there are some lessons that can be incorporated to reduce the amount of time needed to appear as a winner. First, appear busy to the clients. Patients question how good a professional is if they can make an appointment at any time on any day they call. It is not misrepresentation to state several available appointment times during the week instead of saying, "Any time you want Tuesday or Wednesday—I'm open." Honesty may be interpreted to represent poor business and poor service for the money. One practitioner found that as she traveled on business and became less available in the office, demand for her services increased because her professional image was becoming more successful.

One practitioner in California, after being in business for three years, had an actual eight-month waiting period for nonemergency patients to get an appointment. Patients must have felt privileged to see such a successful nutritionist. Why else would they have agreed to wait so long? The practitioner now has three associates and the four of them see over 250 patients per week.

When working in a medical complex or clinic area, it is not suggested that a professional regularly take extended breaks in the public areas. Prospective clients and referring physicians take notice of others who appear not to be busy.

A second lesson in creating an image of success is to look successful. The importance of physical appearance and clothes has been discussed and cannot be overemphasized. The locale and office decor are also important. Medical offices and buildings are not usually known for their attractiveness, but they do have good images because of the high status of the physicians who use them. Renting an office in a medical complex usually is more expensive but creates a more successful image than establishing an office in a commercial building or home.

Robert Shook relayed the story in *Winning Images* of a TV repairman who was working out of his home. He decided to rent a small store to increase his work space and found that his business referrals tripled. His clients commented that he must be "good" to have a store and they started referring their friends to him. He had not been aware that his business locale was that significant (1).

Framed diplomas, degrees, or awards displayed on office walls are also a graphic way to show success and accomplishment. Desk sets and trophies have adorned businessmen's offices for years, so there is no reason for plastic food models and free calorie charts to be the only highlights of a nutritionist's office!

The image of success is undoubtedly the most significant reason why many people are able to demand such high prices for their work. The artist, for example, who establishes the reputation of being distinctive and expensive soon gets more for his work than many unknown artists who have as much or more talent. The secret is in his ability to build a winning image, not in his talent to paint on canvas.

It is human nature to feel at times that the more the fee for services, the better the quality (within reason). It is also common to have people wonder how good a "bargain" nutritionist's services are if he charges only half of what the competition does. If the public can afford it, it will usually choose the higher-priced services, especially if the reputation is stable and credible. However, it is important that a nutritionist set the fees for service low enough not to scare people away. A negative image can be created by charging fees that are either too low or excessively high for what the client *feels he receives.*

CONCLUSION

When consulting nutritionists become successful in business, they usually find that other people who could not be bothered before now seek advice and agree with them on the issues. Referrals of new clients and jobs are received with minimum effort as compared to that needed to start the business. Fees are raised easily to improve the profit margin. But more importantly, job satisfaction increases because more professional and personal options open up in the nutritionists' lives.

REFERENCES

1. Shook, Robert: *Winning Images,* Macmillan Publishers, New York, 1977.
2. Molloy, John T.: *The Women's Dress For Success Book,* Warner Books, New York, 1977.
3. Molloy, John T.: *Dress For Success,* Warner Books, New York, 1975.
4. Chenevert, Melodie: *STAT Special Techniques in Assertiveness Training for Women in Health Professions,* Mosby, St. Louis, 1983.

chapter *12*

Assertiveness

According to Webster's Dictionary, being assertive means "to state positively; conviction of truth and willingness to stand by one's statement because of evidence, experience or faith; aggressive; self-confident" (1). Being assertive or aggressive merely shows commitment and resolve, and both are usually better than being passive when it comes to the delivery of health care or when conducting business.

Assertive people are not easily manipulated or coerced. There seems to be an agreement today that it is not only "OK," but advantageous to be assertive in our daily lives and especially while at work.

In her book *Special Techniques in Assertiveness Training for Women in the Health Professions,* Melodie Chenevert, R.N., points out that, "Women in the health professions are often taken advantage of in the name of sweet charity. . . . For years we have literally donated our time and talent, believing we were doing so in the service of others" (2). In nutritional practice, too often patient care has taken a back seat to required paperwork, time and budget limits, and physician or administrator whims. Steps need to be taken to put good patient/client care and dissemination of accurate, up-to-date information as the top priorities in the practice of nutrition. We must not be afraid to go to the people who need our help.

A private practitioner and writer, Sue Rodwell Williams, Ph.D., R.D., has made a statement that should be shared about the private practitioners' new role,

The newly emerging practitioners must shed subservient attitudes and roles of the past and work with physicians as nutrition specialists in their own right, viewing physicians as team peers, not patrons. We do not practice by their leave or permission or 'orders'—the very word reflects the old order of semantic submission. I think it is past time that we accept ethical, moral, and legal responsibility for our own practice as a full professional, collaborating with all other health professionals, including M.D.s, as team partners re: common goals of patient/client care, carrying responsibility for the nutritional aspects of care, and demonstrating a high level of skill and competence. Without such behavior, we will fail.

ASSERTIVENESS IN PATIENT CARE

Private practitioners have found that going into business does not make them suddenly more assertive. They bring with them the behavior and beliefs that they have always had. Initially, it can make a person feel brazen and overbearing to be more assertive, but it gets easier and more fun as it is viewed as the game that it really is. Just as negotiating is a game of wits, so is assertiveness. It's an attempt to have more control and to effect more change. As consultant nutritionists we need good working relationships with our health professional colleagues—but in the best interest of the patient or client. We have not only the right to protect our patients' interests, but the responsibility.

Many practitioners have experienced situations that have called for assertiveness in the interest of good patient care. Here are two situations that illustrate the importance of this responsibility. Consider how you might have reacted under the same circumstances.

Situation A

Eli weighed 254# at 5'9" and was 54 years old. He was referred by Dr. Andrews for diet instruction for weight loss. His physician did not order a sodium restriction although Eli had high blood pressure (confirmed by occasional tests), and he was not taking any medication for it.

After several weeks Eli's weight was coming down at a moderate rate on the lower calorie diet and daily walking. Eli confided in the nutritionist that he thought his blood pressure was bad because of the headaches he was experiencing; he also had a hernia that he couldn't push in place anymore and he was afraid something was really wrong with it.

With Eli's permission, the nutritionist called and made an appointment for Eli to see his physician. She encouraged Eli to tell the doctor what he had just told her and to discuss the blood pressure problem with him. After Eli left, the nutritionist called and talked to Dr. Andrews. She told him that Eli's weight was coming down, but there seemed to be a bigger problem with his blood pressure and a hernia. Dr. Andrews was very cordial and thanked her for her concern.

The next week when Eli returned, he still looked very bloated and red faced. The nutritionist asked what had been done for him. Eli had been bawled out for 30 minutes about his weight; his blood pressure was 240/140, but the physician said his pressure would just go back up again if he ever stopped the medication, so he wasn't given any, and the hernia wasn't checked.

The nutritionist referred Eli to another physician immediately. Eli was given medicine that brought his blood pressure into normal ranges in a week; he lost 12# immediately due to the fluid loss; he purchased a hernia belt and was able to lean forward for the first time in one and a half years.

The nutritionist felt that helping Eli was worth whatever professional risk she had to take. But, had Dr. Andrews found out about the referral to another physician without his permission, he *could* have created such a furor among his colleagues that no one would have referred patients to her again, or quietly discredited her, or just stopped referring patients himself. Reality shows us that a patient's care is not always as important as ego and professional courtesy.

In similar situations other practitioners have reported more recently that they have received increased respect from the medical community for taking action in the patients' behalf. Attitudes toward second opinions and peer cover-up are rapidly changing for the better.

Situation B

Carolyn, a 28-year-old woman who was 3 months pregnant, made an appointment for prenatal diet instruction. She told the nutritionist that Dr. Johnson didn't want her to eat any dairy products and to take calcium supplements instead. Carolyn questioned the diet order. The nutritionist did not know Dr. Johnson, so she called to discuss the diet order and Carolyn's special needs.

To the nutritionist's surprise, she found that Dr. Johnson takes all of his prenatal patients off dairy products and gives them all calcium supplements for calorie control. The nutritionist tried to discuss the other nutritional merits of lower fat dairy products and offered to research a list of the calcium contents in food for the physician so that he would know amounts as accurately as those in supplements. He wasn't very interested, but he would accept the list, and *he knew how the nutritionist felt about his orders.*

The nutritionist instructed Carolyn on good nutrition. She specifically pointed out what Dr. Johnson had prescribed and explained why he felt as he did. However, care was taken to give Carolyn answers to all her questions, including ones about "standard guidelines" on prenatal nutrition.

The nutritionist could have refused to see Carolyn since she did not agree philosophically with the referring physician's diet order. However, the consultant felt that she had the responsibility to let Carolyn know about other opinions on prenatal nutrition. In time, Dr. Johnson began referring more of his prenatal overweight patients and did not require that they avoid dairy products.

If you really care about patients, don't be afraid to ask questions. Stand your ground until you get results, but do it tactfully. Taking reasonable risks is part of the game.

Assertiveness in Business Grows in Time

As Herb Cohen states in his book, *You Can Negotiate Anything,* (3) we actually negotiate several times per day every day of our lives. Whether we need a refund on poor service, a package delivered on time, or the secretary to answer the phone more pleasantly, we are trying to have our wishes met. And, we sometimes have to become more assertive to do it.

To be more effective in your work and to negotiate better contracts and consultant fees, it helps to know when and how to stand your ground. For persons who are not used to being assertive, finding a happy medium between being passive and being overbearing or stubborn is a necessity. Finesse will develop in time. Consider how you would have handled the following situations:

Situation A

Two businessmen called the nutritionist to ask if she felt she had expertise in menu development for their proposed natural food restaurant. They told her they had heard good things about her and wanted her services. They also mentioned that they were well financed and planned to start a concept that could be franchised nation-wide. A meeting was scheduled for the three on the coming Thursday.

The nutritionist was very excited about the concept. At the meeting the two men asked verbally for her confidentiality, and she agreed. They then explained in general terms what they planned to do, where, when, and how successful it would be. The two men were dressed in business suits and were apparently successful and trustworthy if appearances meant anything.

The two men asked to see some of the nutritionist's work in menu and recipe development and she agreed (she had brought her restaurant portfolio on her past client accounts). The businessmen were impressed and told the nutritionist that they might even have a staff or consultant position for her at a very good salary if she would consider taking a chance with them by working on concept development in return for a "piece of the action."

The nutritionist was always willing to pursue new, exciting concepts, but she had heard too many similar proposals before to go blindly into another one. She knew it was her turn to start asking some questions: Who was backing the venture? What experience did the two have in the restaurant business; if it was very little, who was going to be hired to develop and manage the concept? What did they want her to do besides menu and recipe development, some marketing, personnel training, ongoing updating and testing of food items, or whatever? For what amount of time? Also, what did they propose would be her fair share of "piece of the action?" Would it mean she would be a partner or shareholder? Legally, how would it be set up?

The major clue that precipitated this battery of questions was the fact that they had first said they were well financed and then asked her to work without pay at least initially. The questions were probing, but the businessmen were asking her to participate in their business venture in return for nonpayment of her services. She had every right to find out as much as she could before calling her own lawyer and other business consultants to discuss the offer.

Too often less assertive or business-wise nutritionists accept appearances as the truth and unwisely believe that other people always have their best interests at heart. The businessmen were there because they wanted something that they thought the nutritionist could give them (good recipes, expertise, credibility, or whatever)—it's that simple. It is *always* better to try to find out up front if a business relationship is honest and open, than to assume everything is okay and not be paid or be professionally burned by people who misrepresent themselves and their capabilities.

If the two men had offered to pay on a timely basis, the nutritionist would still need to ask: Who would retain ownership of the recipes she had developed on her own time (a license for limited use could be given and legally written with her lawyer's help)? How many different food items did they want developed in each category, for example, entrees, salads, desserts, and so on? How soon would the recipes and menu need to be done? How many people would attend the tasting sessions to determine menu items? What kitchen facilities were available for the recipe development or would she use her own? Could she have an advance to pay for food before each tasting session and be paid biweekly for her work upon submitting an itemized bill? Would they like her to submit a proposal on the approximate development schedule and cost involved and then agree to sign a letter of agreement on the project? This is a business and should be treated like one. Assertiveness is usually necessary to maintain quality output and a well-run business.

Situation B

The Adams Drug and Alcohol Rehabilitation Center called the nutritionist to see if she was interested in consulting for them. The nutritionist went for the interview.

The center had room for 15 adult residents who lived there for 6 weeks while they went through psychological therapy and drying out from drug use. There was a staff of 12 full-time people and several part-time employees. The Center wanted to pass JCAH inspection in 45 days so they could then receive insurance money for resident visits. To pass inspection the center needed proof they hired a part-time nutritionist to oversee their food service, to develop written policies and to assure the kitchen met local sanitation standards. The nutritionist was satisfied with the interview and tour of the facilities and agreed to take the position.

The job would require concentrated effort on writing the policies to meet the JCAH standards and some time on the menu revisions and sanitation deficiencies. It was agreed that the nutritionist would work and be paid for 15 hours per week for the next 6 weeks. She would then cut back to 4 hours per week to interview residents, give inservices and oversee the food service after all of the requirements were updated and met. A letter of agreement was written for one year of consultation by the nutritionist. She was asked if the agreement could be backdated, but when she refused the issue was dropped. The nutritionist was asked to always call the assistant administrator before making a visit.

The center was able to pass the inspection with a modest amount of deficiencies—none in the food area. However, from the time of the inspection on, the assistant administrator would either not return the nutritionist's phone calls or state that their census was down and a visit wasn't necessary that week. After the assistant administrator refused to allow visits for three months the nutritionist sent a letter of resignation, and a documentation of the weekly attempts to schedule visits to the center's administration documenting the problem and sent a carbon copy to JCAH headquarters. The center was then accountable to JCAH for its feigned use of a nutritionist's services.

STEPS IN BECOMING ASSERTIVE

There are some basic steps that can be followed when you want to become more assertive. Having success at being assertive is one of the best incentives for trying it again (2, 3):

STEP 1: Start on small, nonemotional situations where the outcome is not that important to you. Stand your ground next time a neighbor calls and wants to talk endlessly or when a department store clerk checks out other people who arrived behind you. Taking on an overbearing colleague or your mother for the first time is likely to be an emotional experience for you, and one that you may not easily win. Try something that has a better chance at success to build your confidence.

STEP 2: State your feelings or decision clearly, logically, and slowly without emotional involvement. Stand straight, have good eye contact, and try to avoid nervous body movement that might give you away.

STEP 3: If questioned or rebuked, still avoid becoming emotional and clearly restate your position in as few words as necessary. Do not back down at the first sign of conflict. Document your statements and quote higher sources to show support of your opinion.

STEP 4: Listen to the opposing arguments and reevaluate your stand. If you are right, stick to it!

I find that when I am least assertive in my life is when I don't feel on top of things personally. I either am not versed on the subject well enough to feel I should take a stand on it, for some reason my self-confidence is eroded that day. In every instance it is within *my control* to change the way I *feel* about the problem or to *do* something about it.

SELF-CONFIDENCE IS THE KEY

Part of being assertive is feeling good enough about yourself to want to make a statement. At times, we all feel erosion of our self-confidence. The following are some suggestions to improve self-confidence:

1. Focus your attention on your strong points. We rarely focus on the talents and abilities that make each of us special. Think of the things that you have received praise for in the past. What is attractive about your appearance? What personality traits draw people to you?

2. Research subjects thoroughly for yourself and don't always depend on others to make your choices or form your opinions.
3. Set realistic goals and reward yourself when you reach the goals. Too much time is spent waiting for someone else to reward our good deeds. So, do it yourself, and be your own best buddy.
4. Don't try to please everyone—you never will, so it wastes a lot of time. Set your own criteria for what success would involve, and then use it as your own personal guide. It also helps to surround yourself with positive-thinking people who think you are the greatest.

   Positive energy is known to stimulate more creativity and result in the development of inspired thoughts. This may also mean that you must minimize being with very negative individuals or at least not talk to them about your business plans. As Jean Yancey, a Denver small business advisor suggests, "weed out the garden of your life."
5. If you need it, get professional help. Whether it's help in developing self-confidence, assertiveness, a business plan, or determining career options, an outside objective opinion can sometimes add new perspective. Successful business people learn very quickly that they must seek help when it will still do some good. And when time, money, and effort are still available and useful.

REWARDS

When a person thinks about becoming assertive, it is perceived that the risk of embarrassment or being put down will greatly increase, but what often happens is just the opposite. Mature individuals respect other people who have opinions on the issues and who risk taking a stand. It is not uncommon for a business person to find allies among the same individuals who criticized them earlier in their career.

Becoming more assertive will not guarantee more personal advancement or income. It will not assure you of more love, but it may make you more effective, respected, and confident. So, if you feel that you have not asserted yourself as much as you could, try it, you may love it!

REFERENCES

1. *Webster's New Collegiate Dictionary,* G and C Merriam Co., Springfield, MA.
2. Chenevert, Melodie: *STAT Special Techniques in Assertiveness Training for Women in Health Professions,* Mosby, St. Louis, MO 1983.
3. Cohen, Herb: *You Can Negotiate Anything,* Lyle Stuart, New York, 1980.

chapter 13

Ethics, Malpractice, and Libel

The ethical manner in which people conduct their businesses determines to a large extent the loyalty of clients and the support of peers. Clients want to feel that they are being honestly served for a fair price. Our peers expect us to conduct ourselves professionally, honestly, and within the law. We are expected to give accurate information and not engage in questionable dealings that will reflect poorly upon ourselves and, possibly, the dietetic profession.

Unfortunately, historically, professionals too often have been ridiculed and ousted from their professional groups because they tried or believed something that was new and different, but perfectly ethical. For a profession and its members to lead in their area of expertise, exploration of new ideas is mandatory. Some tolerance must be exercised by peers and organizations in judging the merit or ethical nature of a new idea.

Commonly, business people who get into trouble ethically or from malpractice close shop because business becomes so poor. Occasionally, there is that rare instance where the person benefits from all of the publicity and ends up with a booming business. If the breach is bad enough, a lawsuit, loss of license or professional membership may occur.

WHO JUDGES ETHICS?

Ethics in private practice may be "judged" by our professional and business peers, by government agencies such as the judicial system, the Internal Revenue Service, or the Public Health Department, and by business organizations such as the Better Business Bureau and the local Chamber of Commerce. As long as no one complains, no one will probably ever be concerned about you or your business.

That is one good reason to take complaints seriously and follow them to resolution. However, fear of ethical breaches should not paralyze you or make you compromise on all matters that you feel very strongly are right.

Professional Process

If the person is employed or is contracted as a consultant, an ethical matter could be simply addressed in-house. If the person is in private practice, more than likely it will be the local or state dietetic organization that first questions a professional ethics problem. If the matter is serious enough, the House of Delegates Ethics Committee of The American Dietetic Association will review the case in terms of considering censoring or revocation of membership.

Peers have the obligation to handle an ethical review in a professional manner and not commit slander, libel, and character assassination. The accused individual has the basic right to be considered in the right until proven otherwise.

The Individual

Ultimately, of course, it is individual practitioners who must live with their own decisions. We all have varying degrees of restrictions that we place on our actions according to our value systems. We tempt our ethical boundaries every time we don't simply refuse a physician who wants a kickback or when we give less than our best care because we run short of time or when we discuss our fees at the local dietetic meeting (could be interpreted as price-fixing).

WHAT THEN IS ETHICAL?

The American Dietetic Association's House of Delegates Ethics Committee has written Standards of Professional Responsibility for its members. The main components of the standards include the following (1):

- That a member provide professional services with objectivity and with respect for the unique needs and values of individuals
- That professional qualifications are presented accurately
- That conflicts of interest are avoided
- That competency of practice is maintained
- That confidentiality of information is respected
- That controversial material is substantiated and given an unbiased interpretation
- That a member practices honesty, integrity, and fairness

Up-to-Date Knowledge

As professional dietitians, we are expected to give the best quality of work we are capable of doing. To do that, we have an obligation to remain current and up to date in our field of knowledge. Our knowledge is what we have to market.

Therefore, every effort should be made to have our knowledge timely, unbiased, well thought out, and of such quality that the competition cannot compete.

Advertising

Within the last several years it has become ethical to advertise—in a professional manner. Tasteful ads in newspapers, Yellow Pages, magazines, and on the radio and television have become commonplace for professionals. The wording used in advertising is extremely important. It should *not* convey or imply in any way that you are practicing medicine. Ads should not mislead, misrepresent or make untruthful guarantees. When advertising, professional qualifications should be presented accurately. Clients' identities should remain confidential unless you have obtained written permission to use their names, photos or statements in your advertising.

The types of advertising tools you choose and the messages you convey should attract your target markets to use your services, not just attract attention. In other words, handing out promotion calendars with bathing beauties may be ethical and attract attention, but will it attract the right target market?

Self-referrals

Established private practitioners normally consider it ethical to accept new patients who refer themselves for *normal* nutrition consultations. Normal diets would include good nutrition, weight control, wellness, sports, and vegetarian diets and menu planning. We are certainly more qualified to instruct people on diets than the numerous women's magazines, newspaper columnists, and most physicians who have written popular diet books.

A growing number of highly qualified and experienced private practitioners feel that they are ethically able to see *any* patient for *nutrition consultation*— referred or not. The professional relationship is between the patient and the practitioner, similar to when a patient goes to see a family guidance or stop-smoking counselor—no referral is needed. Why should eating food be controlled by a medical referral? The dietitian is the trained expert in the nutrition field, and nutrition is the area of service. The practitioners do not make medical diagnoses. *They make nutrition assessments and provide nutritional care plans.* Patients who need medical care are given the names of competent medical professionals or are referred to the local medical society.

These pioneering practitioners are sometimes met with mixed reactions from the local physician community. However, as people become impressed by the dietitian's quality of service, they drop their resistance. By taking self-referred patients the practitioner is taking action to become an independent, nutrition specialist and peer to other health care providers. Because of the high expectations of the public and physicians, it is imperative that practitioners be highly qualified. The personality of the dietitian and her or his grasp and use of nutritional knowledge are the two major contributors to success.

Practitioners who feel uncomfortable about leaving traditional roles may be reluctant to make this their business policy. That reluctance will disappear as more and more peers take this step.

Prescribing Diets

Prescribing diets for all patients is becoming commonplace in private practice. Most private practitioners find that as referring physicians gain more confidence in them, diet orders change from specific limits to only diagnoses or chemical scores. It seems we have all come to realize it is premature to guess a calorie level before a diet history and assessment are made.

Patient Records

Your patients' records need to be kept confidential. A patient has the right to see his own chart; therefore, care should be taken when comments not related to the patient's nutritional care are made or even repeated by you. If a patient requests that his records be sent to his physician, clinic, or another dietitian, photocopy the materials—keep one copy and send the other. It is recommended that you keep the old patient charts for as long as you are in business. If office storage space becomes a problem, box the charts that have not been used for many years, label the box, and store it at home.

Referrals to Other Professionals

It is considered good patient care to refer patients to other professionals that you feel could help the patients with their problems. This is often done in the cases of anorexia nervosa, when suicidal statements are made, when the patient needs medical care, or when more testing is needed. If the patient has a referring physician, you should try to work through him or her to help the patient.

Referring patients to other professionals does carry some risk with it for you, especially if you only give one or two names. You may be held responsible if the patient is very unhappy with the care they receive from the other professional—both of you may be sued. Therefore, if you give several names of specialists you highly respect, also suggest the patient seek help from the local medical society, the county health department, or look in the Yellow Pages.

It is ethical to suggest to patients to seek a second opinion in matters of health. Care should be taken not to alarm the patient unnecessarily or to condemn their medical care. Consulting nutritionists state that seeing questionable medical care is not an uncommon occurrence. The hope is that it will not be compounded with questionable nutritional care!

Questioning Diet Orders

It is ethical, if not mandatory, for a nutritionist to question a diet order that is not clear, reasonable, or correct. Part of what the patient and the public expects from a professionally trained nutritionist is that decisions are made in the best interest of the patient.

WHAT IS UNETHICAL?

Other than failing to follow the previously mentioned ethical practices, it is also unethical to commit theft, fraud, and other illegal acts. Many unethical acts are open to interpretation, while others are very clearly defined by the local and federal governments.

Price and Territory Fixing

Price fixing is said to exist when professionals discuss in writing or verbally what to charge for services. This includes when current fees are published as examples. Encouraging someone to set their fees by calling around and checking the "going prices" of any allied health professionals is considered price fixing. The concern is that the buying public is not getting the best deal because everyone who provides a certain service is influenced to charge a certain fee—instead of allowing competition to prevail.

When professionals agree to territorial boundaries, where patients can only see the dietitian in a certain area, it is considered territory fixing. This also is illegal. By the way, it is also illegal for someone to try to keep you from practicing in "their territory."

Restraint of Trade

When you are asked to suggest referral names of professionals, there are several guidelines to help avoid restraint of trade:

1. Give more than one name and only suggest people you highly respect.
2. Suggest that the individual check for other names at the local dietetic organization, medical society, public health department, or Yellow Pages.
3. Members of dietetic practice groups should not just give member names. The concern is that the public must be given a nonbiased opportunity to have a variety and actual choice of providers.

Practicing Medicine

Local medical licensing boards and medical societies are very concerned when they feel people are overstepping their professional scopes of practice into practicing medicine. The line is not always clearly defined, but it usually involves making diagnoses, interpreting chemical invasive tests (blood tests, etc.), and representing oneself as "curing" a patient.

Several private practitioners have been accused by local physicians for what they perceived to be practicing medicine. The three known instances have revolved around allergy or nutrient testing, and miswording of an advertisement in another case. Physicians who knew the practitioners were instrumental in having the problems resolved, but only after much trouble and embarrassment. Care must be taken not to insinuate that diagnoses are being made, that tests are being diagnosed outside of a physician's auspices, and that diet prescriptions for medical diets are being made without a medical diagnosis first being made by a qualified physician.

Ordering Laboratory Tests   According to Sue Rodwell Williams, Ph.D., R.D., from California, some private practitioners "order" appropriate laboratory tests for their patients through arrangements made with a local physician. To do this at least two major criteria must be met: first, the dietitian must be a clinical nutrition specialist and be recognized by the medical community as such; and second, sound protocols must be written jointly by the practitioner and a physician and filed with a nearby reputable clinical laboratory. Periodically the protocols should be reviewed and updated by the dietitian and M.D. Additionally, there should not be hesitancy by a practitioner to recommend to a physician that certain tests would be appropriate for nutrition assessment. Mutual respect and good working relationships are prerequisites for this kind of trust to take place.

Misrepresentation of Ownership of Ideas

Ideas have value. That is why the processes of copyrighting, patenting, and trademarking were started by the government—to protect the ownership of new ideas. Most ideas are evolutions or conglomerations of thoughts from many sources. "New" ideas are often better ways of stating or doing an old concept.

As we progress in business, we evaluate our ideas and keep the ones that work and discard the rest. We also evaluate ideas, programs, materials, speeches, and business techniques that we see and adopt what we think will work for us.

Ethically, the important point to remember is that we should respect the protection offered by the copyright, patent, or trademark. There are also many very unique business ideas or concepts that are the pride and joy of another person. If that person feels that by adopting his or her idea, you have "stolen" or infringed upon her or his business, you may be heading for a legal confrontation.

Given the opportunity many people are happy to give a copyright release (See Chapter 14, Figure 14.3) or negotiate some equitable agreement. All too often it seems the very people who become upset when their own work is taken by another, don't give a second thought about photocopying someone else's brochure, teaching materials, or book chapter.

COMMON ETHICAL QUESTIONS

Is it ethical to suggest to a patient to take vitamin or mineral supplements?

Solution: If in your professional opinion, after assessing the patient's present and past nutritional intake, physical state (pregnancy, post-surgical, etc.), medications, food preferences, and ability to obtain the necessary nutrient levels, you determine that supplements are advised, do so.

The question of whether to suggest individual nutrients such as B vitamins or zinc for a specific purpose is not so clear cut. In doses up to the RDAs it should not be an ethical problem at all. Above that level or if claims are made that the nutrients will "cure" anything but a deficiency, the ethical risk becomes greater. If chemical tests are taken under a physician's auspices, as discussed earlier, and the physician/lab pathologist makes a diagnosis of deficiency or greater than normal need, a dietitian can ethically adjust the patient's diet and suggest supplements, if necessary.

Is it ethical for a private practitioner to share office or building space with a health club, physician, or chiropracter who uses "questionable" nutritional practices?

Solution: It is your prerogative to obtain office space wherever you desire. The important issue to be aware of is you and your reputation may be hurt by the "assumed" association that an outsider may draw. Your good, ethical reputation is one of your most valuable commodities; defend it. If, however, you believe in what the person is doing, and you are willing to stake your professional reputation on it, that is your prerogative and a risk you may choose.

Is it ethical to sell products out of my office?

Solution: If you have the proper sales tax license and your lease allows it, it is legal, if what you are selling is legal. The federal government, however, frowns upon a medical professional who leads patients into buying products out of the office for more than a competitive price.

Obviously, it seems that what you sell would be nutrition or health related in some way and something you recommend. If it is a line of vitamins, a new multi-level marketing diet program, or a movie star's exercise video, and you are willing to stand behind your decision to sell it, that is your right. Recognize again that your reputation may be hurt by affiliating with the "wrong" product. And, care should be taken to let patients know that buying the product from you is not mandatory.

Is it ethical for me to promote a product in the media for a client?

Solution: Ethically, it is fine to promote a client's product as long as the public is aware that you represent the company. The statements you make should *not* be construed as an unbiased, professional endorsement.

One point to mention here is that some companies hire professionals at very good salaries to lend credibility to an otherwise lacking product. Closely scrutinize all facets of your association with the product and company before agreeing to do it.

Is it ethical to use neon signs and windshield flyers to promote my business?

Solution: Can you do a neon sign tastefully? If so, I assume you can do it. I certainly predict that it will draw attention.

Whether you should use flyers or neon signs is more of a marketing question than an ethical one. You want to attract a certain target market from the public as clients. That group of people has certain expectations about medical professionals. Your job is to determine what marketing avenues will attract your desired market.

What is a "kickback" and is it ethical?

Solution: As it relates to our profession, a "kickback" is a payment resulting from noncontractual favoritism, usually involving restraint of trade. For example, a referring physician or clinic wants to charge you a fee merely for the referral of a patient, and if you refuse, the referral would be made instead to a competitor. It can also occur when a consultant dietitian awards a contract for food or services for a client account to a company in return for receiving remuneration "under the table." Kickbacks are illegal.

The government feels that patients should not have to pay to be referred for proper care (fees would no doubt be raised to cover the cost of kickbacks). Client accounts should be able to have fair, honest contracts without the negotiator making a profit, unless that was part of the agreement.

A point of clarification should be made here concerning office sharing and paying a percentage of your income for it. If office space and/or services are being exchanged in return for the referral of patients, it is not considered a kickback to pay for the space.

Is it ethical to use someone else's trademark, if I ask them for permission?

Solution: I can't imagine anyone allowing you to use their trademark, unless there is some sort of legal partnership or franchise agreement. A service mark that represents an organization such as the American Dietetic Association seal or the dietetic practice groups' logos or a service mark of another private practitioner is a valuable commodity to that business. Owners may be held liable for any business conducted under their name and logo.

You may feel that you would never knowingly create any problems. But, if you are ever in a dispute, the other party may feel that you and the trademark owner are worth suing. Don't even think about doing it, unless you have a legal agreement on it reviewed by a good lawyer.

Certainly, not all ethical issues have been discussed, just some of the major areas of concern for private practitioners. For answers to other questions, call the appropriate legal or business advisor or the American Dietetic Association.

MALPRACTICE

Nutritional malpractice occurs when a dietitian fails to meet the accepted standard of care, and the action results in harm to the patient. Although there have been only a few cases where dietitians have been sued for malpractice (all known cases have either been dropped or settled out of court), the possibility of more cases in the future is very real. As dietitians become more visible professionally, as they take the initiative to prescribe diets, and as more attorneys use "blind pleading" in suits for their clients where more professionals other than just physicians are implicated, the risk of a suit is more likely (2).

Life and business are not risk free. However, having a basic understanding of the legal system as it applies to malpractice may help to minimize the risk, and its accompanying expense and embarrassment.

Legal Principles

In their article "Malpractice Law and the Dietitian," JADA, October, 1975, Elizabeth and Daniel Reidy state,

> Each person is required by law to exercise a certain standard of care in order to avoid causing injury to the person or property of others. If a person fails to meet that standard and that failure causes harm to another's person or property, then the person is liable for the damage. This is the basic law of negligence. Dietitians—like physicians, lawyers, accountants, and other professionals—must exercise the skill and knowledge normally possessed by members in good standing of their profession. In a like manner, the dietitians' standard of care will probably be a national one, principally because of educational requirements and the recent movement within the profession toward the adoption of uniform practice standards (3).

There is no theoretical minimum harm that a patient has to prove. Simply demonstrating that negligence of proper care on the part of the dietitian caused discomfort or delayed the recovery process constitutes the basis for a lawsuit. However, if the patient does not prove that the dietitian's care caused some injury to him, there can't be a finding of liability against the dietitian (2).

Possible Liability Situations

Whenever dietitians practice their profession, whether or not they are paid for it, they are potentially risking liability and must meet the professional standards of practice. For private practitioners that means that when they do public speaking, as well as when they prescribe a weight loss diet for a new patient—they are first and foremost dietitians who will be held accountable for their advice. Other instances where liability may be tested are in situations where food from a kitchen gives food poisoning, where a nursing home patient dies and/or is diagnosed with malnutrition, and where there are miscalculations on diet instructions, such as protein or potassium on a renal diet (2). Dietitians violating accepted management principles run the risk of being charged with administrative malpractice.

Protecting Yourself Against Malpractice

The best way to protect yourself against the possibility of a malpractice lawsuit is to practice humanistic nutritional care of your patients and clients. According to the Reidys, "Some people theorize that the recent upsurge in the number of medical malpractice suits is partially caused by the depersonalization of medical treatment. These theorists suggest that there were fewer suits in the past because patients knew the people who treated them and were reluctant to sue" (3).

Along with giving good care, a dietitian should stay current with new advances or practices in the field of nutrition. This does not mean that we all have to appear the same; instead we should give out sound advice, but in our own creative ways.

In a court of law documentation of proper care and communication about the patient's poor eating habits to the proper channels is extremely important. Records should show that the proper information was given to the patient, that his progress was adequately followed, or if he did not return or follow it, it should be so stated, and that the referring physician was advised of the patient's progress in writing.

A final way to protect yourself against the cost of malpractice is by purchasing malpractice insurance. Coverage will normally provide for representation by counsel and will cover payment of any judgment up to a stated maximum. While such policies are very necessary for peace of mind, they do not insulate the dietitian from the problems and time loss caused by litigation. Also, malpractice insurance policies will not necessarily cover your business indiscretions or lawsuits of a nonnutrition or nonprofession-related nature, such as damage of rented property or failure to pay for services rendered. If your business risk is high it may be necessary to look into business liability insurance and the incorporation form of business ownership.

WHAT IS LIBEL AND HOW IS IT DIFFERENT?

Legally, libel is any statement or representation published without just cause or excuse, or by pictures, effigies, or other signs tending to expose another person, corporation, or product to public hatred, contempt or ridicule. Calling someone a "quack," or "incompetent" could cause defamation. However, you should not be discouraged from stating the facts as you know them, backed up with scientific evidence. Such subjects as the danger of a severe low calorie diet regime and the nutritional inadequacy of some foods are important to the public, and it is the responsibility of our profession to warn the public.

Don Reuben, an attorney for Reuben and Proctor in Chicago, Illinois, has stated, that in cases where a dietitian makes a public statement about an issue, "A dietitian's key defense against a public person (corporation) or government official who sues for libel is that the suing party must prove the dietitian knew it was libelous at the time of the statement. A dietitian is an expert and professionally trained authority who has the right to express nutrition facts as she sees them under fair comment protection" (4).

Victor Herbert, who is both a physician and a lawyer, has stated, "If a private individual or company sues you for speaking the truth as you see it, without malice, countersue on the grounds of malicious harassment and abuse of process. Ask the court to order the plaintiff to pay your legal fees, as suggested by Federal Judge A. Sofaer in *NNFA* (National Nutritional Foods Association) vs. *Whelan and Stare* (78 Civ. 6276 [ADS], U.S. District Court, Southern District of New York) (1980)" (4).

Betty Wedman, a Registered Dietitian from Chicago, Illinois, who was threatened with a libel suit by a food company for a statement she made, has stated, "From personal experience let me emphasize the need for daily, detailed logs of conversations that could be used in a court of law, if litigation were pursued. Keep records and be widely read; check out your facts with reference books and other professionals, and you need not be intimidated by the foods industry, drug manufacturers, physicians, or patients" (4).

Malpractice insurance coverage will usually cover your court costs and up to a maximum amount for a settlement for nutrition-related libel suits. Check with your insurance agent or policy concerning all items covered.

CONCLUSION

The dietitian's main concern should always be the welfare of his or her patients. Excessive measures need not be taken to practice differently just out of fear of liability. By offering quality, humanistic care and then taking the steps to document their services, practitioners should be able to conduct business with a minimum fear of risk.

REFERENCES

1. Standards of Professional Responsibility, The American Dietetic Association, 1984.
2. Baird, Patricia, and Barry Jacobs: "Malpractice: Your Day in Court," *Food Management Magazine,* February 1981.
3. Reidy, Elizabeth and Daniel Reidy: "Malpractice Law and The Dietitian," *Journal of American Dietetic Association,* October 1975.
4. King, Kathy: *Starting A Private Practice,* Study Kit #3, The American Dietetic Association, 1982.

chapter 14

Protecting Your Ideas and Interests

People who are new to business are especially concerned about how to keep others from taking their ideas and how to protect their property from lawsuits. The better known means of protection are copyrights and insurance, but there are many other options, including written agreements, personal discretion, trade secret protection, and incorporation.

PUBLIC DOMAIN

A distinction needs to be made about what kinds of ideas can be protected legally or claimed for ownership. Any new and original literary, graphic, audio, mechanical, video, process series, or ingredient may be protected as belonging to an individual or company. All items, names, and so on, that are considered common knowledge and nonunique are in the "public domain," and cannot be the *sole* property of any one person or business. Examples of common items are the words "foods," "juice," and "nutritionist," the Basic Four Food Group listings, and the common medical diets (although unique diet manuals can be copyrighted although they use that information). Everyone can use all items in the "public domain."

HAVE IT IN WRITING

To avoid confusion and lawsuits the best advice is *not* to assume anything about even a simple agreement; discuss it thoroughly and have it in writing. Initially, use lawyers to look over all agreements and later use their services especially on all risky, important, and costly agreements. No one should start a job "on good faith" unless he is willing *not* to collect for the services. An agreement between two people can be as simple as a single sheet of paper that states commitment, money, terms, and expectations, such as a Letter of Agreement. If someone is doing a job for you, explicitly state your expectations so that the work performed is what you expected, and so you only have to pay for what you agreed upon (See Chapter 15 on negotiating agreements).

PERSONAL DISCRETION

Many good creative ideas become public property because the originator of the thought talked about it indiscreetly. Exceptionally different and quality ideas are of great value, personally as well as financially, and should be treated as such. Obviously, in the development of the idea more contract people or professional advisors may need to be involved, but there is better legal recourse if any of these individuals take an idea. Business people will tell you that the best way to avoid being fearful in business is to work only with very ethical, honest people who come highly recommended or whom you have checked out through references.

If an original idea must be discussed with another company or individual, have a trusted acquaintance present who could witness the conversation, or ask to tape record the session, or ask that a simple Nondisclosure Agreement be signed (see Figure 14.1). If handled in a tactful manner, no one will be embarrassed or threatened by the precautions.

With time and experience the ability to "read" an individual or situation and evaluate the risk involved will come easily. Through contacts and networking over the years, trusted acquaintances in business and your own savvy will make the development of ideas relatively non-fearful.

Figure 14.1   Sample Nondisclosure Agreement

NONDISCLOSURE AGREEMENT

_____ agrees to maintain the confidentiality of all proprietary information and trade secrets concerning Diet Control, Inc., or Diet Control, Inc.'s products, and printed information of which he or she becomes aware. This obligation of confidentiality shall survive the termination of this Agreement.

Diet Control, Inc.

_____

Agreed and Accepted:

_____

Date: _____

TRADE SECRETS

Trade secrets (ideas and materials that make the business unique) may be protected in four major ways: (1) by not telling anyone about it or not using it (which may hinder its usefulness), (2) by copyrighting, (3) by trademarking, or (4) by patenting it.

Copyrights are issued by the U.S. Copyright Office for books and pamphlets, for *new* diet programs with original elements that have not been used before, and for other artistic, musical, or literary creations.

The copyright notice should appear on all published works that are distributed to the public. The use of the copyright notice is the responsibility of the copyright owner and does not require advance permission from the Copyright Office. The notice should be on the copies "in such manner and location as to give reasonable notice of the claim of copyright." The required copyright generally consists of three elements: (1) the symbol "©" or the word "Copyright," or the abbreviation "Copr."; (2) the year of first publication; and (3) the name of the copyright owner. An example of a typical copyright is "© 1981 Nutrition Daily." Anyone failing to comply with the copyright notice requirements may lose some copyright protection, and unless it is corrected within five years, the right to copyright will be lost. In books, pamphlets, and other publications a printed reminder is usually added that states, "This material may not be copied or reproduced in any manner without the written permission of the author."

Lawyers who specialize in copyright law suggest that newly published material with the copyright notice be sent to someone by certified mail. The postage receipt will show when the copyright was first used. In case of a copyright dispute the documented date may prove to be significant.

Copyright forms and information may be obtained by calling or writing: Register of Copyrights, Library of Congress, Washington, D.C. 20559 or a local federally authorized library. It is usually advisable to initially contact a qualified lawyer who can answer questions on the subject. The copyright application filing fee is $10 plus at least one copy of the completed work. The form is simple enough for most persons to fill out (see Figure 14.2).

For works created after January 1, 1978, the copyright term will be effective for the life of the author and 50 years after the author's death. Works created for hire, and certain anonymous and pseudonymous works, can be copyrighted for 75 years from publication or 100 years from creation, whichever is shorter.

The copyright owner, not the government, is responsible for protecting the use of the copyrighted material. If the copyright is abused, the owner or his lawyer can send a "cease and desist" order to the infringing person or organization to ask that use be stopped. Going to court is costly but could be used as a last resort.

As an example of how a copyright infringement can be handled, one consulting nutritionist found out that one of her contract OB-GYN clinics was photocopying her copyrighted prenatal brochure and handing it out to all new patients. She made an appointment to discuss the situation with the clinic director. She stated that the contract agreement did not allow uncontrolled use of her copyrighted materials. The clinic agreed to purchase the brochures at a bulk rate from the consultant with 500 brochures being the minimum order.

Figure 14.2 Application for Registration of a Copyright

(*Source:* U.S. Copyright Office.)

FORM TX
UNITED STATES COPYRIGHT OFFICE

REGISTRATION NUMBER

TX TXU

EFFECTIVE DATE OF REGISTRATION
(Month) (Day) (Year)

DO NOT WRITE ABOVE THIS LINE. IF YOU NEED MORE SPACE, USE CONTINUATION SHEET (FORM TX/CON)

1 Title

TITLE OF THIS WORK:

PREVIOUS OR ALTERNATIVE TITLES:

If a periodical or serial give: Vol. ..... No. ..... Issue Date .....

PUBLICATION AS A CONTRIBUTION: (If this work was published as a contribution to a periodical, serial, or collection, give information about the collective work in which the contribution appeared.)

Title of Collective Work ..... Vol. ..... No. ..... Date ..... Pages .....

2 Author(s)

IMPORTANT: Under the law, the "author" of a "work made for hire" is generally the employer, not the employee (see instructions). If any part of this work was "made for hire" check "Yes" in the space provided, give the employer (or other person for whom the work was prepared) as "Author" of that part, and leave the space for dates blank.

1
NAME OF AUTHOR:
Was this author's contribution to the work a "work made for hire"? Yes ..... No .....
DATES OF BIRTH AND DEATH: Born ..... (Year) Died ..... (Year)
AUTHOR'S NATIONALITY OR DOMICILE:
Citizen of ..... (Name of Country) or Domiciled in ..... (Name of Country)
WAS THIS AUTHOR'S CONTRIBUTION TO THE WORK:
Anonymous? Yes ..... No .....
Pseudonymous? Yes ..... No .....
If the answer to either of these questions is "Yes," see detailed instructions attached.
AUTHOR OF: (Briefly describe nature of this author's contribution)

2
NAME OF AUTHOR:
Was this author's contribution to the work a "work made for hire"? Yes ..... No .....
DATES OF BIRTH AND DEATH: Born ..... (Year) Died ..... (Year)
AUTHOR'S NATIONALITY OR DOMICILE:
Citizen of ..... (Name of Country) or Domiciled in ..... (Name of Country)
WAS THIS AUTHOR'S CONTRIBUTION TO THE WORK:
Anonymous? Yes ..... No .....
Pseudonymous? Yes ..... No .....
If the answer to either of these questions is "Yes," see detailed instructions attached.
AUTHOR OF: (Briefly describe nature of this author's contribution)

3
NAME OF AUTHOR:
Was this author's contribution to the work a "work made for hire"? Yes ..... No .....
DATES OF BIRTH AND DEATH: Born ..... (Year) Died ..... (Year)
AUTHOR'S NATIONALITY OR DOMICILE:
Citizen of ..... (Name of Country) or Domiciled in ..... (Name of Country)
WAS THIS AUTHOR'S CONTRIBUTION TO THE WORK:
Anonymous? Yes ..... No .....
Pseudonymous? Yes ..... No .....
If the answer to either of these questions is "Yes," see detailed instructions attached.
AUTHOR OF: (Briefly describe nature of this author's contribution)

3 Creation and Publication

YEAR IN WHICH CREATION OF THIS WORK WAS COMPLETED:
Year .....
(This information must be given in all cases.)

DATE AND NATION OF FIRST PUBLICATION:
Date ..... (Month) (Day) (Year)
Nation ..... (Name of Country)
(Complete this block ONLY if this work has been published.)

4 Claimant(s)

NAME(S) AND ADDRESS(ES) OF COPYRIGHT CLAIMANT(S):

TRANSFER: (If the copyright claimant(s) named here in space 4 are different from the author(s) named in space 2, give a brief statement of how the claimant(s) obtained ownership of the copyright.)

- *Complete all applicable spaces (numbers 5-11) on the reverse side of this page*
- *Follow detailed instructions attached*
- *Sign the form at line 10*

DO NOT WRITE HERE
Page 1 of ..... pages

Other ways to discourage misuse of your copyrighted material include the use of odd size paper that does not easily fit on a photocopier, use of blue or beige ink that does not photocopy well, and use of the new paper and inks that do not reproduce at all on a photocopier.

Formerly employed dietitians are usually in a quandary about who owns the materials and programs they developed while employed. Lawyers usually agree that no former employer can keep you from practicing your profession or using your expertise. However, if you were a paid employee when you developed materials for your employer, unless you have another prearranged agreement, he owns it. You can revise, rewrite, and then republish similar material. But care should be taken not to have the material so similar that it could be confused easily with the original work. The possibility can always arise if you become extremely successful or if your former employer questions it, and you may have to prove your right to ownership.

If you want to use reprints or copies of other persons' copyrighted material, articles, newspaper stories, and so on, you should request permission first. An example of a Copyright Release Form is shown in Figure 14.3.

Trademarks are issued by the U.S. Patent and Trademark Office to provide national recognition of a word, name, symbol, or device used by manufacturers or merchants to identify their products or services. Examples of common product trademarks include: Coca Cola, Vivonex, Kleenex, and Crayola. When a trademark stands for a service offered by a business instead of a product it is referred

Figure 14.3   Sample Request to Reprint Copyrighted Material

Dear _____:

I am preparing an educational exercise and nutrition booklet for the patients at the Medical Treatment Center, Garland, Texas. May I please have your permission to include the following:

Unless you indicate otherwise, I will use the following credit line:

I would greatly appreciate your consent to this request. For your convenience a release statement is found below. Please sign and return this letter to me. A copy has been included for your files.

Sincerely,

Jan Jones, R.D.
1010 Harland
Garland, TX 75075

Permission is hereby granted for the use requested above.

_____   _____

Signature   Date to as a "servicemark." Examples of common servicemarks include: the seal of The American Dietetic Association, McDonald's name, and the name Outasight Optical.

A trade or commercial name is a business name used to identify a partnership, company, or other organization. Incorporation of the business will protect the company name from use by others in the original state and where the business legally expands its markets. There is no provision in the trademark law for the registration of trade names used merely to identify a business. However, the name of a company may be included in a trademark or servicemark, such as "Texaco" is a servicemark for Texaco, Inc.

To establish rights to a trademark, the mark must be applied in some manner to goods (a diet manual or new food item) or their packaging, and the items must be sold or shipped (at least once initially) in interstate or foreign commerce. Document the sale with a postage receipt and/or dated bill of sale. The mark must continue to be used in commerce to maintain the owner's rights to it.

Trademark rights are protected under common law; in other words, the mark belongs to the first user as soon as it is used, whether or not it is ever registered. However, registering a trademark does have its advantages: it shows official claim of ownership and exclusive right to use the mark on the goods mentioned in the registration. There is no time limitation on when an application for registering a trademark can be filed.

Before filing an application, a search of trademarks should be made in the Search Room of the Trademark Examining Operation located in the Crystal Plaza Building No. 2, 2011 Jefferson Davis Highway, Arlington, Virginia. Any trademark that is too similar to one already filed will not be accepted for registration. The search can be done by any individual. Trademark lawyers have contacts with persons who can do the research for a fee. You can also call Yellow Page information in Arlington, Virginia, and get the names of several trademark search companies that will research a trademark for around $30.

Applications and more information can be obtained from the Patent and Trademark Office, Washington, D.C. 20231. The completed application must be notarized and sent along with 5 copies of the mark as it is actually used (a label or letterhead) and the $175 filing fee (see Figure 14.4). The term of the trademark registration is 20 years from the date of issue, and it may be renewed at the end of each 20-year term as long as the mark is still used in commerce.

The owner of the trademark, not the government, is responsible for protecting the mark from being used by others. In hopes of fooling the public, some companies create products with trademarks that are very similar to older, well-known trademarks. In these cases, the established company hires lawyers to start legal proceedings to stop the infringement.

Several private practitioners have had identity problems because words in the "public domain" were incorporated in their servicemarks, such as "nutrition consultants" or "diet services" and this caused logos with similar initials and somewhat "generic" business names. If you are going to go to the trouble and expense of trademarking a name, make it distinctive as well as meaningful.

Figure 14.4 Trademark Application

(*Source:* Patent and Trademark Office, U.S. Department of Commerce.)

TRADEMARK APPLICATION, PRINCIPAL REGISTER, WITH DECLARATION (Individual)	**MARK** (identify the mark)
	CLASS NO. (if known)

TO THE COMMISSIONER OF PATENTS AND TRADEMARKS:

NAME OF APPLICANT, AND BUSINESS TRADE NAME, IF ANY

BUSINESS ADDRESS

RESIDENCE ADDRESS

CITIZENSHIP OF APPLICANT

The above identified applicant has adopted and is using the trademark shown in the accompanying drawing[1] for the following goods: _____

_____ ,

and requests that said mark be registered in the United States Patent and Trademark Office on the Principal Register established by the Act of July 5, 1946.

The trademark was first used on the goods[2] on _____ ; was first used on the goods[2] in
_____ commerce[3] on _____ ;
(date)   (type of commerce)   (date)
and is now in use in such commerce.

4

The mark is used by applying it to[5] _____

_____

and five specimens showing the mark as actually used are presented herewith.

6

_____ .
(name of applicant)
being hereby warned that willful false statements and the like so made are punishable by fine or imprisonment, or both, under Section 1001 of Title 18 of the United States Code and that such willful false statements may jeopardize the validity of the application or any registration resulting therefrom, declares that he/she believes himself/herself to be the owner of the trademark sought to be registered; to the best of his/her knowledge and belief no other person, firm, corporation, or association has the right to use said mark in commerce, either in the identical form or in such near resemblance thereto as may be likely, when applied to the goods of such other person, to cause confusion, or to cause mistake, or to deceive; the facts set forth in this application are true; and all statements made of his/her own knowledge are true and all statements made on information and belief are believed to be true.

_____
(signature of applicant)

_____
(date)

Form PTO - 1476 (**Rev. 10-82**) (Instructions on reverse side) (over)   Patent and Trademark Office - U.S. DEPT. of COMMERCE

Patents are issued to inventors to help protect inventions from being used without the inventor's permission. To be patented, an invention must have a useful purpose for existing and it must have some new, never before patented element that makes it unique. A new patent can be issued on a new process, machine, composition of matter, or any new and useful improvements on an old patent.

A patent is effective for 17 years. Thereafter the invention is considered to be in the "public domain" and anyone can use it. Because of this fact some inventors decide not to patent a product that cannot be duplicated so that they own it exclusively. The owners of Coca Cola chose not to patent their product many years ago so that the formula (which has not been chemically deciphered) will remain a company trade secret.

Patent designs must be researched either at the Patent Office or at one of the federally designated libraries across the United States. An attorney who is qualified in patent law is a necessity when obtaining a patent. More information and an application can be obtained from the Patent and Trademark Office, Washington, D.C. 20231.

INSURANCE

Insurance was originally devised as a means of spreading the risk of having bad luck through a group instead of being shouldered by one individual. It has always been common to insure material possessions, but when starting a private practice, insurance to pay salary in case of disability and malpractice insurance are recommended. The cost of business insurance premiums is deductible as a business expense.

Malpractice insurance is available to privately practicing dietitians and nutritionists as well as those who are employed. The main reasons a professional would carry this type of insurance are because of the high cost of legal representation and the high incidence of threatened and actual lawsuits against not only physicians, but all persons who come in contact with the patient. Malpractice is discussed in detail in Chapter 13.

Disability insurance pays income when the insured person becomes ill or disabled, and is not able to work up to capacity. It is encouraged for sole supported, self-employed people because they are not eligible for workman's compensation, unemployment benefits, or sick time except through programs set up by their own company. Social Security disability insurance requires six months of no income before payments can begin. No income for an extended period could mean loss of the business as well as personal property.

Office insurance would include fire, theft, and liability coverage. This coverage is common and can usually be obtained from a practitioner's existing home insurance company. Office coverage is necessary because many medical buildings' insurance policies do not cover tenants' furnishings, possessions, loss of business, or visitors' accidents. When working out of your home, it is still necessary to carry extra insurance for times when it is used as an office.

Auto insurance on business-owned vehicles is common and necessary. In case of an accident involving the business car, the liability coverage should be especially good because the public believes that a business has more assets, and the possibility of a lawsuit after an accident may be greater. The cost of the coverage is comparable to personal auto insurance unless younger members of the family or persons with poor driving records are allowed to drive the car.

INCORPORATION

Many persons choose to incorporate their businesses to reduce the risk of losing their personal property for business dealings. A corporation is a complete, legal entity separate from its shareholders with its own assets. If all business is conducted in the corporate name and under its umbrella, the corporation's assets alone are at jeopardy for the business' failures, and lawsuits (see Chapter 5 for more information).

HOW MUCH RISK IS THERE?

Private practice and starting in business are not risk free endeavors. In fact, they require an individual to constantly be confronted with numerous important decisions, to initiate new untried ideas, to counsel patients on medical-associated nutrition programs, and risk financial loss.

The best ways to protect oneself are to be ethical, to ask advice of people who are successful in business, to make well-thought-out decisions, to document all important agreements and client visits in writing, and to learn from experience. Most people who have been in business for some time suggest that a person "take reasonable precautionary measures and then go on with business and living."

chapter *15*

Negotiating Agreements

Historically, negotiating was seen as an arena where one person was the victor and the other was the victim. Stronger individuals used negotiations to control the opposition. As a result, the final agreement usually heavily favored the victor. The victim accepted the agreement, but later often either did not produce in good faith or learned to manipulate or sabotage to gain back lost ground.

WIN-WIN NEGOTIATING

In the last ten years or so a new era of negotiation strategy has evolved in business —win-win negotiation (1). With this strategy both parties feel they benefit from the agreement. Now with the win-win philosophy everyone can become quite adept at representing themselves and their ideas and expecting the other party to negotiate in good faith. Some compromise may be necessary on the part of both parties.

When negotiations are stalled on an unbalanced or unfairly weighted agreement, it is not uncommon today to hear the "victim" try to bring the other party into a win-win agreement. This can sometimes be done by stating, "I can't see how I will benefit from this agreement as it stands. Would you be willing to compromise on . . . ?" or, "We have tried to be very fair and negotiate in good faith. You haven't offered any inducements or compromises that show that you feel the same."

SUCCESSFUL NEGOTIATIONS

There are many good books published on the art of negotiation. (See the references at the end of this chapter.) In reality, though, the only way to gain expertise is through experience. One session of negotiation prepares you for the next. One often learns as much by a session that went poorly as by one easily won that lacked challenge.

Negotiation should be seen as a game of minds each vying for its needs to be met without having to give up too much in return. When taken in this light, negotiation can be fun and challenging, worthy of thorough research and time to develop the strategy.

When negotiating, don't share all of your information up front. Clarify each point during your discussions. Document each concession as it is made so opponents can't renege later. Determine who the other party's leader is as soon as possible; it may not be the person speaking. And consider the following points to avoid (2).

- Don't be overwhelmed by the successful position or status of the other party.
- Don't worry about the end results.
- Don't negotiate over the phone.
- Don't oversell and push too far.
- Don't appear to be up tight, but don't relax!
- Don't "lose your cool" and get angry unless it's needed for dramatic effect.

Advantage Points to Remember (3)

- Try to set up the negotiations on your own ground or somewhere neutral where you feel comfortable. The other party's home ground or office may be intimidating.
- Wear your "power" outfit so that you feel comfortable and in control. Overdressing in business attire for the occasion may also prove to be successful in some instances.
- Don't say something you are later sorry about: don't quote figures and offer services until you have a chance to think about them—once spoken they may be difficult to change. If you don't know what to say, try, "I am very interested in what you're suggesting. Let me research it and get back to you tomorrow."
- Be aware of your body language. Sometimes it gives information that may be to the other party's advantage. Nervous movements may sabotage an otherwise strong presentation.
- If you are not comfortable with negotiating for yourself, hire a qualified lawyer or other business advisor to go with you to help carry the session. Or, have them coach you before you go into the negotiation session.

STEPS IN NEGOTIATING

Step 1 Qualify the other party. Is the other party a "middle man" who can only pass on information or the one in charge? Are the businesspersons who want you to write restaurant menus truly solid and well financed? Does the fitness center have any intention of contracting with you after you share your nutrition proposal with them? How do you know that the other party is worth your investment of time, effort, and money?

The best answer to all of the above questions is to ask tactful, straightforward questions of the other party. Don't be so caught up in trying to impress them, that you fail to evaluate them! Another method of qualifying someone is to ask for references or a financial statement (when appropriate). The reputation of a business or its owner can also give a clue whether they are credible and honest.

Step 2   What are the other party's "needs" and are they "over a barrel" for some reason?   By knowing as much as you can about what the other party "needs" from the negotiation, and any reasons that they are motivated to contract with you, you have a better negotiating position. Examples could be that the Health Department has given them a 30-day ultimatum to clean up the food service, or that nutrition consultation is required for the up-and-coming JCAH inspection, or that business is poor and your name and reputation will draw more clients.

Use this information to your advantage, but don't always share the fact that you know their problems. One of the greatest challenges in negotiating is to evaluate the other party and decide how open you should be and how much *not* to share.

Step 3   Are there any "desires" that are strong?   In some instances people or businesses may be motivated more by what they would like than what they need. They may *want* to be the first hospital to offer corporate wellness in the city and may disproportionately allocate funds to it. Or, the team coach may *want* a nutritionist to work with the players. Or, a restaurant owner may *want* to try appealing to a larger clientele by offering nutritious menu items.

Step 4   Determine your "bottom line."   What do you need and want from the negotiations? Determine your financial breakeven point and the amount of profit you will need to make the project worth your time. Develop statistics, illustrations and logical arguments to support and defend your views. What can you ask for, but be willing to give up as a concession? Never ask for the least you will accept up front. Ask for more and then expect that the final agreement will probably be a compromise.

Step 5   Do you have a "Sears Plan" ready?   Jean Yancey, a small business advisor in Denver, Colorado, counsels people to offer the "Sears Plan": good, better, and best alternatives. If the other party doesn't like one alternative you offer, have another ready to go. The best offer would be the most comprehensive and costly; the better offer is a good compromise; and the good offer will at least get your foot in the door or provide an option in case negotiations stall.

Step 6   Determine what other items besides money you will ask for in the agreement?   What interim payments and reports will you want? Ask for regular monthly payments, or for some projects, perhaps one-third up front, a third at midpoint, and the final payment on completion. What about royalties for as long as your materials are used? What about editorial or revision rights when programs

Q & A

Negotiating a Consultant's Fee

What can I use for arguments to substantiate why as a consultant I should be paid $45 per hour? I am competing with dietitians who are willing to work for $12 per hour.

First, realize a few things about our profession and our marketplaces. Professionally, we are in a state of transition from being somewhat passive home economics majors who only work for employers to more assertive nutrition experts who initiate programs and ask a competitive fee for service or as a wage. We are making the transition according to our own timetables and by what our lifestyles dictate. If someone loses a job to a more flamboyant peer or suddenly becomes the family's sole support, awareness and attitude changes evolve more quickly.

Next, not every client or consultant position is willing to pay the higher fee, no matter how good you are. In other words, you won't get every job, nor will you want every job you go after. In some instances if you really want the position, your only other option is to negotiate to do all of the required work in fewer hours for the same total income. For example, if there is $350 budgeted for nutrition consultation each month, sell the client on the idea that that money is a flat fee paid to have the job completed and not tied to being on the job physically for 29 hours or whatever. You will complete all the documentation and counseling or menu review required and be at the job 8 to 15 hours per month or whatever is needed. *You will have to use your time well* and produce for the client, but the pay is better ($23–$43/hour), and you didn't lose the job. The client will have her or his nutrition needs met and still be within budget.

If a prospective client is comparing your consultant fee against that of a $12 per hour employee, there are some good points that may help your case, but first and foremost you must realize that the client must *believe* and be convinced that you are *worth* that fee or no amount of logic will sway him otherwise. Possible selling points are:

- When the cost of fringe benefits and Social Security, etc., are added to the hourly wage, the amount increases by one-third to one-half.

- As a consultant, you are not paid for meal times and breaks. And you come prepared for the job and can produce better work in a shorter period of time. You will even agree to fewer hours (at the higher fee).

- As a consultant, you are bringing your own teaching materials, films, weight loss program, and previously successful seminars. The client does not have to pay for development time and hit or miss programming.

- If you have been marketing well and using the media or other types of exposure to build recognition of your name, this is a selling point that may help attract more business to the client.

- If you have expertise in computers, kitchen layout, marketing, eating disorder programs, or you know people who could also be beneficial to the client's programs or staff, try sharing enough to interest the client in the additional benefits you could bring to the job.

Once a "sell" is made to the client, realize that your arguments cannot be just campaign promises if you want to keep the position. You promised short-term excellence and the client will expect you to deliver.

become dated? Travel, office, and phone expenses—are they included? What staffing or support services will you expect? What marketing support will you request? (See proposal writing, pp. 214–217.)

AGREEMENTS

Agreements or exchanges of promises between two parties can take several forms. The more common are a verbal agreement, a bid, letter of agreement, or contract. Some forms do not offer the business novice much protection in case the other party does not perform as expected. Contracts are more detailed, but are sometimes too complex and expensive to be useful. The best agreements are between two reputable people who have adequately discussed their expectations of the other person.

Verbal or Gentleman's Agreements

Verbal or gentleman's agreements for fees and services are usually considered legally binding and are very common. Professional consultants and advisors often quote their fees for certain services and we agree to them verbally. We may agree to consult at a physician's office or a health club on a handshake. Verbal agreements are fine when you know the other party, and both of you know what is expected and perform accordingly. But in cases where there are misunderstandings or one person does not produce as expected, a verbal agreement can prove to be inadequate protection.

Q & A

Keeping a Successful Account

I am negotiating with a physician to offer nutrition consultation in his office. I am willing to work hard, take a financial risk, and build the program. But what guarantees do I have that as soon as I have become successful financially, I won't be replaced? How can I protect myself before I make the investment?

If the physician is a fair and honest person there are ways to avoid problems. If she or he is not, the situation will probably be out of your control. First, realize that it is only a good deal if you both feel you have been fairly compensated for what you have each contributed. So get out in the open what you each are offering the other. You may be offering time, effort, and some money, and the physician is offering client referrals, facilities, and some money.

Later on as you succeed the possibility of being replaced is reduced if the following have taken place:

- You are closely identified with the nutrition program, and if you go so will the program and client load.
- Each of you feels fairly compensated. Also, incentives should be built in so that extra work or effort on your part is rewarded.
- You developed the teaching materials on your own time and copyrighted them. The programs can only be used as long as you are a consultant there.
- You have a working relationship with the physician and the staff and you are considered an asset.
- Finally, before beginning, you and the physician should put your agreement in writing. At this time try to add a simple partnership buy-out agreement in case the physician wants the program, but wants to replace you.

You may be surprised, it may be the physician who fears you leaving more than the other way around.

Bid

A bid or cost estimate for a job is legal and it can be a good agreement if it is specific as to quality and date of completion, and both parties agree to any changes in writing. The most common shortcomings of bids are too little shared information and when the buyer does not pay as expected (a problem with any agreement). Bids may also be accompanied by an explanation or sample of a similar finished product or a proposal (see Figure 15.1).

Letter of Agreement

A letter of agreement is also legally binding, but less formal or complicated than a contract. For many people a letter is also less intimidating. To be good this form of agreement must be comprehensive and may include the following information:

- What the agreement is for, i.e. services, product, etc.
- Who is providing it
- When
- Where
- For how much
- How often *(List continues on p. 179.)*

(List continues on p. 179.)

Figure 15.1 Sample Bid

SMITH & JONES NUTRITION SERVICES, INC.
2530 Ridgeway
Tucson, AZ 85728

BID

Development of a diet manual for EARTH GROWN FOODS on lacto-ovo vegetarian diets for the following limitations:

Low Calorie
Low Cholesterol
Diabetic
Low Salt

The manual will include sample menus, nutrient charts, references for recipes, and a brand-name food guide. The finished manual will contain approximately 100 pages.

Completion date: One (1) month from the acceptance of this bid.

Project cost: $10,000

_____

EARTH GROWN FOODS

_____

DATE

_____

Figure 15.2 Sample Letter of Agreement

This is an agreement for nutrition services between Jan Jones, R.D., and the Houston Sports Medicine Center.

Jan Jones, R.D., will provide:

- Individual nutrition consultations to Sports Center clients and patients by referral
  Fees to clients will be:
  $55 Nutrition Assessment and Consult with Computer Nutrient/Diet Analysis
  $40 for Individuals referred for Nutrition Consult
  $20 for Follow-up Visits (approx. 20 minutes)
- Printed nutrition teaching materials (list attached)
- In-services to staff, if desired
- Free consultation to the management on nutrition-related matters
- Future group weight loss programs, etc., will be negotiated separately

The Houston Sports Medicine Center will provide:

- Marketing to promote the new services on an ongoing basis
- Private counseling area for individual consults and meeting room for any group classes
- Reception and scheduling services
- Payment of any collected fees will be reimbursed to Jan Jones, R.D., bimonthly

It is understood that the Houston Sports Medicine Center is offering no fringe benefits or guarantees.

Jan Jones, R.D., agrees to represent herself only as a Nutrition Consultant, not an employee of the Houston Sports Medicine Center. She will carry nutrition malpractice insurance and only provide nutrition information deemed sound and healthful by peers and current schools of thought.

It is understood that all nutrition materials, programs, and teaching tools provided by Jan Jones, R.D., remain her property and cannot be reproduced or used in any manner without her consent.

Both parties agree to remain flexible during the development of the systems and schedules necessary for the success of this program. Further, they agree to provide the time, effort, and resources necessary for development of a successful nutrition program.

This agreement will be in force for one year. It may then be renegotiated yearly. This agreement may be cancelled with 30 days written notice by either party.

_____   _____
Houston Sports Medicine Center   Date

_____   _____
Jan Jones, R.D.   Date

- Who is paying for it on what schedule or by what process, i.e. billing, monthly fee, etc.
- Any additional provisions
- Term of the agreement
- Termination clause by either party

A letter of agreement may be written in the form of a short exchange of promises (see Figure 15.2). It may also be in the form of a business or personal letter that outlines what the agreement is as the writer understands it (see Figure 15.3).

Figure 15.3   Sample Personal Letter of Agreement

THE WOMAN'S HOSPITAL
7600 Jones Street
Atlanta, GA 30303

January 19, 1987

Ms. Stephany White, R.D.
Nutrition Consultant Services of Atlanta, Inc.
7800 Fannin, Suite 203
Atlanta, GA 30310

Dear Stephany:

This letter is to confirm our telephone conversation of January 18, 1986, regarding your letter of January 16, 1986.

As agreed in our conversation, your firm will provide its services to this hospital according to the following provisions:

1. The hospital agrees to pay $45 per consultation to Nutrition Consultant Services of Atlanta, Inc.
2. This agreement shall be for thirty (30) days and automatically renewable at the end of each period of thirty (30) days.
3. Requests for services shall be coordinated by the Food Service Department and Nursing Service.
4. Statements remitted by Nutrition Consultant Services of Atlanta, Inc., shall detail each consultation.

Thanks for your assistance. If you have any questions concerning the agreement, please do not hesitate to contact my office.

Sincerely,

Cary D. Henry
Administrator

Q & A

Selling an Invention

I have invented a good product that I want to sell to a manufacturer. How do I go about it?

There are some important points to recognize before approaching any company. First, manufacturers are contacted by thousands of people each year who have "good" ideas for new products. So don't be discouraged if you have to sign forms stating that the manufacturer does not owe you anything unless they use your idea and had not thought of it themselves first. Also, most large manufacturers have their own Research and Development (R&D) departments that come up with new ideas, and they often discourage their bosses from buying an idea that could be developed in-house.

If you cannot patent your product (in other words it does not contain any new ingredients or process or outcome), then often its value is not as great because other companies can copy it legally and exactly, if it becomes popular. Also, if you have an unrefined product that still needs work or one that is only for a small select population, such as for patients with high uric acid levels, or one that has never proven itself on the market, it is usually not worth as much to the manufacturer. Today, because of the cost of introducing a new product on the market, many companies would rather buy out a small profitable company with products that are selling than try an unknown product on their own.

Charlie McCann, a former new products manager for Coca-Cola of New York, once told me that it costs two to three million dollars for his company just to test market a new product. He also stated that the only way a small, underfinanced company can make a lot of money on a new idea is as the granola inventors did it. Come out with a product that sells like wildfire and then sell out to General Mills or Kellogg before everyone else jumps on the bandwagon and puts you out of business. Charlie felt strongly that if a product is *really* a good idea, some company should be intrigued enough to buy it. If no one is, seriously consider *not* manufacturing it yourself unless you do it just to create local grass roots interest.

Along with product samples, a "package" to interest a manufacturer could include a proposal with a market analysis and the product positioning, plus a label or packaging design, and trademarked name and logo. The positioning entails determining who this product is designed to sell to, and why they would buy it.

When you have a product developed that you are proud of, it is time to contact a patent and contract lawyer to get feedback on how to protect your specific product and how to determine what you want from an agreement with a manufacturer. A business person with experience in this area is also very valuable, especially in determining whom to contact and how.

If you have any contacts with someone who could open doors for you or introduce you to the right people, use them. In some instances you may choose to use someone as an agent who knows the industry and offer him a finder's fee if he brings you a buyer who signs with you.

From my own experience, I would suggest that you try to keep control of the product and negotiations as much as possible. Do not expect someone else to do the work as well as you could do it.

When a manufacturer shows more than a casual interest in your product and wants to offer a 90-day contract to look it over or to go with an outright sale or license-use agreement, call your counselors and involve them in securing the contract. I agree with the business people who say, let an experienced negotiator represent you and your interests. Sellers can be so emotionally involved with their products and the negotiations can be so heated that hard feelings may be generated, which could affect working relationships later on. Do not allow the product to be used in any way, if you don't have a signed agreement.

It is suggested that both parties sign the agreement. However, courts of law will usually stand behind a letter that was sent by certified mail (return receipt requested) when no rebuttal was made, and the work was allowed to progress as if the agreement were accepted.

It is highly suggested that you consult with your lawyer concerning the provisions you should include in your letters of agreement to cover your particular business. After you are more familiar with this type of agreement, you will seldom need legal input except in cases of higher risk.

Contracts

Contracts are usually used when the risk is greater, the money is higher, and/or when more control is needed. Legal input is highly suggested for the development or review of all contracts before one is signed.

A contract may have any number of provisions and limitations, and the contract is usually biased to the advantage of the side that writes the contract. Included provisions may or may not be reasonable, so read them carefully. Most items of a contract are negotiable, especially if the other party is highly motivated to get a signed contract.

Figure 15.4   Sample Contract

AGREEMENT

AGREEMENT dated the 20th day of October, 1988, between DIET SERVICES IN FOOD AND NUTRITION, INC. (hereinafter called the "Corporation"), and JAMES GORE.

WHEREAS the Corporation is in the business of providing consulting services and assistance normally associated with clients and

WHEREAS from time to time the Corporation may require outside assistance in rendering said services; and

WHEREAS JAMES GORE wishes to provide said services from time to time when required by the Corporation; and

WHEREAS the Corporation and JAMES GORE desire to set forth herein their understandings and agreement:

NOW, THEREFORE, in consideration of the foregoing, the mutual promises herein set forth, and other good and valuable consideration, the receipt and sufficiency of which are hereby acknowledged, the parties hereto, intending to be legally bound, hereby agree as follows:

1.   PREVIOUS AGREEMENTS CANCELLED

All prior agreements, whether written or oral, between the parties hereto are hereby cancelled and of no further force and effect.

2.   ACTIVITIES OF JAMES GORE

During the term of this agreement, specified in Section 4 hereof, JAMES GORE shall undertake for and on behalf of, and to the extent specifically requested in writing by, the Corporation, subject to his availability and the other limitations set forth herein, to provide the Corporation with systems and other services normally associated with projects for clients of the Corporation.

3.   COMPENSATION OF JAMES GORE

The Corporation hereby covenants and agrees to pay JAMES GORE at the rate of $300 per day and to reimburse him promptly for all travel, telephone, and other expenses paid or incurred by him in connection with the performance of his activities, responsibilities, and services under this agreement, upon presentation of expense statements, vouchers, or other evidence of expense and receipt of payment from the client by the Corporation for such out-of-pocket expenses. Payment for services will not include travel time to a client's location unless client has agreed to pay the Corporation for such travel time. JAMES GORE will submit invoices and time sheets to the Corporation on a monthly basis.

4.   TERM

The term of this agreement shall commence as of the date hereof and shall continue until terminated by either party at any time upon thirty (30) days' written notice to the other. Notwithstanding the foregoing, JAMES GORE agrees that he will complete in a timely manner any project in progress at the time of said notice of termination.

5.   INDEPENDENT CONTRACTOR

JAMES GORE shall at all times be an independent contractor, rather than a co-venturer, agent, employee, or representative of the Corporation.

6.   DISCLOSURE OF INFORMATION

JAMES GORE recognizes and acknowledges that the list of the Corporation's customers, programs, designs, or products, as they may exist from

Figure 15.4 *(Continued)*

time to time, are valuable, special, and unique assets of the Corporation's business. JAMES GORE shall not, during or after the term of this agreement for a period of three (3) years, solicit the Corporation's customers or disclose the list of the Corporation's customers or any part thereof to any person, firm, corporation, association, or other entity for any reason or purpose whatsoever, without the written consent of the Corporation. In addition, at and after any termination, JAMES GORE shall not utilize the Corporation's programs, designs, or products for any purpose without the express written consent of the Corporation. In the event of a breach or a threatened breach by JAMES GORE of the provisions of this paragraph, the Corporation shall be entitled to an injunction restraining disclosing, in whole or in part, the list of the Corporation's customers, or from rendering any services to any person, firm, corporation, association, or other entity to whom such list, in whole or in part, has been disclosed or is threatened to be disclosed. Nothing herein shall be construed as prohibiting the Corporation from pursuing any other remedies available to the Corporation for such breach or threatened breach, including the recovery of damages.

   7. BINDING EFFECTS; ASSIGNMENT
       This agreement shall be binding upon and shall inure to the benefit of JAMES GORE and the Corporation and their respective heirs, executors, or administrators, personal and legal representatives, estate, legatees, and successors. The obligations under this agreement may not be assigned by JAMES GORE without the prior written consent of the Corporation.

   8. NOTICES
       All notices and other communications hereunder or in connection herewith shall be deemed to have been duly given if they are in writing and delivered personally or sent by registered or certified mail, return receipt requested and first-class postage prepaid. Unless notice of change of address is given to either party by the other pursuant to the provisions of this section, all communications shall be addressed:

       (a) If to the Corporation:
               DIET SERVICES IN FOOD AND NUTRITION, INC.
               1967 Sage Circle
               Golden, CO 80401
       (b) If to the consultant:
               Mr. James Gore, R.D.
               JAMES GORE ASSOCIATES
               1414 Clarkson
               Denver, CO 80218

   9. GOVERNING LAW
       This agreement shall be governed by and construed under the laws of the State of Colorado.

   10. MISCELLANEOUS
       No modification or waiver of any provision of this agreement shall be valid unless it is in writing and signed by the party against whom it is sought to be enforced. No waiver at any time of any provision of this agreement shall be deemed a waiver of any other provision of this agreement at that time or a waiver of that or any other provision at any other time.
       The captions and headings contained herein are solely for convenience and reference and do not constitute a part of this agreement.

Figure 15.4 *(Continued)*

JAMES GORE agrees to provide his own insurance coverages and to indemnify and hold harmless the Corporation from any injury or liability arising out of the negligence, misfeasance, malfeasance, or omission in the performance of services to or on behalf of the Corporation.

JAMES GORE agrees to execute any agreement required by a client of the Corporation in order to protect the secrecy and confidentiality of past, present, and future plans, provisions, designs, forms, formats, procedures, methods, customer data, employee data, technical data, know-how, research and development data and programs, financial data, legal data, marketing data, and other technical and business data belonging to said client of the Corporation.

IN WITNESS WHEREOF, the parties hereto have set their hands and seals this 20th day of October, 1988.

DIET SERVICES IN FOOD AND NUTRITION, INC.

_____   _____
Signature   Date

JAMES GORE

_____   _____
Signature   Date

One item of great concern to consultants or subcontractors is the non-compete clause in a contract. If one is used, it must be reasonable. Most non-compete clauses state that clients provided by the contractor are not be be taken or approached for one to two years after the consultant or subcontractor leaves and/or that no directly competing business can be started by the consultant within a 5-to-10-mile radius for one year. If the consultant (it may be you in some cases) signs the agreement but then does not uphold it, the contractor can sue. Lawsuits are costly, so it is best to first reconsider signing such an agreement, or whom, as a contractor, you ask to sign it.

When you are the one who must generate a contract, recognize that it is potentially expensive and time consuming. The better prepared you are concerning your needs, fears, and the provisions to include in a cᴏntract, usually the more reasonable the legal bill will be. Be aware also that unless cautioned otherwise, some lawyers may produce a document that is so long, detailed, and intimidating that no one else will sign it. Contracts should be practical, easily understood, and complete enough to protect your reasonable interests (see Figure 15.4).

Q & A

Subcontracting

I have a private practice that is going fairly well after two years, and other dietitians have contacted me wanting to work for me. I would like to expand my business and eventually make more money. How do I do it?

Expansion is not to be taken lightly. It must be well planned, adequately financed, and you must be willing to accept new additional responsibilities, especially management and leadership. Your accountant, lawyer, and business advisor(s) need to be consulted before any steps are taken in this direction.

The major component that must be present is a larger volume of business, more clients to sell nutrition to. Consult your business advisors to see if there are any untapped public relations or marketing avenues that you could pursue to increase the flow of clients. Why bring on consultants to help you, if only your needs are presently being met? Don't jump prematurely. Many business advisors suggest that a professional have enough work for one and one-half full-time people before a part-time associate is added. The other option is to have a consultant work as needed to free your time to go out and pursue new client accounts, and to interview potential subcontractors (when you are ready for them). First, more business, then subcontracting—in that order.

The dietitians who own businesses that subcontract to other dietitians report it is a big challenge. You cannot expect that other practitioners will have the same dedication as you do to your business. Many practitioners do not know how to work adequately with the clientele seen in private practice settings. Olga Satterwhite, R.D., states that out of every 25 people who interview, 24 will ask what Olga can give them and one will sell her on the flair and expertise she or he can bring to the business (1). Guess which one gets the position?

If you think subcontracting to other practitioners will make you a lot of money fast, think again. It takes years to build the contacts where you will place subcontractors. You will spend more time in overseeing accounts and personnel, and thus may have a resultant loss of income. Overhead expenses will increase for local travel, bad debts, added secretarial service, telephone, printed materials, bookkeeping, attorney fees and so on. After expenses, your 40–50 percent share of the subcontractors' fee may only generate a 10–25 percent net for all of your efforts. That isn't very much when you consider your earlier loss of income. The only way to increase your income potential is through volume (of accounts, clients and subcontractors) or through subcontracting at lower but guaranteed rates. It has worked well for some business owners to offer subcontractors a more stable income (fee per contract or total hours) instead of offering a more risky percentage of the income generated. When the risk is greater a sub-contractor usually expects more income.

In his book on entrepreneurialism, Joseph Mancuso discusses how to choose the team members that work best with an entrepreneur (2). The best choice is not an energetic person like the owner. This person may become frustrated and refuse to take orders or become an in-house competitor instead of an aide. You want to choose a "lazy, bright" person who benefits your company through good ideas and team spirit.

After a subcontractor is chosen, take time to make sure that she or he is adequately trained in your office and billing procedures, philosophies, successful teaching methods, and so on. She or he will be a representative of your business and as such could be a financial and professional blessing.

A contract or letter of agreement should be signed between you two and reviewed by your lawyers. If a subcontractor is placed with a client's account, have the client agree to it in writing and visit the client every four to six weeks. Replace the subcontractor if the client is unhappy instead of losing the account. Keep business as business, but remember if you made a good choice in a subcontractor, give her or him room to use his or her freedom, maturity, creativity, and expertise to both of your advantages.

Advisors will tell you that the advantages of having subcontractors over employees or partners are numerous:

- No employee benefits or taxes required, although you may wish to offer some benefits eventually.
- Subcontractor hours can be cut back more easily when business is slow.
- Subcontractors pay for their own malpractice insurance.
- There is less paperwork using subcontractors than with either a partner or employee.
- Decisionmaking is usually more expedient than when a partner is involved.

References

1. Satterwhite, Olga, President, Nutrition Consultant Services of Houston, TX.
2. Mancuso, Joseph: *How to Start, Finance and Manage Your Own Small Business,* Prentice-Hall, New Jersey, 1978.

CONCLUSION

Underlying this discussion on negotiating and agreements should be the awareness that usually the best outcomes evolve when both parties feel they benefit from the agreement—also, when both parties are honest and produce work in good faith. Learning how to "read" the other party and keep control of your advantage points becomes easier with experience and trial and error.

REFERENCES

1. Warschaw, T. A.: *Winning By Negotiation,* McGraw-Hill, New York, 1980.
2. *Negotiating Tricks,* International Entrepreneurs' Association Special Report No. 200, Copyright 1978 by Chase Revel, Inc.
3. Cohen, Herb: *You Can Negotiate Anything,* Bantam Books, New York, 1980.

chapter 16

Jobs with Physicians and Allied Medical Persons

Becky McCully, M.S., R.D.

Presenting a professional image is imperative if an entrepreneur is to work success-fully with other professionals. This includes a positive attitude, the ability to clearly communicate without distracting gestures or habits, a neat and tailored appear-ance and dress, consideration, cooperation and tact. Showing respect for another professional's expertise and expecting others to respect yours is important.

MAKING CONTACTS

Making contacts to find work or to network with professionals can be accom-plished in many ways. Remember to keep visible and audible. Be seen in public frequently. Be careful not to limit opportunities. Be broad-minded in thinking and explore all possibilities as future contacts. Develop a filing system or use your computer to record all contacts. Include names of individuals, what was dis-cussed, the reaction of the person contacted, telephone number, address, date, and a recommended follow-up procedure (see Figure 16.1).

When making contacts, always have business cards available. Anything else with your name and phone number such as handouts, fliers, brochures, and so on would be helpful to leave. Remember to keep visible!

Who Should Be Contacted?

The number and type of contacts one chooses to make are essentially unlimited. Below is a list of potential organizations and people to approach, but the list should be individualized according to your interests.

Figure 16.1 Sample Record of Networking Contacts

Person contacted _____Date of contact _____

Company or organization _____

Address _____

Mailing address _____

_____

_____

Telephone _____

Referred by _____

Contacted _____ by letter _____ by phone _____ in person

Discussed _____

_____

_____

_____

Reaction of person contacted _____

_____

_____

Accomplished _____

_____

_____

Follow-up plan _____

_____

_____

- Professional health organizations and associations, such as American Heart Association, American Diabetes Association, American Lung Association, Arthritis Foundation, etc.
- County and State Medical Associations
- Education centers (vo-tech schools, community colleges, nursing schools, etc.)
- Clinics and hospitals
- Women's groups (business and professional women's organizations, home extension groups, etc.)
- Fitness centers
- Sports facilities
- Individual physicians

How To Make Contacts

Basically there are three ways to make an initial contact—an introductory letter, a telephone call, or a personal conversation—and each can be appropriate for different situations.

Introductory letters   Although a letter is not as personal as a conversation, it is an effective way to introduce yourself and what you have to offer. It allows time to preplan and edit the message. The letter should vary according to the particular needs of the person being addressed. Keep the letter simple, clear, and concise (see Figure 16.2). Additional information about yourself such as a resume, brochure, or letter of reference could be included. Brochures are also available from the Consulting Nutritionist Practice Group of The American Dietetic Association, which explain the services provided by a nutritionist.

Telephone contacts   Whether networking or marketing your business, decide what needs to be said and outline the points to be emphasized before making the call. It may not be possible to talk directly to the individual in charge. Be concise and yet give enough information so the person will want to schedule an appointment for you. Be flexible in offering times to meet. Offer to go to the physician's or owner's office, or suggest a luncheon meeting at your expense. If the individual is interested, an appointment time will be arranged. If not, neither of you has invested much time.

Be conscious of voice tone on the telephone. Voice sound and the spoken message are the only tools for making a first impression. Speak clearly and slowly.

Personal conversations   Whenever possible personal contact is most beneficial. You are seen, heard and have the opportunity to leave printed material.

Plan and organize the entire presentation. Dress appropriately. When contacting a physician a business suit would be appropriate. Even if the meeting is with an individual at a sports or fitness center, your dress should still present a professional image. Dress to feel comfortable for the specific interview.

Body language speaks loudly. Practice role playing and, if possible, have a friend film it. This allows you to observe individual mannerisms, gestures, and

Figure 16.2   Sample Letter of Introduction

Date

John Smith, M.D.
3621 N. Perry, Suite 245
Oklahoma City, OK 73124

Dear Dr. Smith:

I am a registered dietitian with specialized training in working with patients having nutritional problems. As a consulting nutritionist in private practice, I counsel patients on an individual or group basis to develop nutrition care plans tailored to meet their nutritional needs as well as their lifestyles.

There are so many special dietary needs, ranging from those for patients diagnosed with obesity, hypertension, and cardiovascular disease to those for patients with extremely individual needs such as food allergies or enzyme deficiencies.

As you are aware, the services of a consulting nutritionist are an important and necessary part of medical treatment for many patients. Please consider adding the services of a consulting nutritionist as a part of the care your patients receive.

I will call your office next week to see about setting an appointment to discuss with you how my services could help your patients.

Respectfully,

Rebecca L. McCully, M.S., R.D.
Consulting Nutritionist

---

body movements. Constant movement such as swinging a foot, shifting weight, wringing hands, and so on are distracting and will take away from the presentation.

It's a good idea to take pertinent materials that can be left with the person contacted. For example, if contacting a physician, include a business card, diet prescription blanks (see Figure 16.3), samples of progress notes designed to provide patient information to the physician, newsletters that you have prepared, a list of types of services provided, and so on. If the physician specializes, it would be helpful to include articles on nutrition intervention related to the specialization.

When approaching an owner of a fitness center or clinic director about providing group services, present a brief overview of the particular program. For example, if you are offering a weight reduction class, show, but do not leave, a schedule of class topics, a brief summary of information to be presented in each

Figure 16.3 Business Card and Diet and Prescription Blank
(*Source:* Reprinted by permission of Rebecca L. McCully.)

Rebecca L. McCully, M.S., R.D.

Consulting Nutritionist

Cardiovascular Clinic Office
Pacer Development Center
3300 N.W. 56
Oklahoma City, Oklahoma 73112

Rx

CARDIOVASCULAR CLINIC
Becky McCully, M.S., R.D.
Consulting Nutritionist

Patient's Name

Patient's Number

Diagnoses:

Additional Information:

_____ M.D.
Physician's Signature

Diet Recommendations:
_____Cholesterol Reduction Diet
_____Diabetic Guidelines
_____ _____Calorie Diabetic Diet
_____Mild Sodium Restriction (2 grams)
_____ _____mg Sodium Diet
_____Calorie Control Weight Reduction
_____PSMF
_____Low Sodium PSMF
_____Other: _____

Educational material to send patient:
_____Cholesterol Programs
_____Diabetic Programs
_____Hypertension Programs
_____Weight Control Programs

class, and handouts which would be distributed to class participants. You could leave a brief list including the purpose of the class, fee structure, facilities needed (such as available space, blackboard, etc.), and what will be required of the participants.

OPTIONS FOR WORKING WITH PHYSICIANS

There are many viable options for working with one or a group of physicians. A creative arrangement with a physician allows you to get a taste of what private practice is all about without the risk of opening a free-standing practice initially.

Besides individual consultation on therapeutic, normal, and sports nutrition diets, suggested programs could include weight control groups, diabetes education programs, seminars on specific diseases such as cardiovascular disease and hypertension, wellness and prevention programs, cooking classes for various types of diets such as low calorie, low sodium, and diabetic.

Development of handouts, information sheets, newsletters, and articles is also a part of a well-designed nutrition program. Although these are not directly income producing, they are effective educational and advertising tools and, therefore, indirectly produce income. Such creative tools are enriching to a program. Be sure to include your name, address, and telephone number on all printed materials. They will become very inexpensive advertising.

The attorney who assisted in the preparation of the simple physician agreement (see Figure 16.4) strongly suggests that in cases where long-term association with a physician or clinic is envisioned, that the nutritionist consult an attorney for preparation of a formal contract. The investment in a more detailed contract may pay for itself many times over.

Figure 16.4 Sample Physician Contract

CONTRACT

This agreement entered into this _____ day of _____ , 19 _____ , by and between _____ , hereinafter referred to as "Nutritionist," and _____ , hereinafter referred to as "Physician."

It is agreed by the parties hereto that Nutritionist shall provide professional services to the clients and patients of Physician.

COMPENSATION. Nutritionist shall be compensated for professional services provided pursuant to this contract at the rate of _____ dollars ($ _____) per hour.

PROFESSIONAL SERVICES. "Professional services" as used herein shall be defined as being provided on a contract labor basis and shall consist of the following: (a) nutritional consultations with Physician's patients; (b) development of literature; (c) development of nutritional programs for patients; and (d) public speaking engagements on behalf of Physician.

HOURS. Nutritionist shall perform the above-enumerated services in the office of Physician between the hours of 1:00 P.M. and 5:00 P.M. Monday through Friday each week unless modified in writing.

DURATION. This contract shall be in effect for a period of one year from the date of execution and may be renewed by agreement of the parties.

_____   _____
Nutritionist   Physician

An Employed Position

If the physician strongly desires your services for his or her practice, it is possible the physician will be willing to take considerably more financial risk than if there are questions regarding the importance of nutritional services. The physician may work out an arrangement to hire you as an employee. Although this is different from opening a practice, it can be advantageous. There is virtually no risk to the nutritionist, and it gives the opportunity to try consulting with patients and developing programs for patients before opening a practice.

If the physician hires the nutritionist as an employee, benefits such as health insurance, malpractice insurance, paid vacation, use of office space, equipment, office supplies, and receptionist and/or secretary are usually offered. The patients are financially responsible to the physician and the physician pays the nutritionist a salary. Although this type of working relationship may be beneficial in gaining experience, it has many limitations.

The nutritionist is dependent upon the physician to refer enough patients to use the nutritionist efficiently without open blocks of time. (Other physicians are not apt to refer their patients to a nutritionist who is employed by a physician.) With this arrangement the nutritionist may be expected to see patients when they come to see the physician and, consequently, will not have much control over the daily schedule. The physician may or may not have specific nutrition guidelines the nutritionist is expected to use. The nutritionist may have to compromise personal philosophies to work for the physician.

Independent Contracting with a Physician

It is common for practitioners to work as independent contractors in a physician's office. This arrangement gives much greater flexibility of time and scheduling and more opportunity to control your business, but may also involve more financial risk or investment of personal capital.

Practitioners contract with physicians in a variety of ways. A contract may be for a predetermined number of hours per week or it may vary with the patient load. Another option is to have a percentage of the nutritionist's fee be charged for the use of the office space. And, finally, the nutritionist may pay the physician a flat rental fee for the use of the office and facilities. The physician will certainly continue to refer patients to the nutritionist but incurs no financial responsibility if the patient does not show (see Chapter 9 for more discussion).

Working with a Group of Physicians

It is also possible to work as an employee or independent contractor with a group of physicians in a medical complex. This option offers more variety and sometimes more professional challenge as one works with the different philosophies of physicians. Be sure the physicians specialize in areas of medicine compatible with your interests. Generally speaking, family physicians, cardiologists, internists, diabeticians, obstetricians, and allergists will be able to utilize the services

Q & A

Not Making it in a Clinic Setting

I work "as needed" for a local medical clinic. I see about two or three new patients plus about ten follow-ups each week. There are a dozen physicians who could refer patients, but only two actually do so regularly. What can I do to change this obvious unsatisfactory situation?

First, let's discuss what needs to be done right now, and you will see how to avoid this situation in the future. Since you didn't mention any marketing tactics you have tried, we will start from scratch. The problems as I see them (which results in too few patients) are the following:

- Lack of physician support caused by unawareness of the benefits you and your service could give, or not buying into the need for nutrition, or negative feedback from patients.

- Lack of support (and referrals) by other staff members (nurses, lab technicians, receptionists, etc.) caused by the same reasons as for physicians.

- Lack of demand by the patient population probably due to lack of awareness you and your services exist and no encouragement or referral to use your services.

Assuming that you would not be working there still if there had been negative feedback of any significance, the major problems seem to be that no one knows who you are or what you are doing there. The solution is to make everyone not only aware of you and nutrition counseling, but also to sell them on your services so they wonder how they ever got along without you.

Before I give you tactics to try, first understand that if you truly want to make some changes toward becoming more successful, you and your approach have to be part of the change. I have never seen a brochure, poster, or business card alone make the dramatic improvements in sales that you need.

The areas to evaluate and improve if necessary are:

1. *Services you now offer the clinic*
   Are they successful? Do clients/patients alter their food behaviors? Do your clients seem anxious to work with you and return for revisits? Do your counseling skills need improvement? Could you start a group weight loss class or give a diabetic or healthy heart cooking demonstration? Could you

develop programs to attract healthy individuals: athletes, adolescent weight loss, pregnancy, eating disorders, etc.? When necessary, involve other specialists to give broader focus, credibility, and better client care.

2. After you have identified potential new or upgraded services, develop your marketing plan.

A. *Physician support and involvement*

Ask to attend a monthly staff meeting to present your proposed plan for "Improved Nutrition Services at Midtown Clinic." Propose to involve individual physicians as "invited specialists" at group sessions. Ask for support and propose the names not only of a present referring physician, but also of at least one whom you would like to start referring. Discuss and provide a short written outline of typical group and individual consultations. Educate the physicians on how to "sell" nutrition to the patient when a referral is made.

After this session continue to stay in close contact with the group and each individual physician. Communicate in writing and in person. Announce all new classes, and when significant results or attendance occurs. Consider writing an in-house nutrition newsletter to improve communication and promote your services.

B. *Staff Support*

Ask to be a noon speaker at a "brown bag" lunch. At this "in-service" discuss the programs you proposed to the medical staff. Solicit feedback and support. According to their specialties, ask several staff members to be guest speakers at group sessions. Discuss the referral process and how to excite clients into wanting to attend.

Keep in close contact and publish class schedules well in advance. In fact it is best to have the staff keeping a waiting list of clients ready for the next class to begin. Let everyone know that class size is limited.

C. *Client Population*

Now it is time to use brochures, posters, client bill stuffers, and newsletters to promote your services. Use mail-outs to former clients, as well as patients identified for medical reasons by the staff. To improve the quality of your programs, always hand out anonymous evaluation questionaires at the end of group sessions. Then promote the strong areas and improve the weaker ones.—Kathy King Helm, R.D.

of a nutritionist more fully than specialists such as surgeons, urologists, and dermatologists. Orthopedic specialists who work with athletes are a growing market also.

WORKING WITH REGISTERED NURSES

Numerous types of programs benefit from combined efforts of various health professionals. Consider combining the consultation services of a registered dietitian with a registered nurse. One example would be a diabetes education program. The expertise of each specialist can mesh beautifully to form a well-rounded program. A diabetes program could be designed in a variety of ways including a two- or three-hour class, a weekend seminar, a series of classes meeting daily for a week, or a weekly class meeting for a specified number of weeks. This program could be presented in a clinic, hospital, community service program, or on a college campus.

The nurse could cover information about the disease itself, the mechanisms of oral hypoglycemic agents and insulin, insulin injections, and complications of diabetes. The dietitian could present the principles of the diabetic diet, recipe conversion, eating out, traveling, and shopping for the diabetic diet. A cooking demonstration would also be helpful.

Another program that could be developed by a registered nurse and a registered dietitian is a hypertension control program. This could be offered through a clinic, a hospital, or made available for individual patients to be held in a centralized location such as a church, hotel conference room, school auditorium, clinic, and so on.

Suggested topics to be included in a hypertension control program to be discussed by the nurse are the disease process of hypertension, medications and how they work, complications of uncontrolled hypertension, and instructing people in how to take their own blood pressures. The nutritionist could present various aspects of nutrition intervention with hypertension including sodium restriction and calorie control. Film strips, pamphlets, and dietary flashcards are good tools for teaching specific dietary principles. Discussion of seasoning foods without the addition of salt, how to cut calories, and eating in restaurants would all be applicable.

Pregnancy programs developed by nurses and nutritionists have numerous possibilities. The nurse could present information on pregnancy, delivery, and caring for an infant. The nutritionist could discuss nutritional needs during pregnancy and lactation, as well as infant nutrition.

Another component of a pregnancy program could be an exercise specialist. This person would plan exercise programs for women during pregnancy and after delivery.

WORKING WITH FITNESS SPECIALISTS

There are various areas of fitness involving specialists who could work well with nutritionists. Examples of these specialists include physical therapists, physical

Q & A

Working with a Dietetic Technician

I would like to have a Dietetic Technician work part time for me in my private practice. Has anyone ever tried this and did it work?

Yes, it has been tried and from what I understand, it works well. The Dietetic Technician knows accurate nutrition information, and he or she has skills compatible with a private practitioner. Much of the work needed to run a practice could be delegated to a Dietetic Technician such as marketing to prospective clients by phone or in the office, conducting initial interviews or assisting with interview forms, assisting with group sessions, bookkeeping and filing, and scheduling and reconfirming appointments.

As a private practitioner, you sometimes have the tendency to spread yourself too thin. You don't always need the expense and expertise of another dietitian. You need someone to support your efforts and relieve you of some of the nondietitian level work. Who better than a trained Dietetic Technician.—Kathy King Helm, R.D.

education specialists, and exercise physiologists. Each of these specialists focuses on different areas of fitness and may be located in institutions such as hospitals, fitness centers, nursing homes, or physical rehabilitation facilities. These specialists could utilize a nutritionist as a consultant or partner to develop coordinated nutrition/fitness programs. Health clubs, public school systems, senior centers, wellness programs, corporate fitness centers, and facilities designed to teach educators are all marketing outlets for your programs.

YWCA/YMCAs and community groups may also contract with a nutritionist. Programs for weight control, preschool or teenage nutrition problems, sports, and wellness are all possibilities.

Contact the person responsible for coordinating all programs to determine the primary age groups and the needs of people who primarily utilize the facility. Get feedback pertaining to the types of programs the coordinator feels would be most appropriate.

OTHER GROUPS

There are numerous opportunities for development of nutrition programs with people not in the health profession. Examples include directors of cooking schools, libraries, and recreation centers. Consumer specialists who work for grocery stores and restaurants are also potential clients.

Cooking School Directors

A director of a cooking school may be interested in offering a variety of health oriented cooking classes. These classes could include cooking for your heart, low sodium cooking, low calorie cooking, diabetic cooking, low cholesterol cooking, healthy snacks to prepare, and so on. Consider preparing descriptive introductions for the classes you would like to offer to give to the director. The following is an example for a diabetic class.

I am diabetic and looking for some interesting and different foods. Are there any classes for me?

    Solution: If you are a diabetic gourmet, this is the class for you! A wide variety of foods will be prepared—herbed mushrooms, liver pate, polynesian shrimp, teriyaki chicken kabobs, and other delights —all calculated into the diabetic exchange system and all low in calories.

    When setting your fee, consider the mechanics of the class. Will you only be teaching and cooking, or will you be doing the preprep and clean up also? Will you help advertise the class or will the cooking school absorb this cost? These factors must be considered before quoting a price for conducting the class.

    If doing a series of classes, one should design a creative logo and style of writing recipes. This helps to establish an identity. Again, be sure your name, address and telephone number are on each recipe.

Libraries

Frequently libraries offer classes to patrons on various subjects. Consider doing book reviews on diet books, having discussion groups on various nutrition topics, conducting weight control classes, diabetic classes, and so on. These classes may not prove to be financially lucrative, but your name will be exposed to the public, and this may be a good referral source. Remember to keep visible!

Recreation Centers

Recreation centers frequently attract people interested in exercise and good health. Consider approaching recreation centers with the idea of offering some

Q & A

Networking

What is networking and why should it be important to me?

Networking involves establishing informal lines of communication and support with people around you. By informally talking to people on all levels and in all types of businesses you can increase your awareness of how businesses operate, how decisions are made, and how power is used. You can use this information to help your own business or career by patterning or avoiding common pitfalls. You can better forecast trends and learn of new opportunities in the market place. By the time most information is published and hits the media, it is present or past history. To really be effective in the marketplace, you need to catch and be a part of trends before they hit it big. Networking can help you keep in touch with that pulse.

Through meeting new people both inside and outside of the dietetic and medical fields, you can extend your sphere of influence and become known to new markets. Other people who respect your work can open doors for you and suggest your name when a nutritionist is needed. If they really like your work, they may even create nutrition components to programs so you can be involved. When you look good, that makes the person who suggested you look good, and bonds of support begin to grow. You can also have your own network of specialists who complement and support your programming.

By networking through friends of friends, and using names to open doors, your opportunities in life are greatly expanded. Because we all have so many people vying for our attention, we develop criteria for evaluating what and who will get our time. One very effective means of determination is, do we know and trust the person? If not, do we know and trust the person who referred him? If so, do you allow the referred person an interview? There is a good chance that you will, or you might refer him on to someone who could benefit him even more. That same system can work for us. It is out there waiting to be used.

Building a Network

Most of us already have functioning networks around us, we just need to expand them. Networking is an attitude—one of wanting to help others as well as be helped.

You can build a network by joining or volunteering your time to groups and organizations. You can simply talk to people around you in all walks of life and start a relationship by offering your business card and a few kind words. Successful networks are created by keeping in touch with people you meet in professional situations—at meeting, seminars, as coleaders of group programs, at former jobs, etc. Many cities have executive or women in business or entrepreneurial clubs created specifically for networking purposes.

Considerations–Precautions

Where there are good ideas there are also a few precautions to consider. First, use your time and money wisely—you can waste a lot of both joining groups and becoming "involved" just to meet people. Critically evaluate the benefits you receive against the investment you pay. Second, realize that other people don't usually mind giving if they have the time, but be respectful of their time. In return you don't have to allow others to hang on to you and drain your energy in the name of networking.—Kathy King Helm, R.D.

Reprinted by permission of The American Dietetic Association, 1986.

fun activities centered around nutrition such as nutrition crossword puzzles, quizzes, and games. These could be incorporated with healthy snacks to be served at the center.

Grocery Stores

Many grocery stores now make nutrition information available to customers. This may be in the form of a series of nutrition booklets, healthy recipes using ingredients sold at the store, or creative advertising of new products that can be worked into special diets.

Consider suggesting color coding products in a store according to the nutritive value, sodium content, caloric content, and so on. Another idea is to provide nutritious food demonstrations in the store. Again, this could advertise many of the products available at the store to be used in special diets.

Other Dietitians

Involvement with the local and state dietetic association and Consulting Nutritionist Practice Group is important. It provides support from other dietitians and keeps one visible as well as helps keep one up to date with what other dietitians are doing. Sharing information and working with other dietitians is extremely helpful.

chapter *17*

Selling and Promotion

A commitment to marketing is essential in any business small or large. Lack of sufficient marketing and promotion is one reason so many businesses stagnate or fail to attract customers.

All too often, an entrepreneur assumes marketing falls under the heading of selling and promotion or advertising. In fact, it is the other way around. Selling and promotion are key elements in a marketing plan, but on their own they are only short-term tactics (1). Tactics alone may boost you in your chosen market today, but market assessment and long-range planning prepare you for the new markets.

MARKETING AN INTANGIBLE PRODUCT—NUTRITION COUNSELING, MANAGEMENT

Marketing is concerned with getting and keeping customers. Product intangibility has its greatest effect on the process of trying to get customers. How do you propose to sell something like nutrition counseling or consulting that a customer can't hold in his hand, feel, or see?

Intangible products can seldom be tried out in advance. Prospective buyers are generally forced to depend on surrogates to assess what they will probably get. They can look at before and after pictures of weight loss patients. They can talk to current users of your services. They can see and hold your elegant calling card, brochure, or business proposal in its leatherette binder.

Similarly, companies develop elaborate packaging to best show off their products and not only entice the buyer but also reassure him. Theodore Levitt relates in his article "Marketing Intangible Products and Product Intangibles" that,

> The product will be judged in part by who offers it—not just who the vendor corporation is but who is the corporation's representative. The vendor and the vendor's representative are both inextricably and inevitably part of the 'product' that prospects must judge before they buy. The less tangible the generic product, the more powerfully and persistently the judgment about it gets shaped by the packaging—how it is presented, who presents it, and what's implied by metaphor, simile, symbol, and other surrogates for reality (2).

It is easy to understand why banks build large, sturdy buildings and hire articulate consultants in dark vested suits. Also, why proposals are in "executive" typeset and leather bindings, and why architects laboriously draw renderings of their buildings. It explains why insurance companies offer "a piece of the rock," put you under a "blanket of protection" or in "good hands."

SELLING

A sale takes place when a client or patient pays for a service or product. To survive in business, sales must happen. Of course, everyone wants to offer products that are in such demand that they "sell themselves," but that is a rarity.

Dietitians can increase their sales by improving their sales presentation skills and by better taking advantage of sales opportunities. Constantly be aware of instances where your nutrition services can be appropriately sold.

The Sales Presentation

The sales presentation includes four major components, each with a specific purpose (3):

1. Introduction. The purpose of the introduction is to establish with the prospective client how you are different from all the others waiting to sell the same product. You do this by making statements that either focus attention, specify direct benefits, or warn of danger.
2. Investigative Phase. This phase is one of the most important in the modern-day sales process. Get the buyer to define his or her other needs, wants, and expectations. Do this by asking open-ended questions and by listening to the answers. The information obtained in this exchange will help you personalize your presentation and perhaps think of new products to sell.
3. Presentation Phase. During this phase present facts carefully chosen for their effect on your client. Show how his or her needs will be met by what you have to offer. Buyers base their decisions on fact and emotion. Garner emotional support for you and your services. If you see that the buyer is drifting or does not appear to understand, go back to the investigative phase and refocus attention by asking more questions. You

need to be flexible. The outcome of this phase should be a natural progression to the close.

4. Closing. This is the time to bring the presentation to closure, either by asking for a sale's or other commitment. This can best be accomplished by summarizing the client's needs and identifying solutions that you have to offer. Ask when you can begin or how you can provide more assistance or when you can provide more information. Your purpose may have been to only introduce yourself and explain your services. Even if the client is not interested in your services at this time, leave the session as friends and on a positive note. Don't give up. Look for the next opportunity to present this product or new ones to that prospective client.

After the sales call, drop a note into the mail thanking the prospect for his or her time.

PROMOTION

Promotion is actually the communication you use to help others become familiar with you, your services or product. Promotion is becoming more important than ever before because of the changes in the marketplace.

First, consumers are now shopping around to find the best nutrition services and products for their money. Second, there is confusion today in the public's mind about who to believe in the nutrition field. Finally, dietitians aren't the only legitimate players in the nutrition arena. Where we may have had ownership in the past in some market areas through default, today that is no longer the case. Nutrition is in demand by the consumer; it is therefore a competitive area of business (4).

Dietitians often neglect to plan and oversee adequate promotion for programs, not realizing that poor attendance or tasteless promotion reflects back on the program. Actually, it shows lack of foresight and follow-through if a practitioner devotes total attention to the development of an excellent program that could produce client satisfaction and yet fails to insure the program success through adequate promotion (4).

Promotion will attract far more clients to our doors than any form of legislation. Because the health-care focus is evolving to more health promotion and to attracting the "well" individual, dietitians must accept that their services are one of many nutrition-information options available to each consumer. Therefore, dietitians must learn how to promote themselves.

PROMOTION TOOLS

There are many tools that can be used in promotion. Which techniques you select are usually determined by the target market, your budget, and the degree of competition.

Some promotional tools are far more effective in reaching the target market, but may (like television or color ads in magazines) also be very expensive. Other techniques may better meet the expectations of the target markets, for example, tasteful brochures mailed to clients' and physicians' offices. Medical professionals have been slow in using less traditional promotion tools such as billboards and neon signs because of their own value judgments and what they perceive would be their potential clients' reactions.

Some forms of promotion may make your peers uncomfortable because they are new. If your peers are not your buying market, then you must keep their disapproval in perspective. To play a viable role in the marketplace, dietitians must continually innovate or they will be left behind. Innovation, quality service, and promotion are the lifeblood of success in business (4).

When trying to evaluate which forms of promotion to use, public relations experts suggest that you go down a list of the promotion options and hypothetically try to fit the service or product to it. Look for ideas that are creative, unique, and in good taste.

Promotion is most successful when a plan is designed for multiple exposure of the name or message to the target market over an extended period of time. Example: For a fitness center weight-loss program, promotion could include newspaper and radio advertisements, free newspaper publicity, direct mail promotion and in-house newsletter promotion to members, give-away gym bags printed with the program name and logos given upon payment of the registration fee, and program T-shirts awarded when fitness goals are met. These are just a few promotion ideas; there are dozens more.

There are advertising and public relations firms and individual consultants that can create promotional campaigns for a fee. For most dietitians with numerous projects, that is not always an affordable option, but it may be a wise investment for selected projects. Promotion costs should be seen as part of the necessary expense and investment made to create demand for nutrition services. The challenge is to choose wisely and be cost effective when investing in promotional programs. The question could be asked, "Can you afford not to promote?"

Following is a listing and brief overview of promotional tools that are commonly used to market dietitians services and products:

One-to-One Communication

One-to-one communication can be your most effective form of promotion. It affords the opportunity to speak, hear, see, and exchange viewpoints face to face. As the promoter, you have the opportunity to read the body language and expressions of your listener and then adjust your presentation for best impact.

Satisfied customers are walking promoters of inestimable value. Through word-of-mouth advertising, listeners may be more influenced to try a dietitian's service because the promoter lends credibility as a satisfied customer.

Business Name

A good business name can be a marketing asset to a practitioner. Business consultants suggest that the name be distinctive or descriptive.

Many practitioners use their own names for their business name. They find that as they become better known, people remember both them and their company since they have the same name. Other consultants choose descriptive easy-to-remember business names such as Nutrition Consultants, The Nutrition Group, or Gourmet Services. Less common are names that do not give a clue to the type of business such as Creative Concepts, Midtown Associates, or Lifeline, Inc. Potentially, names could also indicate the area of specialty: Sports Cuisine, Nutrition Communicators, or Kitchen Designs.

In time all practitioners become identified with their business names—if the name is used regularly. Don't waste your time on trying to come up with a creative name, if you end up using only your personal name on promotional materials and when conducting business. Also, it is costly to change your business name, so be sure to research it well before advertising under it.

Logo

A logo is a symbol. If it is used to identify a product, it is called a trademark. If it is used for a company, it is called a servicemark. Logos can be fun and very comical or highbrow and sophisticated. Or somewhere in between. Logos are used to draw attention to whatever they are used on, such as stationery, posters, calling cards, brochures, or billboards (see Figure 17.1).

Business Owner

Private practitioners are potentially their own best marketing asset. Your personality, image, communication and business skills, and expertise in nutrition will be ultimately responsible for attracting and keeping clients.

Business advisors suggest that business people use at least the following four practices to help promote their business. First, use the phone and all of its marketing potential, in other words, talk to clients regularly, confirm appointments, respond to referring physicians, and call for more interviews to let people know about your business. Use the phone to interest new prospective patients into coming for an appointment. Take the time to show an interest in their needs, to tell them briefly what you have to offer, to let them know what you will expect from them, and to discuss an appointment time and your fees. By taking time to market your services instead of just to schedule an appointment, the client will become excited about the expected personalized care.

Second, use your writing skills to correspond with people on a timely basis and to publish. For those who feel weak in this area there are adult education classes, books, and editors or writers for hire to help you (see Chapter 23).

Third, use public speaking to make yourself more visible in your community and to interest people in nutrition. Speaking to clubs, community groups, PTAs, and at conferences will make people recognize you as a nutrition specialist.

Fourth, become involved in several local or national organizations that

Figure 17.1 A Selection of Logos

(*Source:* Reprinted by permission of the business owners.)

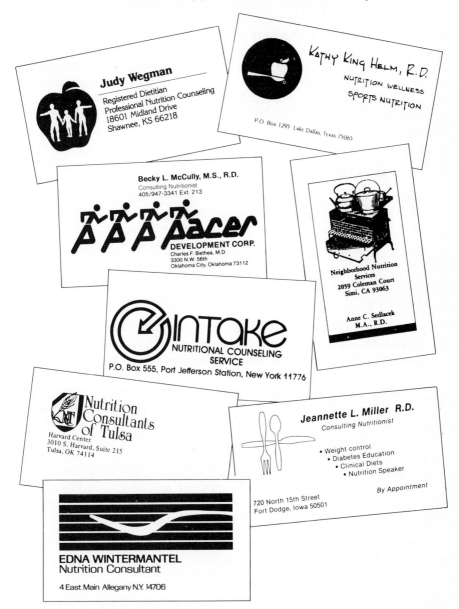

could benefit you personally and/or professionally. Attend meetings, support activities, and run for offices. Dietetic organizations, including Dietetic Practice Groups need input from active, assertive dietitians on their way up. Small business owners' groups, executive clubs, Toastmasters, and local political groups offer opportunities to become involved.

Writing for Publication

Writing is an ideal medium for practitioners to distinguish and promote themselves by communicating with the public or their peers. Writing for lay periodicals or books provides the opportunity to reach a potentially large audience, to share your views, to be paid for your work with more frequency, and to become known.

Writing for publication in professional journals does not pay directly, but it helps establish you as a knowledgeable, qualified professional and excellent resource. Articles may also lend credibility to your programs and services. This type of promotion also may attract more business in the form of referrals, or consultation opportunities.

PROMOTION MATERIALS

Promotion materials are an extension of you and your expertise. Buy the most attractive ones that will serve your purpose and upgrade them as you have the money to do so. Visit several printing shops to see what papers, inks, bindings, turnaround times, and other services they have to offer at what price. Work closely with any artist that you hire to make sure you get what you want.

Business Cards

Business cards should always be carried and handed out. They can be powerful marketing tools and one of the least expensive. Other peoples' cards should be saved and used the next time you want to network or you need some information or service.

Business cards should list your name, credentials, business name, phone number with area code, and full address. If additional information is needed, a good typesetter can usually arrange the lettering and adjust the size type.

Some considerations to think about: Do you want to print appointment information on the back of the card? Does the card look too cluttered as it is laid out? Can everyone read the typeface (script and Old English are difficult to read)? Since card sizes are fairly standard, will choosing another size card make your card stand out or be thrown away? How can you best use color, style, paper, and design to attract attention to your card? (See Figure 17.2.)

Letters

Letters that are well written and to the point have boosted the careers of many businesspersons. All too often we overlook the contribution that impressive correspondence can provide. As important as the content of a letter is, its neatness and grammatical correctness can influence a reader just as much. Letters with numerous corrections or misspelled words are poorly received (see envelope address layouts in Figure 17.3).

Busy people will often refuse to read obvious mass mailings, such as those

Figure 17.2 Sample Business Cards

(*Source:* Reprinted by permission of the business owners.)

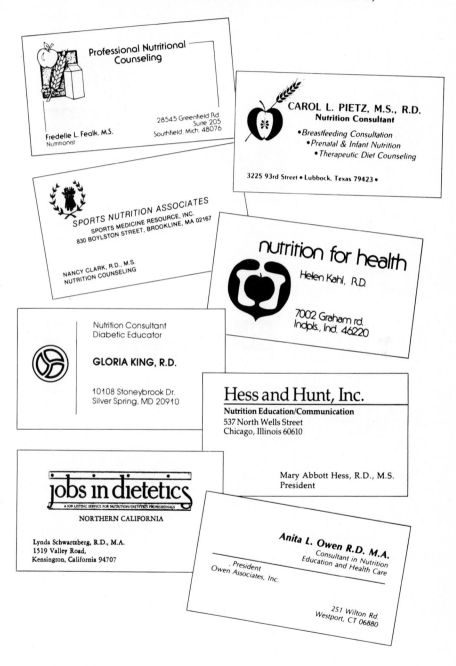

Professional Nutritional Counseling

28545 Greenfield Rd.
Suite 205
Southfield, Mich. 48076

Fredelle L. Fealk, M.S.
Nutritionist

CAROL L. PIETZ, M.S., R.D.
Nutrition Consultant

•*Breastfeeding Consultation*
•*Prenatal & Infant Nutrition*
•*Therapeutic Diet Counseling*

3225 93rd Street • Lubbock, Texas 79423 •

SPORTS NUTRITION ASSOCIATES
SPORTS MEDICINE RESOURCE, INC.
830 BOYLSTON STREET, BROOKLINE, MA 02167

NANCY CLARK, R.D., M.S.
NUTRITION COUNSELING

nutrition for health

Helen Kahl, R.D.

7002 Graham rd.
Indpls., Ind. 46220

Nutrition Consultant
Diabetic Educator

GLORIA KING, R.D.

10108 Stoneybrook Dr.
Silver Spring, MD 20910

Hess and Hunt, Inc.

Nutrition Education/Communication
537 North Wells Street
Chicago, Illinois 60610

Mary Abbott Hess, R.D., M.S.
President

jobs in dietetics
A JOB LISTING SERVICE FOR NUTRITION/DIETETICS PROFESSIONALS

NORTHERN CALIFORNIA

Lynda Schwartzberg, R.D., M.A.
1519 Valley Road,
Kensington, California 94707

Anita L. Owen R.D. M.A.
Consultant in Nutrition
Education and Health Care

President
Owen Associates, Inc.

251 Wilton Rd.
Westport, CT 06880

Figure 17.3 Sample Envelope Layouts
(*Source:* Reprinted by permission of the business owners.)

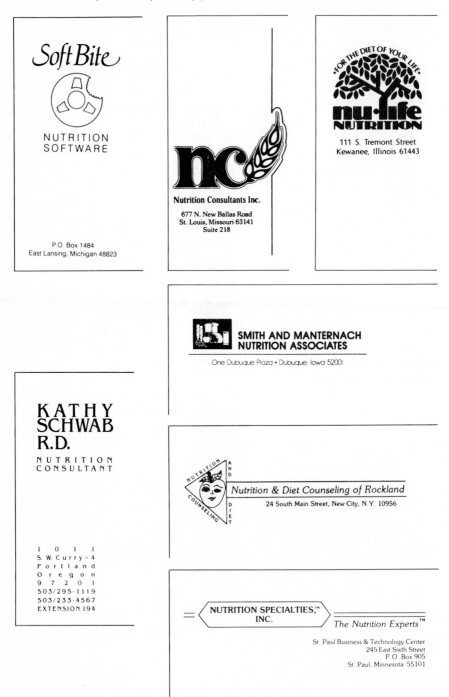

addressed to "Dear Sirs" or "Dear Philadelphia Physicians" or those that are poorly photocopied. Creativity, time, effort, and money must be invested to ensure that your letters are read. Business consultants suggest that even on mass mailings, the signature and heading should be individualized whenever possible.

Direct Mail

Direct mail is used when you know specifically whom you want to contact (usually either potential clients or referral agents) and when you want to increase your chances of attracting a higher-percentage response.

Direct mail should be personally addressed instead of "To whom it may concern." Personalizing mail as much as possible increases the readership.

Direct mail is used for marketing surveys, announcements of a new office location or new services, and to acquaint potential clients or referral agents to your services. Membership lists of your local medical society or national dietetic practice groups, the Yellow Pages, and shared business cards are good sources of names and addresses. Many organizations ask for a fee and an explanation of how the membership lists will be used before use is granted.

Resume

As discussed in Chapter 2, a resume can be a very effective marketing tool. It should highlight the aspects about you and your experience that best qualify you for a position you are seeking. In other words, you may need several different resumes. Resumes also can be used along with letters of introduction in business or to establish credibility in a proposal.

Typeset resumes look impressive, but are expensive to update. In certain instances, the typeset look may be worth the extra expense. Word processing can make updating a resume very easy. Business managers state that on the whole, good quality typed resumes are just as impressive. There is hope that content may actually count.

Letters of Reference

Letters of reference written by prominent people who know you personally or professionally are impressive. They help establish credibility and may help open doors for you. Keep the original on file and use good prints or photocopies.

Brochures

Brochures are used to introduce and promote. It is not imperative that a private practitioner have a brochure, but many have found that attractive, clever ones attract business and easily pay for themselves.

The three most important things to remember about a brochure are to make it attractive, simple to read, and interesting. It is not necessary to state every service you have to offer. It may be more interesting to the reader to include a picture of yourself, quote statements from satisfied customers, or offer your nutrition philosophy.

Brochures seldom list fees because it dates them and sometimes makes them poorly received. Your name, business name, address, and phone number should be highlighted. It is highly suggested that brochures be typeset and printed on good quality paper. (See brochures in Figures 17.4, 17.5, 17.6, and 17.7.)

Portfolio

There are times when private practitioners want to show the scope of their creativity and samples of their work such as creative menus, educational materials, media work, or catering ideas. When a business is new and its reputation and yours are unknown, a portfolio may be the marketing tool you need.

A portfolio is similar to a scrapbook or a slide show designed to show graphically what you have to sell. The portfolio may be in a commercially available portfolio folder, on a tripod display with charts, on slides or on audio or video tapes for dietitians who do media work. Presenting a portfolio to the client helps make the intangible promise tangible, enticing, and clearly defined.

The cost of a portfolio can vary greatly, depending upon what is included.

Figure 17.4 Sample Brochure
(*Source:* Reprinted by permission of Kathy King Helm. No portion of this brochure may be reused without permission.)

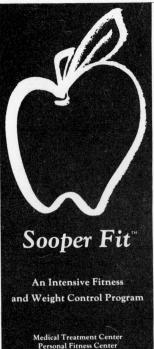

Sooper Fit™

Everyday more Americans and businesses are recognizing the importance of good health and wellness. However, health care costs are increasing faster than inflation. Insurance premiums rise at a rate of 15% per year. Obesity has become the nation's number one malnutrition problem with 80 million Americans — one third of our population — overweight.

The *Sooper Fit*™ Program is an intensive eight week program individualized to each person's needs in the areas of nutrition, fitness and lifestyle habits. Each participant will be individually cared for, evaluated and followed. The spouse or family will always be welcome to attend counseling sessions and will occasionally be requested to participate when home or environment changes are desired.

The program emphasis is on the overweight adult, teenager or child wanting permanent weight loss as well as the person wanting weight gain and muscle building. Athletic individuals can use this program to improve their eating and training habits in preparation for competition or for rehabilitation from injury.

This comprehensive program will include:

- Two months of intensive evaluation, therapy and individualized care

- Eight weeks of nutrition consultation by a Registered Dietitian

- A Physician consult and evaluation

- Before and after fitness evaluations and individualized exercise program by a Physical Therapist

- Two months of supervised aerobic and Nautilus exercising at the Personal Fitness Center

- Blood chemistry screening

- Computer analysis of your diet

- Wellness/Lifestyle Appraisal

Call 530-1123

Sooper Fit™

An Intensive Fitness and Weight Control Program

Medical Treatment Center
Personal Fitness Center
5120 N. Jupiter Rd., Garland, Texas

Figure 17.5 Sample Brochure Cover

(*Source:* Reprinted by permission of Judy Wegman, 1983. No portion of this brochure may be reused without permission.)

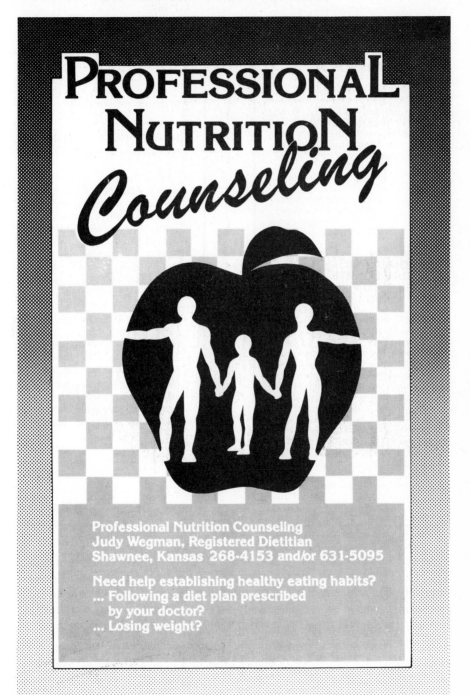

Figure 17.6   Sample Brochure
(*Source:* Reprinted by permission of business owner, Jan
Shore-Lewinsohn, R.D. No portion of this brochure may be reused without
permission.)

OUR MISSION. .

NUTRITION DYNAMICS is dedicated to the overall health and well-being of the individual by working in partnership with physicians and other health professionals to provide the highest standards of professional care in nutrition.

Our nutritional services are offered strictly through consulting nutritionists.

WHAT IS A CONSULTING NUTRITIONIST?

A consulting nutritionist is a registered dietitian (R.D.) dedicated to providing quality nutrition counseling to people of all ages, to help them understand and cope with their individual nutritional needs. A consulting nutritionist works independently of any health care facility to provide nutritional expertise and guidance to patients, through a physician's private practice. A consulting nutritionist may also counsel hospitals, nursing homes, community health agencies and professional health associations.

HOW CAN A CONSULTING NUTRITIONIST HELP YOU?

Being specially trained in such a vital area of preventative and maintenance health care, a consulting nutritionist can relieve a physician from the task of developing the individual diet instructions for his/her many patients. The consulting nutritionist will develop the physician's diet prescription into complete meal plans, individualized to each patient's needs. The nutritionist will then counsel each patient to assure a complete understanding of his/her nutritional plan. Being relieved of this task, the physician is better able to apply his/her specialized skills in other areas.

Items may range from professionally produced food photos or renderings to just copies or samples of educational materials, authored articles, menus, snapshots, letters of reference, and newspaper coverage. Occasionally it is worth paying a professional artist or calligrapher to add a special touch. Unfortunately, many of us never use samples of our past creativity to help us win the next contract.

Proposals

A proposal is a comprehensive marketing tool used to present the selling points of an idea. One could be used to interest a corporation in using you in their

Figure 17.7 Sample Personal Promotion Brochure

(*Source:* Reprinted by permission of Hess and Hunt, Inc., 1984. No portion of this brochure may be reused without permission.)

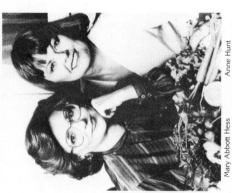

Mary Abbott Hess   Anne Hunt

Hess and Hunt helps the foodservice and health care industry and its agencies. . .
- Meet the needs of consumers who have health concerns.
- Promote nutritious products by providing responsible spokespersons and developing publicity materials.
- Educate the public and health professionals by making presentations and teaching courses.

Hess and Hunt helps foodservice organizations. . . .
- Write menus and expand current offerings of light, healthful items.
- Create effective nutrition promotions.
- Sell products to markets with specific health needs.

Hess and Hunt helps social service and government agencies . .
- Develop innovative nutrition education materials.
- Improve services to the community by teaching staff and client groups.
- Formulate food specifications, menus and evaluation tools to improve program quality and meet federal requirements.

Hess and Hunt helps print and electronic media . . . .
- Obtain responsible nutrition information.
- Inform the public about popular nutrition topics by writing articles and appearing on radio and television programs.
- Translate scientific jargon into language that ordinary mortals can understand.

Since 1979, **Hess and Hunt, Inc.** has provided insightful, professional nutrition expertise for business, industry and government. The firm brings together the broad knowledge of Mary Abbott Hess, a registered dietitian and associate professor of nutrition, and the communication background of Anne Hunt, a food public relations specialist, formerly food editor of *Sphere* (now *Cuisine*) magazine. Hess and Hunt with a support staff of experts in nutrition education, foodservice, marketing and graphic design offers nutrition communications that are both creative and dependable.

Hess and Hunt can translate the science of nutrition into language consumers understand. The firm is experienced in all print and electronic media, as well as in the preparation of booklets, educational programs, brochures, radio scripts, posters, displays, slide presentations, menus and recipes. Hundreds of speeches have been made to professional and general audiences.

Mary Abbott Hess and Anne Hunt were recently honored with the Morris Fishbein Award for excellence in medical writing for their book, *Pickles & Ice Cream: The Complete Guide To Nutrition During Pregnancy* (McGraw-Hill, 1982; Dell Paperback, 1984). Hess is the co-author of *The Art Of Cooking For The Diabetic* (Contemporary Books, 1978) which has sold over 200,000 copies.

Both Hess and Hunt are active in professional organizations, including the American Medical Writers Association and Society for Nutrition Education. Mary Abbott Hess, R.D., M.S., has been elected to leadership positions in the American Dietetic Association and the Chicago Nutrition Association. She is a member of the Institute of Food Technologists and the Roundtable for Women in Foodservice. Anne Hunt is a member of the American Home Economics Association and has served on the Board of Directors of Chicago Home Economists in Business. She is editor of the Nutrition Educators With Industry newsletter.

Mary Abbott Hess has a B.S. from Simmons College in Boston and an M.S. from Northern Illinois University. Anne Hunt is a graduate of Wooster College, Wooster, Ohio, and completed a post graduate course of study in food and nutrition at Mundelein College in Chicago.

wellness program, or to sell an obesity seminar to a clinic director or to interest a financial backer in a new product or business venture.

Proposals can range from a simple one-page typewritten information sheet to a typeset, bound presentation containing a volume of pages, along with a slide show and taste session. The scope of the proposal is determined in a large part by what is expected, what is used by the competition, and what will be impressive enough to make the sell. The use of a proposal should not be reserved only for the experienced practitioner; the novice may find it to be the very marketing boost needed to build the business more quickly.

Proposals should only be long enough to interest the client and make the sell. Care should be exercised so that explanations are not so detailed that clients can carry them out themselves without you.

Proposals usually represent many hours or days of research of the market and the client so that the proposed item to sell is "positioned" correctly—it will fit the client's needs. One may include:

- An introduction or explanation of the scope of the proposal
- An overview of the market and its potential
- A short analysis of the competition
- Background information about the client and his needs
- Your answer to fulfilling the client's needs
- Why you are best for the job (include resume and references)
- Estimates of costs and potential income
- Any final selling points

A proposal should build in excitement and interest as it leads to the answers you have to offer. Determination of which points to use and their order are at your discretion. You want the client to feel that they can't live without *you* and what *you* have to offer.

An experienced negotiator may choose to orally paraphrase the proposal and offer a shorter written copy. Whenever possible, the proposal should be made in person to the entire staff of decision makers. Questions and any confusion can be handled immediately. However, instances may arise when a proposal must be mailed or left at an office. When you are not there to give the introduction and to promote the concept with tact and enthusiasm, a letter of introduction and the written document must do it for you. A phone call should be timed to coincide with the day the person receives the document. If the contact person must sell the concept to others, when preparing the proposal enlist his or her help and ask what selling points, statistics, or other information she or he feels will be needed to impress the others. Ordinarily, the answers you receive will give you great insight into the client company and their real interests.

Most proposals will involve ideas that have been around for a while in which case you are selling the client on using you and your creativity and expertise. There is always some fear about the risk in giving a potential client the opportunity to see a truly unique, clever idea such as an invention or new business concept. You can ask that the client sign a Non-Disclosure Agreement (see Chapter 14). However, some people will take offense to being asked or will refuse to do so on legal grounds (they may have already had plans to pursue the idea). As a safeguard, it is usually acceptable to bring another person with you as an associate (and witness). In many instances a proposal is presented, but only a summary sheet is left with the client. And finally, you can always ask before the proposal is offered that the ideas be considered privy information. If an agreement is never reached, and yet your unique idea is used by the client, you could sue if your case is strong enough (a witness or written agreement may be necessary to do so).

A proposal provides a perfect opportunity to offer the "Sears Plan" to a client: the good, better, and best approach. (See "Negotiating," Chapter 15.) Anticipate that the client may be hesitant to buy the most comprehensive plan you have to offer and be ready to promote the contingency plan of lesser cost and involvement in case the first one doesn't sell. A third "at least you got your foot in the door" plan could be either offered initially, or you could wait and use it if all else fails.

Making a proposal may set the beginning groundwork that will lead to other new ideas or ventures between you and the client. Or it may only help your client decide what he doesn't want to do. Whatever the extent of the agreement to work together, it should be outlined, and all parties should have a copy. If the agreement refers back to the original proposal, a copy of the proposal should be kept with the agreement (See "Negotiating," Chapter 15).

Posters

Using posters to promote seminars and classes has proven to be successful for some practitioners. To save money on printing costs, a large number of poster shells (ones with only partial information) can be printed at one time with the logo, business name, and phone number. The date, place, time, and event can be added as the posters are used. Sometimes a pad is attached with tear-off cards to send in for more information.

If the posters are not too large, most stores, health clubs, beauty shops, and so on that allow posters are willing to let you have display space to solicit their customers. When you use this type of marketing and you want to use the locations more than once, call or stop by when the event is over to take the posters down and check in with the owner.

Press Kits

Press kits are commonly used to interest the media in writing or broadcasting a story to help you promote your services, product, book, or speaking engagement.

The kit may include a variety of items:

- A press release on the service, product, or book you wish to publicize, and/or a program brochure
- A sample of the product or book, or a copy of newspaper articles, advertisements, or critical reviews
- A resume and short biographical sketch
- 5″ × 7″ black and white glossy photo of you and also the product

Press kits should be descriptive, attractive, and to the point. They should explain why the public would be interested in the topic. Although press kits can be very elaborate with printed covers and numerous photos, they can also be as simple as several of the above items placed in a large folder with pockets.

Banners

Banners draw attention and create name recognition. They can be used at a "fun run" finish line, in a lobby during a Wellness Festival, or over the cafeteria door to promote the new line of 'Light and Natural' foods. Banners can be made with paper and paint; however, they can be reused many times if they are made from cloth. They are a great promotional tool for a large area where crowds are gathered and also create a festive mood (4).

Give-Aways

Give-aways (T-shirts, notebooks, mugs, gym bags, etc.) with the program name or logo are popular promotion items. The more useful and practical the item, the more it will be used and the name or logo displayed. (These items are sometimes sold as fund raisers rather than given away.)

FREE PROMOTION

The word "free" means that it is not paid advertising, but in most instances this type of marketing requires a substantial amount of a practitioner's time, effort, and money. Many elements of free promotion have already been discussed under promotion tools and materials.

Public Speaking

Although we encourage practitioners to charge for public speaking there are times when you are just starting a business that you may accept speaking engagements for the experience and exposure, or later, as a tithe of your time. Even when you charge a fee most groups can afford, if you count your preparation time, phone calls, travel, speaking time, and loss of income while away from the office, you will be lucky to break even. So, it is understood that we speak for the public relations value, to gain experience and poise, to educate others, and because we enjoy it.

Speaking does not come easily to many people. Controlling and yet exciting a group while one speaks is even more challenging. Following are some preplanning secrets that will make speaking engagements more predictable and enjoyable for you.

Ask for a speaking fee.   When a group pays for a speaker, it often spends more time and effort in promoting the speech and the turnout is better. When you are paid to speak, you often put the talk as a higher priority, come better prepared, and give a better presentation. If the group fits into the tax-deductible or nonprofit category and is unable to pay your fee (and you want the engagement), for tax purposes agree to donate your fee to their organization in return for a statement to that effect or have them make out a check that you will then return.

Set minimums on the size of the group you will speak to.   If a group in your area wants you to speak and by reputation you know that their turnouts are poor, especially if the fee is low, state that you request groups to have at least 20 people (or whatever number) present. If they still want to have you, they will accept the commitment. We have all had the experience where we drive across town at night to find an obscure building and give an elaborate presentation to three people.

Find out as much as you can about the group you are going to speak to. What is the range in ages? What are the percentages of men, women, and children? What are their educational backgrounds and do they know much about nutrition, weight loss, fads, or whatever? Will other speakers be on the program with you or speak the week before or after on a similar subject? What specifically do they want you to speak on and highlight? What are some human interest items about the group or individuals that will personalize the talk without embarrassing anyone?

Find out about the building, the room, audiovisual capabilities, and reprinting of handouts.   Request a letter of confirmation on the time, date, place, topic, expense reimbursement, and fee. People who speak regularly usually ask that a one week (or two) cancellation clause be added. In case you become ill keep names of substitute speakers available. Be sure to state that you will want to have your business cards, brochures, and order blanks for your booklet or whatever available at the speech.

Before accepting a speaking engagement to school groups, find out about the groups and the school policies.   The last ten years willing speakers have reported frustrating experiences while trying to teach children who were not adequately disciplined or prepared to hear the topic. Substitute teachers are not always welcomed unless someone with authority is also present for the talk. Presentations before children are challenging and enlightening. Props, student involvement, and question and answer sessions are always welcomed more than a straight oral presentation.

Be sure to get the name and phone number of the person contacting you and write the date down in your calendar.

Media

Working with the media—radio, television, and newspapers—gives free marketing exposure to practitioners. One can do years of public speaking and not reach a fraction of the number of people who watch one television program or read a newspaper.

Nutrition, fitness, and health are "hot" topics right now and probably will be for several years to come. Experts in these fields who have a flair for this type of work and have something unique to say are sought after.

Media people are looking for stories and information that will interest their public. It can be classified as controversial, human interest, new research, exposés, practical, or a scoop story, but it has to have a "hook" or a "handle"—some unique element to attract the audience. Working with the media is discussed in detail in Chapter 22.

Before approaching the media it is important that you do your homework. Read the newspaper and listen to programming to become aware of what subjects they cover and how. It is usually impressive to a writer or program director when you can speak knowledgeably about what they already offer and how you could augment it. Also, have ideas and suggestions available for articles or program segments.

Many practitioners got their first start with the media during National Nutrition Time. We sometimes forget that there are 11 other months to work with also. We do not have to wait until we are invited to contribute. If you plan to have a successful private practice, it is imperative that people know about you. Through a phone call, introductory letter, over lunch or at an office interview, however possible, try to talk to the local media program directors and newspaper writers. A private practitioner in Chicago reports that she has been quoted or consulted on articles over 50 times in the last year in local newspapers. She sent her card, introduced herself, and offered to act as a resource person. Eventually, she was credited with a by-line or in the article for what she contributed.

Public Service Announcements (PSAs) are welcomed by the media. The PSA can announce a new series of classes, a seminar, or a new associate's arrival. The announcement must be short, concise, and cover a subject or event *that is in the public interest.* It can be printed in a newspaper or read on the air. Obvious commercial promotions for your business or to sell something are not permitted unless you pay for commercial time or space. The lead time for PSAs ranges from three to eight weeks, so call ahead and plan accordingly (see Figure 17.8).

Radio and television stations support PSAs because of the service they provide to the community and because it looks good on their record when they reapply for their broadcast licenses. Newspapers usually feel that PSAs increase readership.

It is becoming more common for commercial food and beverage companies to hire dietitians as media spokespeople to offer PSAs. The dietitians are trained to provide interviews on an educational topic relating to food or nutrition and to interject the information about the company's product.

Publicity

Publicity is free media coverage of some newsworthy story, program, or event. It is easily recognized as the media coverage of a local Health Fair or of the local school children during National Nutrition Month.

Practitioners can call or write the media with their requests for publicity. For planned events, such as the beginning of weight loss classes for teenagers or a sports nutrition conference, the media should be contacted several weeks in

Figure 17.8 Sample Public Service Announcement

Diet Control, Inc.
Janet Jones, R.D.
2020 Main Street, Suite 30
Rockville, MD 20852

For Immediate Release

SPORTS NUTRITION SYMPOSIUM

Athletes, coaches, parents, and the public are invited to the second annual Sports Nutrition Symposium sponsored by Diet Control, Inc., and Health City Recreation. Well-known speakers will cover the topics of the effects of exercise on food and liquid needs, pregame meals, vitamin supplements, and "making weight."

Registration is free. The symposium will be held from 7:00 P.M. to 9:00 P.M. on Tuesday, April 27, 1988, at the Health City Recreation Center, 1104 Cook Street, Rockville, MD 20852.

For more information, call Janet Jones, R.D., at (301) 597-3558.

---

advance. When planning a special event consider including a local celebrity or co-sponsorship with a philanthropic organization to improve the possibility of media coverage and to attract a larger attendance. Publicity comes for no cost, but it may be sporadic or completely upstaged if a bigger news item breaks the same day as your story.

PAID ADVERTISING

It is ethical, professional, and highly recommended that you consider using advertising. The U.S. government encourages professionals to advertise in hopes of producing more competitive services and better values for the public. Professional organizations are recognizing that it is becoming a fact of life for their members and stress that it be done tastefully.

Advertising is used by some practitioners as an ongoing budget item used to attract clients. Others use it only at times for special events, new program announcements, and at the beginning of seasonal peak periods (September and February–March). Whenever it is used there are two guidelines that should always be followed: first, make it clever and distinctive, and second, plan to have a campaign, not just a single ad. Estimates vary that the average person must see or hear an ad between 5 and 11 times before he or she remembers it, so repetition is necessary.

A good rule of thumb to determine how much to spend on advertising is 5 to 10 percent of the gross annual budget. This is after the initial expense of the campaign to first open the doors. Another way would be to divide the cost of the advertising by the cost of the initial consultation fee. Evaluate if the number of new clients needed to break even on the advertising is *reasonable* (you may have to see 25 new patients/clients per week *just to pay for advertising*). There is a point where putting more money into ads will not bring more clients or profit to your office. When you first begin a business, budget an amount that you can afford to spend and look for other previously mentioned ways to market yourself for less cost.

Most private practitioners cannot afford to compete with the mammoth amount of advertising purchased by commercial weight loss programs and other nutrition programs. For that reason where we spend our advertising money and the distinctiveness of our advertising are all the more important. To help determine what works for you, *ask clients and patients how they heard about your business.*

The Yellow Pages and the media all have free sales personnel that can assist clients in determining the best way to use their advertising dollar and help with ad ideas on a limited basis.

If a practitioner wants help on an overall advertising strategy, plus artwork and a slogan, an advertising agency or public relations firm can do it for a price. Obtain estimates before you agree to have work done because good firms are usually expensive.

Fees often range from $1,500 to $15,000 on up (advertising not included) to set up an advertising campaign with a logo and slogan for a small business. Fees are less if you come up with the ideas and do some of the leg work yourself or limit the items they contribute.

Yellow Pages

The Yellow Pages offer a business the opportunity to advertise to everyone who owns a telephone for a year. Most businesses find this type of advertising to be very productive.

Patients and clients know to look under "Dietitians" or "Nutritionists" to find a consulting nutritionist listing. Occasionally, practitioners also list under such titles as "Reducing and Weight Loss," "Physical Fitness," "Catering," or along with a contract clinic or spa. One listing in the Yellow Pages and white pages is offered when you have a business phone. All other listings, display ads, extra lines, or bold print are an extra charge.

It is highly recommended that a Yellow Pages listing include the words "Registered Dietitian." The telephone company does not police their listings so anyone can list themselves under a title we and the public assume to be ours alone. When a private practitioner chooses a business name that does not indicate that the business is run by a trained professional and there are no credentials listed, there is a good chance that business is lost. Examples would be "Big Pines Consultant Services" or "Moore & Associates, Inc."

To help save money but still have a good size ad and several listings, buy only one larger ad and refer the other listings to it, such as "See ad under 'Nutritionists.' " Put the ad under the listing where you think it will be seen best and where clients would look for your name first (see Figure 17.9).

The Yellow Pages closing date for having your ad ordered is usually three to five months before the books are available. Plan ahead and call and ask for

Figure 17.9 Sample Yellow Pages Advertisements

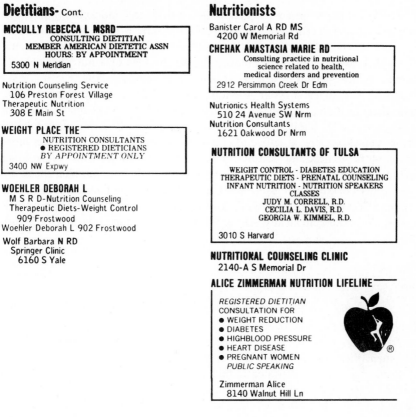

Dietitians- Cont.

MCCULLY REBECCA L MSRD
CONSULTING DIETITIAN
MEMBER AMERICAN DIETETIC ASSN
HOURS: BY APPOINTMENT
5300 N Meridian

Nutrition Counseling Service
106 Preston Forest Village
Therapeutic Nutrition
308 E Main St

WEIGHT PLACE THE
NUTRITION CONSULTANTS
● REGISTERED DIETICIANS
BY APPOINTMENT ONLY
3400 NW Expwy

WOEHLER DEBORAH L
M S R D-Nutrition Counseling
Therapeutic Diets-Weight Control
909 Frostwood
Woehler Deborah L 902 Frostwood

Wolf Barbara N RD
Springer Clinic
6160 S Yale

Nutritionists

Banister Carol A RD MS
4200 W Memorial Rd

CHEHAK ANASTASIA MARIE RD
Consulting practice in nutritional
science related to health,
medical disorders and prevention
2912 Persimmon Creek Dr Edm

Nutrionics Health Systems
510 24 Avenue SW Nrm
Nutrition Consultants
1621 Oakwood Dr Nrm

NUTRITION CONSULTANTS OF TULSA
WEIGHT CONTROL - DIABETES EDUCATION
THERAPEUTIC DIETS - PRENATAL COUNSELING
INFANT NUTRITION - NUTRITION SPEAKERS
CLASSES
JUDY M. CORRELL, R.D.
CECILIA L. DAVIS, R.D.
GEORGIA W. KIMMEL, R.D.

3010 S Harvard

NUTRITIONAL COUNSELING CLINIC
2140-A S Memorial Dr

ALICE ZIMMERMAN NUTRITION LIFELINE
REGISTERED DIETITIAN
CONSULTATION FOR
● WEIGHT REDUCTION
● DIABETES
● HIGHBLOOD PRESSURE
● HEART DISEASE
● PREGNANT WOMEN
PUBLIC SPEAKING

Zimmerman Alice
8140 Walnut Hill Ln

assistance. Evaluate your listings and ad each year and try new ideas that might work better.

Newspapers

Newspaper ads are commonly used by private practitioners with varying degrees of success. The wording and placement of the ad are critical. It must be distinctive enough to catch the reader's eye. The competition to attract attention is very stiff in a newspaper, especially a large daily one. Ads should run on a regular basis in order to be remembered. Scheduling ads regularly also makes the cost of each individual ad more reasonable.

Large daily newspapers have good exposure but are only partly read by most people. Readers go to the sections that interest them most and skim the rest. Fortunately, newspapers know what sections are read most and by whom. Advice columns, horoscopes, cartoons, letters to the editors, sports' scores pages, and, in small towns, the obituaries are usually read closely. Although women's sections are read well, on coupon day that is often not the case, according to a practitioner from Rhode Island who advertised regularly. Request that the ad be placed on a page that is mostly writing so that your ad will stand out and not be lost between the furniture ads.

Small newspapers and weekly papers are usually read more closely and have a loyal but smaller readership. The cost of advertising is more reasonable. The placement guidelines for an ad are the same as mentioned for large newspapers. Also, smaller papers are usually more open to the idea of a nutrition column written by a local person or articles that are contributed locally.

An ad should catch your attention with either a catchy word, phrase, graphic design, photo, or *something.* It should be easy to read and understand, plus be clever. The phone number should stand out. It is not necessary to condense your brochure or calling card into an ad. In fact, you will attract more attention with the headline "Ready for Bikini Season?" than with "Nutritional Consultation by Professional." If you cannot think of an idea you like, check the ads that other businesses are using and see what you like and dislike about them. If you have an idea but need artwork, go to a graphic artist. If you cannot think of a good idea, budget in an advertising firm for the creation of the ad (see Figure 17.10).

Radio

Radio advertising can be geared to a very specific group of the population. Depending upon the type of music played and the time of day, radio stations know from national surveys their listeners' average ages, the percentages of men and women, their approximate income, and educational levels.

Radio ads must be repeated to be remembered. Sales people from stations will offer several "packages" of ad lengths and airing times to make the campaign more reasonable. They often will help with writing the ad and having a station person record it or read it live. Smaller stations have lower advertising fees because fewer people listen to them.

Businesses that can afford regular radio advertising report that it is very successful. Smaller businesses with lower budgets and irregular use of radio advertising report hit or miss success. According to business consultants if you plan to use advertising, you need to commit enough financial support to produce results or you should not do it at all.

TV

A television ad is extremely expensive to produce and to show on the air. Again, it must be repeated to be effective, and target audiences can be determined by the type of programs being shown. Television advertising reaches a large number of viewers, but is so expensive it would be very difficult for a consultant working alone to break even on the number of added customers it would attract. Not enough income is usually generated by one person in one hour to support this expenditure and other overhead too. It may be possible that several consultants working together or working for one person could generate enough added income

Figure 17.10   Sample Newspaper Advertisements
(*Source:* Reprinted by permission of Philomena A. Koulbanis, R.D.)

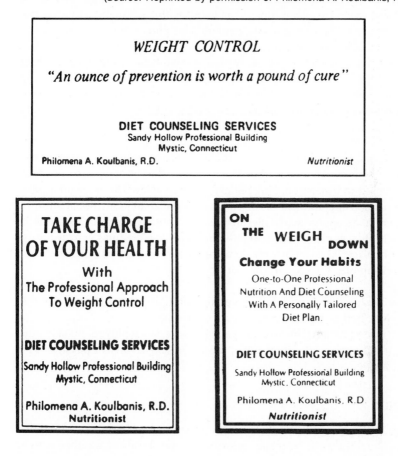

to warrant television advertising, but exhaust all avenues for getting free television exposure first.

KEEPING CUSTOMERS

After you have marketed successfully enough to attract customers, it is important to keep them. Customers are assets for more than just a source of revenue. They are "walking promotion" of your services and an advertising medium of great value. Each person has a sphere of influence that reaches far beyond his immediate family and business peers to a potential of several hundred people.

There are numerous ways to strengthen relationships with clients or referral agents that can be carried out with a minimum amount of effort on your part once the system is established.

Some examples of how private practitioners as well as other professionals have strengthened their relationships with customers include:

For patients Begin having a strong relationship with your patients when the appointment is scheduled and again at the first visit by providing personalized care. Continue with the same quality of care on the follow-up visits so that patients feel your initial concern was genuine. Use phone calls or mail notes to reconfirm appointments. Periodically call patients in between visits to see how they are progressing or when the call would be significant to the patient. Send out announcements when new group classes are forming or to let patients know that you can now do computer analysis of their food intakes. When a new diet program is particularly dangerous and you send a letter to discuss the pros and cons, patients appreciate the communication.

For physicians Follow-up after patient visits can include not only written notes or referral acknowledgment, but also a phone call. Periodic letters or phone calls can be used to discuss ongoing patient progress. Newsletters, regular office visits, or luncheon appointments to discuss new services and nutritional information or research are appreciated. Offering to conduct noon in-service seminars for the office staff has worked well. A thank you card or Christmas card is always welcomed. For special accounts, try delivering gourmet fruit or other food baskets or food samples for special low salt or low fat diets.

For consultant accounts Depending upon the situation, check in monthly with the people higher up and send copies of your reports to them. If appropriate, offer to do inservices, weight loss, or wellness talks to employees outside your regular contract agreement. Use many of the above suggestions for physicians for consultant accounts too.

CONCLUSION

Attracting and keeping clients is necessary to survive in business. Selling and promotion should always be major priorities of any business whether new or established. Private practitioners soon learn to carry a supply of calling cards wherever they go. Stepping forward to shake hands and introduce themselves becomes second nature. Although many things seem awkward at first, after so many hours and days are invested in a project we love, it becomes very easy to talk about it and encourage others to use it.

REFERENCES

1. Mancuso, Joseph: "What Business Are You Really In?" *Success,* New York, September 1985.
2. Levitt, Theodore: "Marketing Intangible Products and Product Intangibles," *Harvard Business Review,* May–June 1981.
3. Rose, James: "The Sales Presentation" in *The Competitive Edge,* The American Dietetic Association, 1986.
4. Helm, Kathy King: "Promotion Strategies" in *The Competitive Edge,* The American Dietetic Association, 1986.

four

DEVELOPING YOUR PROFESSIONAL PRACTICE

chapter *18*

Office Policy and Dealing with Clients

There are many other factors beside the quality and amount of nutrition information given to clients that influence their opinion of your services. Clients are usually expecting their association with you and your office to be courteous, organized, efficient, reasonable in cost, and timely. Actually, our clients' expectations are no different than our own.

SETTING UP A SMOOTH OPERATION

Competition is growing for the public's dollar and a business owner cannot afford to turn clients off with sloppy service. *Personalized* care of clients should begin when they first call to either inquire about your services or make an appointment. Attempts should be made to impress clients with the nondietetic functions of your operation.

Establish office hours and days and try to follow your schedule as closely as possible to help develop an image of stability and continuity.   As long as clients can leave a message for you, it is not necessary to be available in the office, in person, five days a week. In fact, in the beginning condense your patient instructions and interviews with other clients to only a few days per week. The remaining days can then be used to help market your business, to write, and to take time for your personal life.

Telephone coverage for your business is extremely important. The telephone is your clients' major link with you. During normal business hours Monday through Friday, clients should be able to either reach you by phone or leave a message with a secretary, answering service, or recorder machine. If you cannot answer the phone yourself, be sure to take the time to instruct the secretary or answering service in exactly what to say and what information to ask for. Have someone call to check for you occasionally just to see whether your instructions are being followed. Messages on telephone answering recorders should be well prepared—keep trying until you record a message that people will not only listen to but, most importantly, respond to. Also, clients and patients appreciate it when you return their calls promptly.

Some hints that may be important to you concerning your telephone answering service include:

1. Do not allow your services and fees to be given to clients by people who are not trained to properly "market" your business. Have them state instead that they will be very happy to take the clients' name and number and have the nutritionist call them back.
2. Have your service or secretary be cautious with information about your private life, such as your home phone number, address, and when you are out of town.
3. When you are out of town, instruct your answering service to tell people that "She (or he) will be in the office to return your call on Monday, July 10; can she (or he) call you back at that time or is this an emergency?" If it is an emergency, leave the number of another dietitian or the local hospital clinical nutrition department. If it is a personal message, leave a number where *your answering service* can reach you or leave a message.

When scheduling appointments with new patients, use the conversation as an opportunity to "market" your services. Explain what the patient will receive in the way of individualized care and information. Take the time to ask several questions about the patient's nutritional needs, pertinent lab values, and referring physician's name. Request that a copy of the most recent lab results and if applicable the physician's written referral be brought to the appointment. It is suggested that you also state approximately how long the appointment will take and how much it will cost. Make sure that the patient knows the directions to your office, the suite number, where to park, if it is a problem, and the date and time for the appointment. Request that the patient try to give 24 hours' notice if the appointment has to be changed or cancelled.

The office setting should be quiet, comfortable, and professional. The office furnishings are usually not as important as the atmosphere, hospitality, and service provided. However, because of the image they want to portray and their clients' expectations, some private practitioners spend extra for more affluent looking office space and interiors.

The chart system for your office can be as expensive as the color-coded systems, or as simple as a manila folder for each patient, or just the patient interview sheets kept in one notebook. Because of the importance of documentation of a patient's progress, it is best to have the patient's nutrition chart available for all visits. The patient's medical chart is usually only available when you work in a medical office.

The information to include in the patient's chart is name, address, work, and home phone numbers, their physician's name, the referring physician's name (if different), and a copy of the diet prescription, if available, pertinent lab values, a diet evaluation, action plan, and goals. The follow-up sessions should have any changes in lab values and other objective measurements listed, as well as more subjective comments, both pro and con. After the initial instruction and when something significant happens to a patient, the referring physician should be notified, and the contact documented.

Handouts and printed materials can add a lot of distinction and improve your image of success if they are well prepared. As was mentioned earlier, it is probably not necessary to copyright your diets, unless you feel it would keep clinics, physicians, and clients from photocopying them. Any booklets, programs, etc., that you write should definitely be copyrighted.

The cost of handouts and diets is usually incorporated in the fee for the instruction and is not charged separately. Many consultant nutritionists keep a supply of books, booklets, and other educational items they know patients are interested in buying. However, in most states, whenever a sale is made sales tax must be collected, and a sales tax or even vendor's license may be necessary.

An easy way to have diets that all use variations of the exchange lists is to print one style of the lists and change the top cover page. It is suggested that the paper size be a standard $8\frac{1}{2}" \times 11"$ or $8\frac{1}{2}" \times 14"$ to reduce the cost of printing. The typeface should be easy to read, not script; some people with poor eyesight also have trouble reading single-spaced elite type. Printing 100 pages at a time on white paper with black ink usually is the most economical, compared to colored ink and paper and small batches of printing. However, many practitioners feel the flair of color is worth the added cost.

The tendency of many private practitioners when they first start their businesses is to load patients down with every free booklet that even vaguely covers their diet limits. What evolves in time is an awareness that the majority of patients and their families: (1) get confused by material that is not specifically for their diet, and (2) can only absorb a small amount of information on a new subject at any one time, and patients lose sight of the most important points of the diet when so many new points are made in the additional booklets. Save the less specific material and the larger number of booklets, for the few clients who want them and will use them appropriately.

Many practitioners report that their patients were impressed when they started using folders to hold materials. The folder usually has pockets on the inside to hold the diet and any booklets. On the outside of the folder, the company name or logo is printed for easy identification of the contents and for advertising purposes. A calling card is usually attached to the folder to provide the consultant's address and phone number.

Diet manuals are readily available to all practitioners today. In writing your own diets, you may choose good ideas from several manuals and from your past experience. If you are unaware of your local medical community's nutritional biases, try to purchase diet manuals from the local hospitals or make an appointment with a hospital dietitian to discuss them. Pages should not be photocopied directly from a manual unless it was designed for that purpose or you request permission from the copyright owner.

In private practice it is not necessary to have a large variety of different diets, such as in the hospital. Practitioners report the most common diets are weight loss, diabetic, hypoglycemic, low salt, low cholesterol, hyperlipidemia diets, allergy, high potassium, normal pregnancy, and good nutrition for the healthy individual. Specialties in your medical community may dictate that other diets be developed.

DISTINCTIVE SERVICE

Private practitioners feel that their handout materials, consultative sessions, and instructional guides need to be different and better than those provided by free hospital clinics or by physicians' office personnel. Practitioners must create this difference or patients and clients will balk at paying the fee. The key words are "quality," "individualized," and "personalized."

Many practitioners, though not all, think it is important to use different terminology in private practice from that used in acute care settings: "diet" could be "nutritional care plan" or "food plan," and "diet order" could be "nutrition prescription." Some practitioners call the people they instruct "clients" instead of patients, especially in more wellness-oriented settings. Always remember, care should be taken to differentiate patients from their illness. In other words, a person is not a diabetic or a hypertensive, but instead, *a person with diabetes or hypertension.*

COLLECTING FEES AND ENDING A SESSION

The end of the interview is a good time to talk about rescheduling a visit, or to discuss why it is not necessary. This is a good "ending" subject and lets the client know that the visit is over. As you are winding up, be sure to incorporate some system to collect the fee. You may simply state, "I will make out your receipt now—how do you want to pay for your instruction?" or "The fee for the initial visit is $———— and revisits are $————. I will give you an itemized receipt that you can attach to your insurance company's form along with a copy of the referral slip from your doctor. You can try to get reimbursed for our visit." If you have a secretary or receptionist, be sure to train her or him on how to collect fees.

If a patient continues to linger after the closing of the session and you have

Q & A

Patients Aren't Returning

My patients aren't returning after the first visit. What might be wrong? What can I do?

There are numerous reasons why patients don't return. Some reasons are in your control; others are not. The reason physicians overbook and some dentists and psychiatrists charge for no-shows is because a certain number of patients will not keep appointments. That point known, there are still professionals who do not have as bad a problem as others, and there are times when each of us experiences it more frequently.

After allowances are made for weather (snow, ice, etc.) when driving is hazardous, business advisors will tell you that it is significant whether patients don't show at all or they call to reschedule. Not calling or showing is of course more symptomatic of a problem.

Some of the more obvious reasons patients do not return are:

- They feel no commitment to the care plan because they were not involved in developing it, or it did not fit their true lifestyle. It was not their choice to make the appointment and they only gave lip service while there.

- The patients did not understand the importance of follow-up and how it would improve their chances for successful behavior change.

- They followed the suggested guidelines and did not get results —or they got results without following it.

- They were not impressed with either you or the consultation, or something about the office visit. (Some patients will not take advice from traditional-thinking or young and/or inexperienced counselors.)

- The fee was too high for what they felt they received or for their present income.

- The consultation style and approach may have been too threatening, embarrassing, or too familiar to suit the patient. (We do not always hit it off with every patient.)

- The instruction materials may have been too confusing.

- The patient may believe his present habits fit his needs better, and he is not willing to change. Maybe the suggestions weren't reasonable—or maybe they were but not at this time.

Areas you may want to evaluate and improve if you deem them a problem are:

- Are you marketing and describing your services well over the phone when the patient calls for an appointment? Fees should be mentioned up front along with what you have to offer and what commitment is expected from the patient. The patient should feel he knew what to expect.

- Are you impressing upon your patients the importance of follow-up visits?

- Is the patient's visit a pleasant one? Is he greeted and given good, timely service?

- Are you up to date and knowledgeable in nutrition and counseling? Can you offer a variety of solutions and are you flexible enough to make changes when they are needed? Are your counseling sessions organized and professionally handled?

- Do you have the appearance of a credible, competent, stable professional? Can you change your appearance to look more like what is "expected" by your clientele?

- Are your fees too high or low for what you offer or for your local community? Could you offer more, package it better, or offer a sliding scale? Should you change your fees?

One of the best ways to take the mystery out of this process is by calling all patients a day ahead to remind them of the appointment and to ask how they are doing. Some practitioners will call patients a day or two after their first appointment to show concern, answer questions, and make adjustments in the care plan. Calling a patient can serve several purposes: the patient may feel more at ease about stating a problem, he may decide to make a greater commitment because of your apparent interest, or he may cancel future appointments on the spot.

other commitments, you can try standing up and walking slowly toward the door to show him out and simply state, "I want to thank you very much for coming. I am sorry to rush, but I have another patient waiting."

EMPLOYEE CONSIDERATIONS

If you decide to budget an office employee into your business, there are several considerations to think about:

1. How will the secretary/receptionist spend her or his day—write a job description.
2. In the beginning can he or she work mornings or a short week to help keep overhead lower.
3. Determine how much you can afford to pay—remember that it may be worth paying a little more to keep someone who speaks well on the phone and is courteous and efficient in the office.
4. Determine what skills are most important for the running of your office before you start to interview applicants.
5. Talk to your financial advisor about what "perks" if any to offer as present or future incentives to your employee.
6. Discuss with your CPA the difference in costs to you for an employee versus contract labor, such as, payroll taxes, social security, workman's compensation, added paperwork, pension plan, etc.

To assure that the person represents you well, take adequate time of your own to train your new secretary well. You should decide whether to teach him or her how to market your business on the phone or just to take messages. Some practitioners have had a problem with their enthusiastic secretaries trying to do diet counseling over the phone, using their own remedies. To help avoid this problem, office policies need to be determined and procedures established to carry them out. A poor employee can harm your business, so do not hesitate to terminate someone who does not work out. (See Dietetic Technician, page 198.)

Although there is added expense in having an employee, a person who can perform such duties as typing, mailing, screening phone calls, confirming patient appointments, scheduling new patients and revisits, collecting fees, and greeting clients can be as valuable as your right arm. It may take time to find the right person, but it is worth it, if in the long run you generate more income and a better-functioning business.

CONCLUSION

Other than having a good background in nutrition, it is just as important that a private practitioner have good management and business skills in order to succeed. A practitioner should strive to produce distinctive service and provide up-to-date information with a flair.

chapter *19*

Counseling Expertise
Paulette Lambert, R.D.

The role of the nutrition counselor has changed. No longer can we provide lists of foods to avoid along with a sample menu and feel that we have functioned as a professional counselor. A receptionist with no training can do as much; we have to do a lot more.

Our success as consulting nutritionists depends on our ability to help clients learn and apply new information and skills. What transpires in what we call the "counseling session" determines our success. Dietitians entering private practice as counselors need to realize that their level of counseling expertise determines the quality of their output. When consulting nutritionists have problems getting their businesses established it may be for several reasons. One reason may be their lack of counseling skills.

Developing high quality counseling skills is a time-consuming, complex task. It often means changing old well-established but unsuccessful counseling habits or beginning with no applied experience. Not everyone has the personality and patience to be good at counseling. Do not expect yourself to achieve perfect skills within a few weeks or months. It takes time to practice the new techniques learned through course work, seminars, and self-study. There will always be room for improvement and a need for continual change.

This chapter intends to share some of the newest techniques and resources for producing successful counseling sessions. Successful practitioners each have their own style of patient counseling. The amount of information, number of sessions, commitment to wellness, behavior modification, or psychology is a counselor's decision and varies with each patient.

QUALIFICATIONS OF A CONSULTING NUTRITIONIST

Nutrition consultation, as a specialized skill, requires a rich background of experience in the profession. Skills are needed in more than one area. And must be studied and practiced. These include academic, clinical, administrative, behavioral therapy, psychology, and interpersonal communication skills.

Clinical judgment is imperative to good nutrition counseling. The American Diabetic Association's position paper on consultation emphasizes a minimum of three years experience in clinical, administration, and education. Without this practical experience, a clinical nutritionist has not been able to practice long enough to be proficient at counseling or to have developed sound clinical judgment. A consultant must be aware of common drugs and their side effects, know how to perform simple assessment tests, and be aware of the laboratory chemical values as they relate to nutrition.

Relationship-building skills are necessary for effective counseling. In the dynamics of counseling, before counselors can develop plans for a client's behavior change, the counselor needs to understand the client's needs. (1) The development of a "helping relationship" that projects empathy, understanding, and trust needs to precede any development of plans and strategies.

The nutrition counselor understands the client's concerns because he or she encourages them to talk about themselves and their feelings. A client needs to feel safe in reporting failures in order to adjust the care plan to make it more successful.

Being a good nutrition counselor involves possessing interpersonal skills that promote positive outcomes in counseling. A successful counselor is one who genuinely cares about and is committed to her or his patient. Three attributes are desirable: warmth, genuineness, and empathy.

A word of caution must be mentioned here; although a counselor wants to be warm, caring, empathetic, and so on it is important that the counselor remain professional. There is a point in counseling where becoming very close and familiar with patients may jeopardize your ability to act as a counselor to them. Occasionally, having a patient as a friend is certainly no problem, but if you notice it happening with a large number of clients *with a resulting decline in counseling effect,* reassess your needs as a counselor. Several solutions may keep your private and professional lives more separate; spend more time making or seeing friends in your personal time, or seek help—read about handling this counseling problem or talk to a counselor yourself.

Several other traits are helpful in being successful in nutrition counseling. A positive attitude keeps the client and you interested in continuing to work together. Changing eating behavior is difficult, with many barriers to overcome. One needs to be positive and even tempered to deal with the phenomenon on a day-to-day basis. Being assertive in a caring way and not being afraid of dealing with issues that inhibit progress is important. Nutrition counseling is not passive but a very active procedure and is doomed if otherwise.

Behavioral therapy skills are important to counselors.   Along with the ability to dispense information, a practitioner needs to be able to promote behavior changes in clients. Nutrition counselors need to be proficient in skills in behavioral therapy. As Ohlsen has commented, "true dietetic counseling must involve discrete counseling skills, not merely dissemination of information" (1). The focus of behavioral therapy is to do something to actually promote a change in behavior. Behavioral therapy skills include being able to define a problem, design plans and strategies to treat a problem, and to evaluate and make necessary changes. Behavioral therapy uses various techniques such as behavior modification, stimulus control, and cognitive restructuring to assist in helping the client change his behavior.

An understanding of psychology is important to a counselor.   By understanding peoples' motivations for different behaviors, a good counselor can then offer alternative suggestions for satisfying needs in non-self-defeating and food oriented ways. An appreciation for psychology also helps in perspective—in other words, the counselor becomes part of the solution, not part of the problem. As an example, if the counselor fails to comprehend a patient's frustration with weight loss and lectures him or her, any possibility of helping the client may be lost.

Teaching skills help ensure that the patient learns the new information.   The content must be geared to the patient's level of understanding. A patient is often "turned off" by language and nutrition information that is either over his head, or too elementary and thus unchallenging and uninteresting. Presentations should be organized, since random discussions are hard to recall. A good teacher knows how to help patients reach their goals by using a variety of teaching methods. As a patient's needs change a good teacher should be flexible enough to adjust the patient's care plan to handle new problems.

The ability to sell is a vital skill often overlooked.   Selling is based on meeting the client's needs. Selling means convincing someone of the importance of something to them. For example, a client may not realize why the physician wants him to lose weight in relationship to decreasing his blood sugar. The counselor needs to convey benefits to the client.

In her book, *The Woman's Selling Game,* Carole Hyatt defines selling as skillfully negotiating, persuading, influencing, and enlightening people to change behavior (2). In nutrition counseling you sell the client, his family, the physicians, and all others involved in counseling. You sell the program and the changes the client needs to make in order to be successful. If you look at the many fad diets that materialize each year, you soon realize the power of the ability to sell.

THE ROLE OF THE NUTRITION COUNSELOR

Traditionally, the role of the dietitian was to be an educator, a teacher. With the role expanded to nutrition counselor, we now need to see ourselves in a more complex role: that of a trainer. The trainer role includes both consideration of the client's needs and the application of training technology. Together they produce a change in behavior.

The nutrition counselor is more effective today than in the traditional role. Training involves active, not passive learning. The client actually does something. Traditionally, we used to give out information and hope the client would change his eating habits. Now, the trainer provides information, has patient interaction, patient practice, and the client responds. Emphasis is on the benefit to the client. The trainer's role is to guide, not dictate the consultation. Training is a balance between client- and content-focused instruction. The following example (See Table 19.1) compares traditional, content-focused teaching to trainer, client-focused instruction (3).

When counseling is totally dominated by client requests and tangential topics, little behavior change will take place. A session totally dominated by counselors who provide only information, without listening to client concerns, can be equally unproductive. The ideal is a mix of client and counselor interaction (4). A very good book on the subject of counseling is Linda Snetselaar's *Nutrition Counseling Skills;* please refer to this resource for more in-depth discussion.

Client expectations of what the counselor will be like can greatly influence how receptive he or she is to counseling. If a client expects the counselor to be domineering and antagonistic or friendly and helpful, the client may react to the counselor as if he were actually playing that role (4). Through experience counselors learn to perceive what the client is expecting from them. Qualified counselors then try to correct or validate clients' preconceived beliefs.

Table 19.1 **TRAINER VS. TRADITIONAL INSTRUCTION***

Trainer (client-focused)	Traditional (content-focused)
1. Information given determined by assessment of individual needs.	1. Information given is determined by availability.
2. Practice is provided—active learning.	2. Information is given—passive learning.
3. Only needed information is given.	3. An abundance of information is given.
4. Success is determined by the ability of the client to function independently.	4. Success is determined by how much and how well content was delivered.
5. Instruction is based on premise that virtually all people learn what they need to learn, allowing for adequate time.	5. Instruction is based on the assumption information was delivered, and only some clients will be able to learn material.
6. Learners' mastery is practiced and then observed.	6. Learners' mastery is assumed.
7. Instruction is paced according to the individual accomplishments.	7. Instruction paced according to subject matter.

*An instruction is never totally client- or content-focused but a balance between the two.
Source: R. Shortridge: *The Percepteur,* A manual of training behavior for professionals, Dairy Council of California, 1980.

Clients also come to nutrition counseling sessions with feelings about themselves that may act as barriers to behavior change. A young obese woman may say that she wants to lose weight, but may be so fearful of the attention she may receive from men when her weight goes down, she puts up barriers (regains lost pounds) to keep her "safe." A man with hypertension may come for instruction because he knows he should be careful with his food intake. However, he may choose not to be responsible because of his relationship with his wife. For example, he may want her to feel responsible. A counselor learns to perceive a client's needs so that those needs can be either satisfied or altered. The client is then motivated to change and take *responsibility* for his own *constructive* behavior.

Counseling Theories

Counseling theories and personal philosophies influence the way in which a counselor conducts a session. Snetselaar lists four theories commonly used in nutrition counseling (4):

1. *Client-centered therapy* assesses clients' needs and perceptions and changes behavior through promoting more positive, confident, and realistic attitudes about self. Realistic, attainable goals are set to build clients' self confidence.
2. *Rational emotive therapy* encourages clients to confront and alter their inner self-talk and self-thoughts to ones that promote positive behavior. Clients learn not to punish or belittle themselves for less than ideal behavior.
3. *Behavioral therapy* believes that clients' environments shape their behavior; therefore changing experiences and role models should alter the clients' behavior.
4. *Gestalt therapy* emphasizes confronting the barriers to behavior change so that clients can regulate their actions with present needs. Clients identify and confront the "deeper" reasons why they believe and act as they do.

In practice Snetselaar feels that most counselors use a combination of theories and determine what to use according to the clients' needs or their own biases.

In addition to these theories counselors are very concerned about being able to "read" clients and "speak their language" in order to establish or enhance communication. Study of body language and nonverbal communication is imperative to achieving good counseling skills.

Some counselors use the techniques outlined in *Frogs into Princes,* called Neurolinguistic Programming (NLP) to better interpret how a client communicates (5). Some individuals speak in terms of wanting personal attention or wanting to "feel" better; others want to "look" differently or want written directions; and still others want "verbal" input and feedback. Telling a "visual" person who wants to look thin that he will "feel" so good when his weight is down may not interest him nearly as much as working with him on imaging.

Wellness Approach

A counselor may also choose to incorporate emphasis on the "wellness" approach in nutrition consultations. This approach believes that nutrition information should not be separate from other life-style decisions. Counseling sessions could include evaluation and discussion of the client's fitness and exercise program or referral to a fitness specialist.

The counselor may identify a client's inability to handle stress or a dependence on alcohol, drugs, or smoking and encourage the client to consider a change in behavior and referral to a program or specialist who could help him or her. To be qualified to discuss these other topics a nutrition counselor must be familiar with health risk factors and their effect on health. A counselor should also take course work and seminars on wellness, health education, and exercise physiology.

VARIOUS APPROACHES ALL "SELL"

Experienced nutrition counselors bring a wealth of practical knowledge when they begin their own businesses. Counseling sessions are usually a mixture of what has worked in the past along with a few ideas that the counselor has always wanted to try. Here are examples of different approaches:

- Many practitioners do not feel that a dietary program should be given at the first counseling session. They feel that the initial session should be used to collect data, teach patients how to measure foods for computer analysis, make assessments, and determine habits and needs. A later session is used for more formal instruction. One practitioner's program consists initially of three, one-hour sessions over several weeks, followed by short sessions scheduled as needed. Another practitioner sees a patient initially for 30 minutes to instruct him or her on filling out the computer food intake record then begins counseling at the next session.
- Some practitioners set limits on the total number of sessions a program includes. A weight loss program may be eight weeks of individual or group sessions. All clients may be limited to a designated number of sessions so that patients know they must be independent and self-reliant soon.
- Other practitioners provide written nutrition instructions at the first visit of approximately one hour and schedule follow-up visits every one to two weeks and set no limitations on the duration of therapy.
- Practitioners may incorporate a variety of activities in their programs: computer nutrient analysis, menu planning, grocery shopping, skinfold analysis or impedance body analysis, individualized fitness program and workout, and long-term follow-up. Sometimes the nutrition consultant handles all of these functions and other times he is in association with a fitness specialist.
- Practitioners sometimes choose to send their patients questionnaire/interview sheets in advance or ask that they arrive a little early so that session time is not spent filling them out. Others want to fill out the questionnaire with the patient in order to better interpret insinuations and body language (see Figures 19.1 and 19.2).

Figure 19.1 Sample Nutrition and Medical Evaluation Form

Name _____ Date _____

Address _____ Phone _____

Physician _____ Diet _____

Age _____ Sex _____ Marital status _____

Height _____ Weight _____ Percent body fat_____

Desired weight _____ Recent change in weight?_____

Occupation_____Hours work/day _____

EXERCISE

At work_____ During leisure_____
Discussion:

MEDICAL DATA

Personal history: (List any medical problems, past or present.)

Family: (List major medical problems of family members.)

Medication: (List any medications taken recently, include vitamins, antacids, aspirin, birth control pills, etc.)

BIOCHEMICAL DATA

Hct_____ Hb_____ Albumin, serum_____

Fasting blood sugar_____mg% GTT_____

Chol._____ Triglycerides_____HDL_____LDL_____

Other:

Figure 19.1 *(Continued)*

NUTRITION HABITS

1. Are you on a special diet?_____ If so, which one?_____

2. Is your appetite good_____ fair_____ poor_____ ?

3. Who prepares your meals?_____

4. Whom do you eat your meals with?_____

5. How many times per week do you eat out?_____

6. Where do you eat out?_____

7. How many alcohol drinks per week?_____ Kinds?_____

THE SESSIONS

Before beginning with a new patient, a counselor should prepare for the role of diagnostician by reviewing all available data on the patient (4). If the patient's chart is accessible, it should be reviewed. However, in private practice it is usually necessary to start your own chart and put the chemical scores, intake analysis, anthropometric results, interview sheet, progress notes, etc., in as you have them (see Figure 19.3, p. 245).

The Introduction

The patients' first exposure to you and your office begins to form their opinion of your ability to help them. Trust and respect for the counselor are important motivators to patients.

Small, fairly simple actions on your part can help engender good feelings in your patients. Try to start counseling sessions on time. Be sure to introduce yourself and be friendly. It sounds so elementary, but many counselors and medical professionals are so consumed with their counseling or the patients' diseases that they forget that it's the *person* they are working with (4).

The Interview

The session begins with an explanation of the counseling relationship describing enough so that the client knows precisely what will take place (4). If the client has other expectations, this is the time to have them known.

During the assessment phase, the counselor acts as a diagnostician and evaluates the client's nutrition status and relates food intake data to behavioral indicators (4). Assessments can be made of many categories of information (also see Figure 19.4, p. 246) (7):

- Biochemical studies
- Anthropometric studies   *(List continues on p. 245.)*

Figure 19.2 Sample Food Intake Form

PRESENT FOOD INTAKE

Morning Time:	Noon Time:	Night Time:	Between Meals Time:

DIET PRESCRIPTION

	Amount	Carbohydrate	Protein	Fat	Calories
Milk					
Meat					
Eggs					
Bread					
Fruit					
Fat					
"A" Veg.					
"B" Veg.					
Total					

DISTRIBUTION OF EXCHANGES

	Breakfast	Lunch	Dinner	Snack

Comments:

Figure 19.3   Model for Nutrition Counseling

(*Source:* Linda Snetselaar, *Nutrition Counseling Skills.* Reprinted with permission of Aspen Publishers, Inc. Copyright © 1983.)

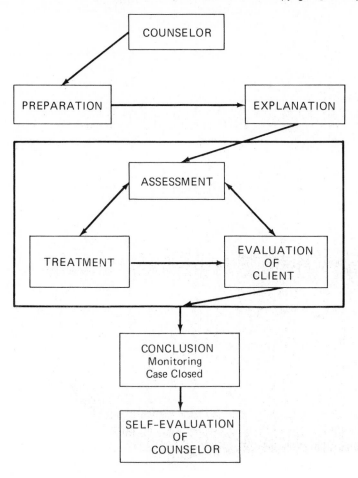

- Vital and health statistics
- Food consumption patterns
- Socioeconomic data
- Additional medical information

A client's behavior must also be assessed (4, 8):

- General health practices
- Health, attitudes, beliefs, and information
- Physical activities
- Educational achievements and language skills
- Economic considerations
- Environmental considerations
- Social considerations

Figure 19.4 Possible Factors to Include in an Assessment
(*Source:* Reprinted by permission of The American Dietetic Association.)

Anthropometrics	Laboratory (can include)	Diet and Nutrition
1. Height in cm	13. Serum albumin in gm/100 mL	22. Protein intake in gm
2. Weight in kg	14. Total iron-binding capacity (TIBC) in μg/100 mL	23. Caloric intake in kcal
3. Usual weight in kg		24. Nitrogen balance in gm
4. Sex (male/female)	15. Serum transferrin in mg/100 mL [Trans = (0.8 × TIBC) − 43]	25. Obligatory nitrogen loss in gm
5. Ideal body weight (IBW) in kg		26. Net protein utilization
6. Weight as percent of IBW	16. Lymphocytes as percent	27. Basal energy expenditure (BEE) in kcal/day
7. Weight as percent of usual weight	17. White blood cell count in no./mm³	28. Caloric intake as percent of BEE
8. Triceps skinfold in mm	18. Total lymphocyte count	29. Skin test results in mm
9. Arm circumference in cm	19. 24-hour urine urea nitrogen in gm	
10. Arm muscle circumference in cm	20. 24-hour urinary creatinine in mg	
11. Triceps skinfold as percent of standard	21. Creatinine height index as percent of standard	
12. Arm muscle circumference as percent of standard		

Motivation must also be assessed since it is essential for compliance. Motivation is the desire to change (behavior, in this case) in return for perceiving a positive gain. In order to counsel effectively, we must pay attention to the content of the instruction as well as how well we motivate our clients. Clients are motivated by their own needs more than by the counselors' desires (3). Therefore, in order to motivate clients, we need to perceive their needs appropriately and the clients need to perceive the changed behavior as important to them. Clients also become motivated when they see results. To that end it is important for the counselor to identify and set intermediate, more easily reached goals with the client.

Nutritional care or treatment plan can be developed once assessments are made and problems are identified. In the treatment phase the counselor assumes the role of both expert and mutual problem solver (4). Most novices at counseling tend to follow one extreme or the other—expert or empathizer. Patients may be overwhelmed by the counselor who knows everything and makes all of the decisions. On the other hand, as mentioned earlier, counselors may become ineffective if they become too friendly or liberal with clients and their diet limitations. A good balance of the two roles is optimal.

In the treatment phase problems, behaviors, inconsistencies, and wrong beliefs are matched with possible solutions or alternatives. Desired changes or goals are prioritized and a program for step-by-step counseling is developed by the practitioner. For many reasons if the counselor determines it's necessary a patient may be referred to another health professional.

When assuming the training role, the nutrition counselor works hard to interpret the identified problems to the patient. In an orderly fashion, solutions are offered that would be acceptable to the patient—considering all that is known about him now. The patient has ample opportunity to react and provide input of his own.

Good counselors attempt to keep instructions as simple as possible. People remember more of the information they hear in the beginning of the instruction so top priority items are discussed first.

Behavior or belief changes are discussed with the patient (and his family) in a manner that will produce positive results for that individual. For some patients it may mean confrontation in order to fully explore underlying reasons for present actions or beliefs (8). Other patients respond well to logical explanations of cause and effect; as long as they agree with the logic they will try to make changes. Patients may sometimes need to be led initially when they don't trust or believe anything. In this instance the counselor says, "Let me show you how it will work for you, if you take responsibility for yourself and follow the steps I suggest to you." Most patients who come to see private practitioners have already decided to give the counselor "a chance" to help. The important determinants are whether the patient and his family understand and respect what the counselor says, and whether the changes are reasonable given the patient and his lifestyle.

Factors associated with compliance

- Belief that following a diet is necessary for good health
- Supportive family members
- High level of concern over consequences of noncompliance
- Eagerness to reject the sick role
- Feeling comfortable about ability to cope with the diet

Factors associated with noncompliance

- Living alone
- Lack of symptoms that belies need for diet regime
- Failure of consultant to communicate purpose of diet treatment adequately
- Multiple restrictions that require changing one's lifestyle
- Poverty or unemployment

When teaching nutrition information, a counselor produces his best results when he uses a variety of tools and methods (9):

We remember 10 percent of what we read, 20 percent of what we hear, 30 percent of what we see, 50 percent of what we see and hear, and 80 percent of what we ourselves say. To increase compliance combine visual aids, verbal instructions, written instructions, and learner feedback.

Counselors determine on a patient-by-patient basis whether to use an exchange list, a point system, or another method. To improve adherence and understanding it is important that the patient receive only the instruction materials and handouts that apply to his lifestyle changes or eating pattern—not every free booklet on low fat foods or diabetes. If the patient or his family expresses an interest for more recipes, etc., at follow-up visits, additional materials can be offered.

To conclude a session it is suggested that counselors summarize the agreed upon goals for the next visit and reiterate the most important points they want patients to remember about the session. Except in very rare cases patients need follow-up visits in order to make permanent changes in their behavior. They also like to be told that they may call with questions or concerns at any time.

Evaluation/Follow-Up

After clients have been counseled, they are ready to apply and practice the suggestions at home and work. Practice gives the patient the opportunity to actually try new ideas and behaviors. Patients may be asked to prepare a week's menu or list the lower sodium entrees on a favorite restaurant's menu. The counselor uses the follow-up sessions as a time to reinforce the positive behaviors and provide immediate feedback on any completed projects, behavior records (see Figure 19.5), or questions. In evaluating clients, counselors once again become diagnosticians (4). If no solution to the problem has been reached, counseling reverts to the assessment or treatment phase. In some cases the clinicians may decide to refer the client to a more experienced practitioner or other health professional (4).

Ending Care

In concluding counseling care, a practitioner and client should come to mutual agreement that the client is ready and/or that any benefits from counseling have been derived. Monitoring the patient with appointments (or phone calls) every three to six months helps identify and solve problems that tend to appear when living in the real world. Again, counselors usually offer to be available by phone or appointment if a problem arises.

Self-evaluation

Since a practitioner's success as a counselor depends to a large extent on the patients' abilities to make lifestyle or belief changes, a counselor needs to evaluate his patients' performances. It is the patients' responsibility, not the counselors to make changes in their lives. The counselor's responsibilities are to make the

Figure 19.5 Sample Meal Record

MEAL RECORD

Name _____ Day of the week _____

Time	Meal	Hunger 0–5	Food Eaten and Amount	Place	With Whom?	Sitting or Standing?	Related Activity	How Did You Feel?

patient aware of the foods and lifestyle habits necessary for good health, to help the patient identify and alter barriers, and to motivate the patient to want to make changes. A counselor can build on past experience to improve present skills.

Documentation

Records should be kept on each patient and his progress. The information is not only important and useful to the consultant, but it may prove essential in case of a malpractice suit. In courts of law the statement is often made that if the service wasn't documented it didn't happen—where is the proof?

Whether a practitioner uses the SOAP method of recording or just states the pertinent facts is not important. The most important point is for objective changes such as improved chemical scores or anthropometric values to be documented along with behavior and belief changes.

CONCLUSION

Creating realistic expectations of what your clients can do and guiding them through the changes are of the utmost importance. Change is difficult to achieve and cannot be done in a short time. The belief, held by many health professionals and clients, that lasting changes in food behavior require only a few interviews is an illusion. Change has a complex nature. Nutrition counselors and clients should not feel as if they failed when a perfect, smoothly functioning set of skills are not achieved in a few weeks. Lasting change, the goal of nutrition counseling, is most likely to occur when the nutrition counselor can teach the client the general steps for learning and problem solving.

Professional commitment, along with hard work, will assist you in refining and improving your counseling skills. The experience should reward you as your professional effectiveness improves.

REFERENCES

1. Snetselaar, L., H. Schatt, L. Iasiello-Vailor, and K. Smith: "Model Workshop on Nutrition Counseling for Dietitians," *JADA*, 1981, 79:678.
2. Hyatt, C.: *The Women's Selling Game*, Warner Books, 1979.
3. Shortridge, R.: *The Percepteur*, A Manual Of Training Behavior for Professionals, Dairy Council of California, 1980.
4. Snetselaar, Linda: *Nutrition Counseling Skills*, Aspen Publishers, Maryland, 1983.
5. Bandler, R., and J. Grinder: *Frogs Into Princes*, Real People Press, Moab, Utah, 1979.
6. Danish, S., M. Ginsberg, A. Terrell, M. Hammond and S. Adams: "The Anatomy Of A Dietetic Counseling Interview," *JADA*, 1979, 75:626.
7. Mason, M., B. Wenberg, and P. Welch: *The Dynamics of Clinical Dietetics*, John Wiley and Sons, New York, 1977.
8. Egen, H., L. Iasiello-Vailor, and K. Smith: "Confrontations: A New Dimension in Nutrition Counseling," *JADA*, 1983, 83:34.
9. "Compliance Dilemmas: The Renal Diet From Patient and Dietitian Perspectives" presented by James D. Campbell and Anne R. Campbell at ADA Annual Meeting, San Antonio, TX, 1982.

chapter *20*

The Wellness Movement

Desiring "wellness" and other self-help information is a megatrend of the American people for the 1980s. People are excited about taking more responsibility for their own health and lives. Health professionals are being seen not only as providers of care but, increasingly, as providers of information. The media regularly offers proof that substantiates that a person's cardiovascular fitness, stress management, and quality of life can be improved through lifestyle changes made by the individual.

WHAT IS WELLNESS?

The term "wellness," although we consider it new and futuristic, is what many people have been saying for ages should be health care's major concern—prevention or keeping well people (the majority of us) well. Wellness involves striving for a state of health that is not just absent from disease, but, rather, optimum. It reinforces that being healthy permits us to enjoy life and shape our own future.

Most wellness leaders assert that wellness is a multidisciplinary approach to health. It is not just exercise or nutrition or stopping smoking or handling stress or making choices better—it is all of these and more. What wellness programs offer depends upon variables such as client needs, available financial support, and the leadership of the program. Typically, wellness programs in the United States include encouraging physical fitness, good nutrition, and healthy lifestyle

Adapted from Chapter 40, "Wellness," by Kathy King Helm, R.D., in *Handbook for Health Care Food Service Management,* James C. Rose, editor, Aspen Publications, Maryland, 1984. Reprinted with permission of Aspen Publishers, Inc. Copyright © 1984.

changes. However, it is not uncommon for only one of these areas to be stressed more heavily, often to the exclusion of the other two.

Advocates of the wellness movement are quick to make the distinction between *wellness* and *holistic* since the latter's reputation is somewhat tarnished by so many questionable "treatments" that have used holistic as a banner. Charles Sterling, Ed.D., Executive Director of Cooper's Institute for Aerobics Research in Dallas, Texas states, *"Holistic* is associated with treatments of all sorts used to attain good health. Wellness is a lifestyle approach to realizing your best potential for physical health, mental alertness and serenity. It is not about extending your life or curing disease" (1).

In his book, *High Level Wellness,* Dr. Don Ardell explains that traditional medicine usually stops treatment when a patient's disability or symptoms no longer exist. But wellness starts taking place when patients become educated about their bodies and good health, when they practice new health habits and take responsibility for their own bodies by keeping them healthy. Dr. Ardell also asserts that besides nutritional awareness, stress management, and physical fitness, wellness includes environmental sensitivity and self-responsibility (2).

The Wellness Mind Set

For traditionally trained health professionals, the wellness concept may require a new mind set about their role as health providers. No longer does the medical professional do all of the work and make all of the decisions for a passive patient. Patients are taught that the responsibility for their well-being is theirs. The health provider becomes teacher, friend, and information specialist, as well as provider.

Wellness doesn't involve quick, curative measures, such as drugs and surgery; instead one works with something much more challenging—the human mind. The medical specialist works with changing habits, giving guidance to people who may feel well, are energetic, and are excited about life. Many health professionals have problems understanding how they are supposed to help this individual since there isn't anything to cure. Many of us have become so dependent upon motivating patients with fear of illness that we are at a loss when trying to motivate someone who isn't sick. The answer lies in the fact that there is a growing public awareness that good health should not be taken for granted. Therefore, when an individual either becomes aware of his own health habits or takes a fitness test, diet, or stress evaluation or health habit appraisal, she or he is often highly motivated by the promise of *continued* good health.

The biggest challenges that nutritionists have with wellness is learning about the normal individual and then making normal nutrition *exciting* to the listener or reader. Good marketing is a must. Merely having fantastic handout information will not have people flocking to the door. The presentations must be interesting, stimulating, creative, timely, and packaged well. And, for the first time in our nutritional careers, our effectiveness may depend 80–90 percent upon our personal skills instead of our knowledge. Successful program directors are aware of that fact and are looking for nutritionists with unique skills in effective leadership, marketing, and public relations.

WHY WELLNESS NOW?

The wellness concept is growing and coming into its own now because of problems in our present medical system and because statistics are finally being generated by reputable sources that show positive results.

The way medicine has been practiced: acute care with passive patients and with little-to-no cost containment has reached its limits in public acceptance. The public is being repeatedly made aware of the fact that some 80 percent of all symptoms will go away given rest and good food. When sick, people want to know if they are in that 80 percent and can go home to wait it out. Many physicians believe that iatrogenic medical care and misdiagnosis may cause far more discomfort to a patient than the flu or infection that precipitated the medical visit. If they are truly ill, most patients want good, prudent state of the art medical care from caring health professionals who involve the patients in the decision making. After the symptoms disappear, patients want to know what they can do to keep the symptoms or illness from reoccurring. Patients and families are usually highly motivated at this time. Family members have become more aware of the relationship of heredity to their own health and are willing to adjust their life habits to help avoid problems later.

According to popular news reports health care costs in some areas of the country have risen between 400 percent and 600 percent since 1965. The cost of health care insurance for employees has become a major concern of employers. The average annual expenditure in 1965 for health insurance was $625 per employee. However, today that average is $1,000–$1,500 per employee. Ford Motor Company calculated in 1977 that it spent $2,100 per employee (3). General Motors reports that it spends more on health care for its employees than on steel for its cars (4). Inflation on cost of goods has been fueled by spiraling insurance benefit costs for employees. Historically, there have been few questions about the necessity of medical care procedures and tests and the overgrowth of hospitals, their equipment, and the length of patient stays. No one, including patients, insurance companies, or businesses, checked the bottom line on cost. As expenses went up, patients still expected care, insurance companies had to raise premiums, and businesses paid them and passed the cost on to the consumer. Now, the entire system is questioning value and necessity for dollars spent.

MEASUREABLE RESULTS

Trying to measure the results of a wellness program has proved difficult. Some changes such as attitude improvement and better quality of life are so subjective that they are not easily quantified. The indices that are used are aerobic fitness, absenteeism, medical claim costs, sick days, accidents on the job, and productivity. However, these indices also involve many variables other than a wellness program.

Companies with employee wellness programs are becoming more plentiful every day. On-going programs are starting to report their preliminary results: Kimberly-Clark reports a 70 percent reduction in accidents (5): Blue Cross of

Western Pennsylvania reports that for 136 persons who used insured outpatient psychiatric benefits, their medical claims dropped from $116.47 to $7.06 per month; New York Telephone showed a one-year medical cost savings of $1½ million; a Goodyear plant in Sweden reports that after offering an employee fitness program, absenteeism by participants fell by 50 percent; and, General Motors Alcoholism program reports a 49 percent reduction in lost work hours and 29 percent reduction in disability costs (5). The results are encouraging and indicate that altering one's lifestyle may produce measurable, as well as very personal, health improvements.

CORPORATE WELLNESS PROGRAMS

Businesses are understandably interested in the boost in productivity, output, and morale that good lifestyle changes can produce. The financial savings produced by some companies are also very impressive, though many other businesses have tried and failed to duplicate such dramatic reductions in costs.

When wellness programs are introduced into the workplace, it is imperative that the employees be approached correctly, especially when unions are involved. The motives for encouraging wellness can be and have been misinterpreted, or in some cases interpreted correctly, as coming from the management for purely financial reasons (instead of their purported humanitarian ones).

Some companies have begun programs that spread some of the savings around. They offer bonus plans when fewer sick days are used, mental health days off, bonuses for exercise participation and stopping smoking, all in the hope of changing lifestyles. Some companies use peer teachers to train and encourage their colleagues, while others use competitions or private professional counseling.

Consulting nutritionists can perform a variety of services for a corporate program: counsel clients, adjust cafeteria menus, teach other staff members, give speeches, write newsletters and brochures, make videos, and so on.

WELLNESS IN HOSPITAL SYSTEMS

Hospital systems are interested in the wellness concept for several major reasons. It offers public relations opportunities to improve the image of the hospital in the community. It may reduce health care costs for self-insured institutions or give premium breaks to those who have an outside insurer. It can offer the opportunity for greater income generated by community and corporate outreach programs. Some hospitals develop programs to placate administration, medical staff, or patients. The bottom line is usually the same in all institutions—eventually, results must be generated that substantiate the value of the program and warrant the capital expenditure and continuing expense.

Creating an in-house wellness program presents many challenges for an institution. Obtaining financing is usually not as difficult as gaining consensus about program staffing and defining *wellness*. Depending upon who runs the program and how involved the medical staff is, program emphasis too often begins to look very similar to the director's philosophy of wellness. A general practitioner wants to screen everyone medically, identifying illnesses and curing them. A cardiologist develops a cardiac rehab and aerobic exercise wellness program, assuming that if your heart is OK so are you. A psychologist emphasizes counseling and stress management and wants us to believe that good mental health conquers all. Many nutritionists emphasize food and exercise, but are often hesitant to forge new roads in programming or philosophical change. The exercise physiologist sees wellness in terms of fitness. Actually, then, the most successful programs use an integrated approach to wellness, treating equally the importance of nourishment, being physically fit, and making lifestyle choices.

The complexity of the hospital staff coupled with the medical hierarchy and the bureaucracy often make the development of hospital wellness programs tedious and complicated. The need for good communication is paramount. Strong leadership is a must. And most importantly, the program developers should never lose sight that it is the *client* who should be at the center of the program. For that reason, it is often beneficial to include a client or two on the development staff. Why create a program that doesn't fit the needs of those it was created for? It is also very helpful as a communication tool to have a business prospectus or plan written that describes the goals, purposes, target audience(s), staffing, plan of action, and timetable for the program.

Hospital Wellness Programs Come in Many Forms

Originally, hospital wellness programs were based in or near the hospital and catered to the hospital employees and the local community. Today, programs also can be found in shopping centers as store front operations and as outreach programs in corporations and health spas and hotels.

Facilities for wellness programs vary from the very elaborate with exercise equipment, pool, jogging track, and meeting rooms to only an office for one or two people to coordinate the programs for a staff of consultants.

Special events offered by wellness programs include sponsoring races, health fairs, and wellness retreats as well as media spots on health topics. Classes and seminars cover topics such as alcohol, stress, and smoking, all facets of sports, making good choices in life, healthful cooking, weight loss, aerobic and strength exercises, wellness nutrition—the prudent diet, vegetarian diets, relaxation, and flexibility exercises.

WINNING A NUTRITION POSITION IN WELLNESS

Most wellness programs assume that nutrition is a necessary component. However, that assumption does not necessarily include having a registered dietitian as the only professional giving out nutrition information. Today, ethical information on basic nutrition is readily available. Dietitians face job competition/encroachment in wellness settings even in some hospitals from at least nurses, social workers, health educators, physiologists, and physicians. However, dietitians who distinguish themselves in teaching skills, program and marketing creativity, and keeping abreast in nutrition knowledge will always have jobs.

Several years ago a hospital in Denver decided to cut expenses at their wellness program and only keep the positions that were generating a profit. That left only the dietitian on staff. Eventually, she built up her staff and wielded much more professional weight because she had demonstrated fiscal responsibility.

Wellness programs are looking for dietitians who have good communication skills (writing and speaking), who believe in and know about wellness and who are innovative and creative in programs, materials, and teaching skills. Dietitians must be assertive leaders while at the same time know how to interact and appreciate what other health professionals working on similar goals have to offer. Appreciation of the team approach is vital. It is also important that dietitians acquire business savvy so that they understand the "larger picture" of the organization, are politically effective, and understand and contribute to financial goals.

Seeking Leads and Making Contacts

Hospitals and corporations are usually very good about advertising available positions on their staff. However, to be associated with a wellness program during its beginning developmental stages, contact should be made early. In other words, it may be necessary to "cold call" on an institution to establish your interest. If you are already an employee at the hospital and want to apply for the job, you may find that you will still have to sell yourself and convince the wellness director that you can do well in the new position.

Tools that can be used to promote yourself for the position include a good resume, written with emphasis on skills and experience that would be useful in a wellness program, copies of published articles, booklets, or teaching materials you've written, copies of newspaper articles, brochures, or flyers that have promoted your public speaking, and, finally, a proposal either oral or written on what you could do for their program. If you do not have enough information to offer suggestions on the first visit, offer to write a simple proposal after you meet outlining what you could do for them. Try to return the proposal within a week so that they feel that your work is timely and efficient.

Dietitians can be hired as employees for the programs and therefore acquire all of the benefits of a salaried person. Many enjoy the creativity of a position at a wellness center, but love the regular paychecks, paid vacations, and medical benefits. They are willing to work in a more structured role and accept the fact that the institution owns the developed materials and programs (unless negotiated otherwise).

Wellness programs can also hire consultant dietitians who do not normally have any paid benefits. These dietitians prefer to take more risk and the responsibility for their own vacations, insurance, and continuing educations, and so on, in return for more money and freedom. Consultants are often paid to bring expertise that is not easily found or creativity that inspires a program. Usually the materials created belong to whoever paid for their development. Some consultants prefer to create them on their own time and then sell the materials or the right to use them to an institution.

Services to Offer

A proposal for a job should include at least three components. First, document what you have to offer that fits the needs of the program. Second, suggest approaches or activities that were not previously discussed (to show creativity and initiative). Finally, in words with which you are comfortable, let them know that you are interested in the position.

Dietitians offer a variety of services to wellness programs. These services include nutrition counseling, presenting classes and workshops, providing in-service classes to the wellness staff as well as other medical people, and conducting weight loss classes with an exercise specialist or psychologist. Others work with the cafeteria to change recipes and menu items to ones lower in fat and sugar and to include more fresh foods—"gourmet natural." Some wellness programs are also interested in dietitians who have media experience and can do media interviews, cable, and video programs. Dietitians with writing skills and experience are in demand by programs that plan to produce educational materials for sale. Computer expertise has opened doors for some dietitians when some wellness programs have wanted to produce their own software. Many hospital or corporate fitness weight loss programs have also employed dietitians.

MARKETING AND PROMOTION ARE MUSTS!

Wellness programs must recognize early on that their competition for clients is in the private sector. They do not have the luxury of a "captive audience"; unlike a hospitalized patient, wellness participants are not ill and do not require immediate treatment. Therefore, employees and the community have to be enticed and excited about the programs being offered or they will go elsewhere, if they go at all.

It will take a while for the image of a center to become established and market itself. The same will happen with individuals, classes, and programs. More time and money must be spent up front to acquaint prospective clients with you and what you offer. It may be necessary to give free introductory "brown bag" talks on the patient floors, visit community meetings, or give a prerace seminar.

To promote an individual program, such as a new weight loss series, marketing tools could include: an easy to remember name and logo, colorful posters, brochures, and folder covers for handout materials, and a personal letter to all physicians promoting the classes. T-shirts could be displayed that will be given out at the class. Paycheck stuffers could promote the program, as well as any other newsletter or communique. Ads could be purchased in local newspapers. Public service announcements are also available to nonprofit organizations through local media, and occasionally, a local newspaper or magazine writer will give an interview and take photographs. Advance time must be used to properly schedule all of the promotion events and allow for delays in orders.

Marketing is so important and critical to the survival of your programs. Don't leave it to chance and don't assume that someone else has it all under control. Stay on top of marketing!

WHY WELLNESS PROGRAMS FAIL

Even wellness programs with good financing and staffs can have problems and eventually fail. In surveys conducted by Robert Allen, Ph.D., and reported in "The Corporate Health-Buying Spree: Boon or Boondoggle?" reprinted from *Advanced Management Journal,* he found six factors that contribute to failure: (1) Fragmentation of effort—timing, organization, or marketing were off; (2) overemphasis on initial motivation—lack of long-term effect or follow through; (3) misdirected emphasis on illness—trying to motivate by avoiding disease instead of encouraging the positive potential of a healthy lifestyle; (4) appeal to individual heroics—there is a need for a supportive environment that is not competitive; (5) overemphasis on activities as opposed to results—a successful program produces lifestyle changes, not just good attendance; (6) a "we will do it for you" approach rather than a "together we can do it for ourselves" attitude —avoid passive programs (3).

THE COMING AWARENESS

The people who are well are seen today as an untapped market and potential source of revenue. Perhaps someday, they will also be seen as the medically exciting and unique individuals that they are. Why should someone have to be ill to be studied and helped to a better quality of life?

REFERENCES

1. Fitness Leadership Program Manual. Cooper Clinic Publisher, Dallas, Texas, March 1983, pp. 21–25.
2. Ardell, Don: *High Level Wellness.* Bantam, New York, 1979, p. 1.
3. Allen, Robert F: "The Corporate Health Buying Spree: Boon or Boondoggle? *American Management Association* (Society for Advancement of Management), New York, 1980. (monograph)
4. Fitness Leadership Program. Cooper Clinic, Dallas, Texas, March 1983, pp. 21–25.
5. "Kimberly-Clark Health Management Program Aimed at Prevention." *Occupational Health and Safety,* November/December 1977, p. 25.

chapter *21*

Sports and Cardiovascular Nutrition

Marilyn Schorin, M.P.H., R.D.

Two of the most exciting areas in which the entrepreneurial dietitian can become an expert are the specialties of sports and/or cardiovascular nutrition. Clients' ages and levels of physical conditioning as well as their motivations will vary substantially, posing a bold challenge to one's professional capabilities. Young athletes may be more interested in maximizing performance with foods and timing of meals. Adult clients may seek ways to become fit, prevent disease, or use nutrition and exercise to control either their weight or illness. This specialty is demanding, but the opportunity to have a salutary effect upon the lives of many individuals awaits those who have the ambition and energetic dynamism to enter this field.

The dietitian who chooses to specialize in sports and/or cardiovascular nutrition today is getting in on the ground floor of a brand new specialty. Five years ago, there may have been only about ten dietitians in the country who possessed expertise in both sports nutrition and nutrition of the cardiovascular system. Today, the Sports and Cardiovascular Nutrition Dietetic Practice Group of the American Dietetic Association boasts about 1500 members! Many, it is true, work solely with either athletes or cardiovascular patients, but a number of dietitians combine the natural interface between fitness and heart disease prevention.

WHO ARE THE CLIENTELE?

Three groups of people provide the best target for *direct* nutrition counseling. The target groups for individualized nutrition counseling are:

259

- School athletes and their families
- Adults with high risk of cardiovascular disease
- Adults with confirmed ischemic heart disease

Athletes

Many dietitians longingly fantasize themselves as counseling Alberto Salazar, Franco Harris, or other top athletes when they choose a sports nutrition emphasis. Of course there are occasional opportunities for reaching professional sports personalities, but almost no dietitians are earning their entire livelihood providing nutritional advice to these elite competitors. Bread and butter must be sought elsewhere.

Legions of athletes outside the realm of the top professional athletes want more information on diet for improved health and performance. Young athletes, of high school age or even younger, provide a wide open market for sound nutritional advice. At this age eating behaviors become entrenched as habits; they are far more difficult to modify in adults. Youngsters today have more money and more freedom than formerly, frequently eating their meals and snacks away from home. Even workout schedules can add to their hectic lives. When swimming practice is held at 7:00 in the morning, breakfast is sacrificed or bought on the run and devoured on the way to school. Other teams hold workouts right after school. Varsity athletes, hungry at 3:30, may grab a snack at the school vending machines to "tide them over" through practice. Many times these high schoolers need help not just in deciding what and how much to eat, but when. Salient suggestions that the nutritionist can offer regarding food choices and timing of meals can make a difference in both their team and academic performance.

The parents of these budding sportsmen and sportswomen also want help. In an era of struggling authority between parents and their teenage children, the dietitian must weigh the needs of a youngster who is striving to eat a high carbohydrate diet against the economic anxieties of the mother and father who complain that every time Junior reaches for a cold drink, a quart of orange juice disappears. The nutrition expert's timely explanations and compassionate intervention may ease some of the diet-related perturbations in the young athlete's home.

High-Risk Cardiovascular Disease

Adults who are at "high risk" for developing coronary artery disease represent the second prominent population to target for individual counseling. Mortality from coronary heart disease has declined by 25 percent in the past 15 years; nonetheless, deaths from heart and vascular problems still count for more than 50 percent of the annual mortality in the United States. Part of the reduced number of deaths can be attributed to better medical care, but a hefty improvement in cardiovascular health has probably resulted from lifestyle changes including, for example, consuming a diet lower in saturated fat and cholesterol, quitting cigarette smoking and getting more exercise (1).

Clients who fall into this second target group will require specific information on shopping for appropriate food and instructions on how to choose food from a restaurant menu to comply with a diet that is low in total fat, saturated fat, and cholesterol, yet high in complex carbohydrates. They will probably also require counseling to moderate sodium intake, balance calorie intake for weight control and physical activity, and find substitutes for sugar and alcoholic beverages to control serum triglycerides. The dietitian's unique knowledge of food composition in combination with an understanding of cardiovascular disease etiology and diet therapy creates a winning combination for the nutritional entrepreneur.

Dietitians who have worked with the Multiple Risk Factor Intervention Trial (MRFIT) and Lipid Research Clinic (LRC) research projects have developed numerous techniques and skills for increasing community awareness of the problems of coronary heart disease (CHD) and motivating clients to make dietary changes. A manual documenting some of their experiences and lesson plans was published by the National Heart, Lung, and Blood Institute (NHLBI) of the National Institutes of Health (NIH). Although the suggestions were developed in a research context, an ambitious entrepreneur will find this book a goldmine of ideas.

Confirmed Heart Disease

The third category of people receptive to personalized nutritional counseling is the group of patients with confirmed cardiovascular disease. These individuals may be convalescing from a myocardial infarction, coronary bypass surgery, or angiography; others may have been diagnosed as suffering from ischemic heart disease, but may be free of acute symptoms. Their dietary requirements include those of the "high risk" client, but the prescription is more stringent, and their compliance may determine their survival. Caffeine reduction may be added to the list of dietary modifications. Depending upon the patient's mobility and the physician's recommendations, exercise may be either prescribed or proscribed; caloric requirements will vary accordingly. Meals and snacks may need to be timed to obtain the most positive response to exercise.

COMMUNICATING WITH CLIENTS

Through a concerted effort to expand one's audience, the sports and cardiovascular dietitian can reach many people via methods less direct than individualized counseling. Communications skills become vastly more important when one does not see the client face-to-face. In direct counseling, the skilled dietitian can determine whether the nutritional recommendations are understood through gentle probing and observation. When the message is relayed through an indirect medium, expertise in writing and public speaking is demanded. Some modes of communicating with clients include:

- Individualized counseling
- Classes on specific topics
- Lectures

- Articles written in lay publications
- Radio and television appearances

One of the most commonly used approaches is to offer seminars or food demonstrations on one's specialty. Classes may be offered through hospitals, adult education programs, junior colleges, or health clubs. Some corporations welcome the opportunity to provide on-site instruction for their employees, set up under the auspices of the corporate health, personnel, or education departments.

Should the nutrition specialist prefer to avoid the constraints of regularly scheduled meetings, lectures offer an alternative avenue for educating the public. Finding an audience for lecturing is usually easy. In addition to many of the same organizations that sponsor classes, a number of local groups seek out lecturers for their meetings. Examples include business and professional women's clubs, men's clubs such as the Elks or Kiwanis, clubs with a religious affiliation (Hadassah, Christian Women), the "Y"'s, clubs focusing upon a specific health problem (Happy Hearts, Make Today Count), or booster clubs (usually associated with major high school sports). Depending upon the site, lecturers may charge admission, be paid by the sponsoring organization, or agree to speak as a public service. (Public service lecturing is not to be sneered at. I advocate that, for carefully selected audiences. It can provide inexpensive publicity for one's service; in addition, expenses are usually tax deductible.)

Other "indirect" avenues of communication include radio, television, and print media. Sports and cardiovascular nutrition are "hot" topics today. A recent poll of a wide spectrum of American adults stated that 72 percent of those interviewed believe that Americans are more interested in nutrition now than they were a few years ago. In the same poll, people reported doing more exercise now than in the past (2). The mass media do not want to know that "a balanced diet that is low in fat may help prevent heart disease." They might get excited, however, if they were offered (1) ten "new" ways to cut down on fat in your food or (2) "why and how to incorporate yogurt in your cooking when you are accustomed to sour cream." The topic of working with mass media is dealt with in greater detail in Chapters 17 and 22.

WHAT KNOWLEDGE AND TRAINING IS NECESSARY?

We are acutely sensitive to the propensity of marginally trained lay people or health care professionals with no background in nutrition to advertise their dubious expertise in our field. It follows, then, that we must be as insistent with our peers, requiring them to be well trained in the nutrition specialties they purport to practice. In fact, the dietitian who is an expert in sports and cardiovascular nutrition must have *at least* a basic knowledge of each of the areas listed below.

Baseline subjects for sports and cardiovascular nutrition specialists include:

- Nutritional science
- Biochemistry

- Physiology
- Cardiovascular disease etiology and treatment
- Sports rules, training, common injuries
- Counseling skills
- Communications skills

He or she is expected to have specialized knowledge or advanced training in at least one of these categories.

Nutrition

First and foremost, of course, is a working knowledge of nutrition science and food composition. Sports and cardiovascular dietitians must not only be conversant with general information about foods taught in most nutrition courses, but must keep tabs on particulars such as which cuts of beef offer the lowest saturated fat content and which vegetable oils are highest in polyunsaturates. They must know food composition in terms of specific brand names. (For example: Which brand of cheese can be recommended for low sodium diets and which local stores carry it? Which sport drinks advertised as complete meals are lactose-free?)

Knowledge of food exchange lists must be second nature, whether they are used for sodium, carbohydrate, or fat exchanges. Although clients do not think in terms of "exchange" lists, this is still one of the best ways to teach diet flexibility.

Biochemistry

Sports and cardiovascular dietitians need a working knowledge of the metabolism of macronutrients and the interrelationships among energy-providing fuels. If they have not kept up with lipid metabolism, they must be sure to either obtain some advanced training or assiduously review this critical and rapidly changing area. The biochemistry of exercise is a fascinating, but complex subject, yet it is essential to grasp its intricacies in order to explain sports nutrition in terms appropriate to each client. It is difficult to advise athletes and fitness enthusiasts on their nutritional requirements without a comprehensive understanding of this field.

Physiology

A clear understanding of muscle morphology is necessary when talking to athletes, coaches, and trainers. Since some medical and exercise specialists talk in terms of white or red muscle, while others distinguish between fast-twitch and slow-twitch fibers, the specialist in this field will need to know both of these classification systems. He or she will be familiar, of course, with digestion from a background in dietetics, but this dietitian will need more *advanced knowledge* of cardiovascular and respiratory physiology as well as hormone physiology.

Cardiovascular Disease

The dietitian whose clientele will be primarily cardiac patients or those at high risk of cardiovascular disease will require greater proficiency in the diagnosis and treatment of heart disease, enhancing interaction with other professionals involved in the patient's care as well as maximizing the quality of client counseling. Ideally, the various drugs used to treat angina, cardiac arrhythmias, and hypertension should be recognized, with an emphasis placed upon familiarity with the nutrient interactions caused by these pharmacological agents. The specialist's effectiveness is increased by awareness and mastery of other modalities of treatment of coronary artery disease and atherosclerosis, such as techniques for stress reduction and smoking cessation.

Sports Knowledge

When confronted with an athlete who plays an unusual sport, the sports dietitian must learn about both the client and the sport during the interview. If a dietitian intends to counsel those who play one of the more common sports, it is best to brush up on the rules of the sport. Get a book; go to the events or games; talk to athletes or fans. Learn something about training schedules: do participants train throughout the year or is there a season? How long do they train per day? How much training is done outdoors? Find out what type of injuries they sustain. Is nutrition generally considered an important adjunct in early recuperation from injury? (This point is very important to professional athletes.)

What are the commonly accepted guidelines for body weight in this sport (or in the various positions on the team)? What data has been collected in regard to body fat for these athletes? What are the typical energy requirements in this sport? Often, the training sessions will require a great deal of energy, but the athlete may spend much of the game itself "on the bench."

Counseling

Finally, the dietitian who concentrates on sports and cardiovascular nutrition needs to have well-honed counseling skills. Like all aspects of dietetics, sports and cardiovascular nutrition counseling achieves its greatest impact when these two factors prevail: (1) the client is highly motivated and (2) the nutritionist knows how to structure the care plan into small, manageable steps. Male and female athletes are motivated by improvements in performance; they constantly seek the competitive edge. Nutrition has been touted to them as a type of snake oil in which anything from carbo-loading to bee pollen may provide that edge. Their motivation is, fortunately, not usually a problem. On the other hand, the client at high risk for cardiovascular disease may feel "fine" and, therefore, resist making any dietary changes. A skilled counselor can dispel resistance, increase motivation, build confidence in the client's ability to make dietary changes, and promote maintenance of positive salutary changes.

Q & A

Consulting for a Local Sports Team

I want to be a sports nutritionist for the local professional basketball team. How do I go about it?

From my experience and observation, nutritionists are chosen or asked to work with athletes because of their acknowledged expertise and experience in sports nutrition. Occasionally, dietitians have had calls out of the blue to consult for professional sports teams, but that is a rarity.

Before approaching a sports team make sure you are well versed and knowledgeable in sports nutrition and its practical application. Then contact anyone who could open doors for you with the team owner, coach, or trainer or call them directly. The trainer is the person who works first-hand with meals on the road and pregame. He or she also works with weight problems, and illnesses or injuries that may call for special nutritional care. However, it is either the coach or the owner who approves of your talking to team members and getting paid, so he or she must be "sold" also.

In several instances dietitians have joined forces with either a physician or exercise physiologist to consult to teams as sports specialists. It also helps to be known in your area by giving talks on sports nutrition to amateur athletic groups and coaches' conferences.— Kathy King Helm, R.D.

WHERE TO GET INFORMATION

Although the demand for adequate formal training is emphasized above, equally important to success in this field is keeping up with new information and materials. Included in this area are professional meetings, reading selected journals, and networking with colleagues in this field. The Dietetic Practice Group on Sports and Cardiovascular Nutrition (SCAN) of the American Dietetic Association represents a broad group of Registered Dietitians who are working in this area. They publish a newsletter, *Pulse,* four times a year which keeps dietitians up-to-date regarding meetings, books, pamphlets, and other dietitians in this field. In addition, most states have physical fitness councils. Dietitians concentrating on this specialty should strive for representation on the council in their state. Perhaps the state dietetic association would be willing to nominate your name for membership on the council or one of its committees.

REFERENCES

1. National Heart, Lung, and Blood Institute, *Proceedings of the Conference on the Decline in Coronary Heart Disease Mortality,* National Institutes of Health, Bethesda, MD, NIH Publication No. 79–1610, 1979, pp. xxv–xxvi.
2. Yankelovich, Skelly, and White, Inc., "Nutrition Vs. Inflation: The Battle of the Eighties," *Woman's Day,* New York, 1980.

SUGGESTED BIBLIOGRAPHY

Nutrition and Sports

Bayrd, Ned, and Chris Quilter: *Food for Champions: How to Eat and Win,* Houghton Mifflin, New York, 1983, $11.95 (hardcover). *Food for Champions,* written for the lay person by two journalists, is an excellent example of a simple approach to a complex problem using scientifically correct information.

Bierman, June, and Barbara Toohey: *The Diabetic's Sports and Exercise Book,* Jove/Harcourt Brace Jovanovich Books, New York, 1977, $2.25 (paper). The authors provide accurate and reassuring advice to encourage many diabetics to exercise. This book is written in an informative style, explaining what may happen when a diabetic exercises and how to avoid any problems.

Clark, Nancy: *The Athlete's Kitchen,* CBI Publishing, Boston, 1981, $9.95 (paper). Nancy Clark combines sound information on sports and nutrition for the average person with a series of tempting recipes.

Coleman, Ellen: *Eating For Endurance,* Self-published (5336 Bardwell, Riverside, CA 92506), 1980. Ellen is an R.D. and exercise physiologist. She has been a competitor in the Ironman Triathalon. Her book contains a wealth of information on the theoretical aspects of exercise, as well as food for sports.

Haskell, William, J. Scala, and J. Whittam (eds.): *Nutrition and Athletic Performance,* Bull Publishing, Palo Alto, CA, 1983, $19.95 (paper). Proceedings of a conference held in 1981 in which many of the researchers and leaders in this field are represented. Written for the professional.

Schorin, Marilyn: "Nutrition and Athletic Performance," in *Nutrition in Clinical Care,* R. Howard and N. Herbold (eds.), McGraw Hill, New York, 1982 (hardcover). In this chapter, I have summarized many of the findings of sports nutrition research and presented guidelines for implementation. Written at the professional level.

Smith, Nathan J.: *Food for Sport,* Bull Publishing, Palo Alto, CA, 1976, $4.95 (paper). Pediatrician Nathan Smith has worked with athletic teams for a number of years. This book is simply written and should be part of every sports nutritionist's library.

Nutrition and Cardiovascular Disease

Feldman, Elaine B: *Nutrition and Cardiovascular Disease,* Appleton-Century-Crofts, New York, 1976 (hardcover). Although Feldman's book is several years old, much of the information is still appropriate. The information and style are oriented to technically informed readers.

Biochemistry

Harvey, Richard, and Pamela Champe, *Biochemistry—Outline Review,* Medical Exam Publisher, Garden City, NY, 1984, $19.95 (paper). This biochemistry book is short and presented in outline form. It will be a good review book to have when you want a reference to material, but do not want to read in great detail.

Stryer, Lubert, *Biochemistry,* Freeman, San Francisco, 1981, $32.95 (hardcover). Stryer's *Biochemistry* textbook is one of many fine basic texts with some clinical applications. It is nicely illustrated and clearly written. This is a general biochemistry text, with no specific applications to sports and cardiovascular nutrition.

Physiology

McCardle, William D., Frank I. Katch, and Victor L. Katch, *Exercise Physiology: Energy, Nutrition and Human Performance,* Lea & Febiger, Philadelphia, PA, 1981, $19.95 (hardcover). McCardle and the Katch brothers have written an eminently readable textbook of exercise physiology. They might have gone into greater detail on specific points about food, but since dietitians are well versed in that aspect, they would read this text for the information on exercise.

Sharkey, Brian J., *Physiology of Fitness,* Human Kinetics, Champaign, IL, 1979, $10.95 (paper). Brian Sharkey is clearly an exercise enthusiast as well as an exercise physiologist. His *Physiology of Fitness* seems to be written as a basic exercise text, but the informal style makes it more appropriate for the well-informed lay person.

Journals/Newsletters

Pulse, the newsletter of the Sports and Cardiovascular Nutrition Dietetic Practice Group, free with $15 annual membership, 4 issues per year. Write for subscription to SCAN c/o ADA, 430 N. Michigan Ave., Chicago, IL 60611.

Sports Nutrition News, Healthmere Press, PO Box 986, Evanston, IL, $18.00 per year, 6 issues per year.

Medicine, Science and Sports, bimonthly, free with membership in the American College of Sports Medicine.

chapter 22

Media Savvy

Health professionals who are comfortable with consultations and public speaking are often unnerved when entering the unfamiliar world of radio and television. Interviews with the print media are usually more relaxed, but there is seldom control over what is quoted. Why then, become involved in something so challenging or risky? Because you want to communicate with a great number of people. How else can you discuss nutrition with a million people for five minutes or warn your entire city about a new diet fad?

First chances, much less second chances, aren't always easy to get in any of the media avenues. Because so many people recognize the value of media exposure there is stiff competition in becoming a guest, especially on national programming. Local media and some cable stations are not so difficult. Jack Hilton, author of *On Television!* states, "The electronic media have replaced print as the basic source of information in this country, and the ordinary person is severely limited in the ability to get before a microphone and camera. In fact, even the extraordinary person has found it difficult to reach an electronic forum with regularity" (1).

Even considering all of the benefits, media work is not for everyone. Radio and television work requires that the person have an original personality and/or something to say, and of course, the ability to say it. The pace is usually quick and just as soon as you feel you are adjusting, it's over. And, there are times when the station or paper never again has time for another interview, and you never know why. They have time for the chef, the fortune teller, the gardener, and the policeman, but not the dietitian. At least not you. Was it something you said? Were you too straight? What could you have done differently?

PRACTICE MAKES PERFECT

Experts usually suggest that you plan, practice, and seek training or professional advice if you are really serious about pursuing the media on anything but an occasional or strictly small-time basis. It also helps to have experience. But how can you get it, if no one will give you a chance to start?

Practitioners have trained by first going to small local radio stations and newspapers to learn the ropes and the style that sells. If writing style is a problem, hire an editor to review your work or follow the other suggestions in Chapter 23. If speaking off the cuff is not comfortable, take communication course work or a seminar, pay a tutor, or practice with another person using a tape or video recorder. It is also beneficial to watch, listen to, or read what is being used on the media. Train yourself to begin thinking of angles that will make your project (or you) more newsworthy. Review media topics below:

Food demonstrations on
- Low-cholesterol cooking
- Vegetarianism
- Sugarless desserts
- Low-salt dishes
- Eating out on a low calorie diet
- Natural food sources of vitamins

Discussion on
- Diabetic diets
- Fiber and cancer
- Obesity in children and adults
- Elderly persons' nutrient needs
- Sports nutrition
- Baby formulas
- Breast feeding
- Allergy diets
- Hypoglycemia
- Hyperactivity in children
- Foods for the storm box
- Snacks for long auto trips
- The importance of water
- Nutrition cultism
- Vitamin supplements
- Caffeine
- Dial-a-dietitian
- Qualifications to become a Registered Dietitian

To prepare for call-in talk shows I read newsletters, such as *Nutrition and the M.D.* and *Tuft's University Diet and Nutrition Letter.* I also read lay publications, such as *American Health, Prevention,* and local or national newspapers, to get a better idea what my audience is reading.

Jack Hilton offers some good suggestions to consider before joining the talk show circuit, even on the smallest scale. He states, "Watch every talk show you can. Get a feeling for the rhythm, . . . for how much can be said. Note how questions tend to be repeated from show to show. Make up a set of questions and answer them in the microphone of a tape recorder. Listen to your voice. If you hear a continuing series of crutch words or sounds, practice talking without them" (1).

Being interviewed by a newspaper writer is usually less stressful, but answering with concise clear statements is just as important. The fact that the interview is more relaxed should not be construed as an invitation to ramble or become too familiar so that statements are made that you *hope* will stay "off the record."

LEGALITIES, LIABILITIES, AND CONTROVERSIES

When you appear on or write for the media on the subject of nutrition, you are representing yourself as an expert and as a member of your profession. Obviously, the better you do, the more credible everyone appears. However, there are legal and liability implications involved that you must be aware of:

1. As a nutrition expert, you have the right (and perhaps civic responsibility) to state the facts on an issue as you know them and as your peers would, given thorough research. If someone sues you for what you say, *they* have to prove that you intended malice to them (See Chapter 13 on ethics, malpractice and libel).
2. If you have been introduced as an officer or representative of your local, state, or national dietetic practice group or professional organization, you are speaking not only for yourself, but also for that organization. It is therefore very important, especially when you want to take a very controversial stand, that you think it out ahead of time. Then either only represent yourself by not implying otherwise or make sure that the organization is in total agreement with your statement *before* you make it.

To help avoid problems with controversial subjects, it is suggested that you research the subject thoroughly and then state fairly both sides of the controversy. Afterward, you can either state your opinion with your reasons or quote a higher source and give their reasons.

A personal experience by the author helps illustrate the viewer interest that can be generated by controversy:

After years of doing media work in Denver on subjects that I thought were interesting and sometimes controversial, I learned a valuable lesson. One week Judy Mazel, the author of the Beverly Hills Diet, was a guest on NoonDay, the NBC TV program where I was a weekly guest on nutrition. She appeared about 15 minutes before my segment and was lively, vivacious and a "media event." After her segment, the hostess asked if I could quickly look over the book and critique it for my segment instead of talking about what I had planned. I told her I needed more time to do an adequate job, but suggested we give a "promo" for next week's segment where I would give a critique. At least people might wait a week before they bought the book.

That next week I spent three times more preparation time than normal in developing my critique of Ms. Mazel's book. I even called several PhDs to get their comments on some of the erroneous statements made on physiology and digestion. The show went very well, but the viewer response to the station was much greater than I expected.

A physician friend, whose opinion I respected, said it was the best show I had ever done, and he gave me a quick review. He stated that the hostess and I first got everyone's attention because we issued a warning about the book. Then my arguments began to crescendo as each became stronger than the preceding one. At the moment when I had everyone's attention I quoted a higher source which lent greater credibility, and the hostess and I made light of the author's poor knowledge of the subject. I hadn't realized what had transpired, but I was glad it was pointed out to me so that I could use it again. My reviewer also told me that I should stop covering such "milktoast" subjects and go after the "hot" or controversial ones.

I took my friend's advice and immediately went after the Nestle issue, Dr. Adkins and other similarly qualified authors, stagnant schools of thought in nutrition, and the Cambridge Diet Plan (our station received its first threatening phone call for my segment on that one). To prepare for the subjects, I called national headquarters to talk to people, requested printed materials, read other professionals' reviews and even had a personal interview with the president of Cambridge International the evening before the televised program on the diet. Phone calls and letters increased to the station and to me, and the station loved it.

BY-LINES AND PROMOTION

Many good opportunities to market ourselves in the media are missed because of our hesitation to ask for by-lines and promotional credits. A by-line is a written acknowledgement in a newspaper, magazine, or other article that you were the author or at least a contributor. A promotion on radio or television usually consists of a short statement that people can contact you directly (presumably for more information) through the Yellow Pages, or a place of employment, or by a phone number offered over the air. It is *not* assumed that any of this will be offered to you automatically and the media person can refuse your request, but at least ask.

DEVELOPING YOUR SALES STRATEGY

There may be many motives for wanting to pursue the media: personal challenge or promotion, business exposure, consumer crusading, or all of the above. Whatever the reason, you must demonstrate that your cause is of interest or benefit to a great many people. But a worthy cause is not enough in itself. Unfortunately, the importance of your cause may be less important than the style in which you sell it.

You must have something new to say about the subject, something you have discovered yourself, engineered yourself, or dramatized in a newsworthy fashion (1). Appearing each March to say that this is National Nutrition Time wouldn't gain much attention if it weren't for the creative dietitians willing to appear on the media or the school children's colorful projects or the "new" nutrition facts used to catch the audiences' attention. Television stations and newspapers love stories with visual content. It doesn't have to be spectacular, just interesting or dramatic.

Becoming involved in "causes" to get media exposure (along with other personal and professional benefits) is a tactic long used by individuals in the know (2). In many business instances our notoriety is often equated with or partially responsible for our effectiveness or our clout. Sometimes doors open to us first because of our popularity or the draw of our name, before our great expertise in nutrition is even considered!

Some suggestions that may help develop a sales presentation include (1):

1. Is there a way to demonstrate a perceived benefit to many people from your cause? The benefit need only be perceived, not real.
2. Is there a way to package your cause that makes it seem new, even if it's old? New research or study results may prove your point.
3. Is there a dramatic way to illustrate your cause (charts, films, slides or testimonials)?
4. Can you demonstrate a particular expertise in talking about a subject of continuing public interest? (This is a favorite ploy of professionals who do not advertise widely, but who like broadcast exposure as a way to build a practice.) (2)

How to Get in the Media

You can always call up and ask if you can be on a show or talk to a reporter. By first doing your homework and observing the media, you should know whom to contact. In radio and television first start with the program host (1). If that person is unavailable or won't talk to you, speak to the producer. At a newspaper ask to speak with the editor of the section most likely to be interested in what you have to say.

If the show or paper prefers to have requests made in writing, keep it to one page and attach a few clippings and your resume to support your point and credibility. Follow that up with a phone call. Try to call at least an hour or more before any show or deadline time so that the person will have time to speak with you.

You will need to let them know your ideas, what you have to offer, and why the audience would be interested. Remain flexible in case the reporters or station people have a new twist or approach that they like better, but that still includes you. If the person doesn't like the idea at all, ask why. Offer to rethink the concept and offer a new proposal. Do not, however, ask for recommendations for other media contacts or approaches for you (1). The information may be offered, but it is not their responsibility to be your public relations counsel.

"Gentle persistence is the key" to finally getting in the media, according to Jeffrey Lant, author of *The Unabashed Self-Promoter's Guide: What Every Man, Woman, Child and Organization in America Needs To Know About Getting Ahead by Exploiting the Media* (2). No one should be discouraged if turned down; just keep persisting until someone is interested or the idea finally proves that it isn't right for you.

Before Arriving for the Media Interview

When you work with the media you are selling yourself and your ideas. It is very important that you be comfortable, prepared, rehearsed, and confident about your appearance. You will not be able to read a prepared speech, so reference material, notes, props, or whatever else you plan to refer to should be accessible, easy to read, and familiar to you.

Many media consultants encourage interviewees to choose only three major points that they would like to emphasize. Props, notes, charts, and so on could revolve around those points. All artwork and lettering should look professionally prepared, not homemade. The possibility of "freezing" or getting off the subject is much smaller when the interview is simplified and your expectations are more realistic. Also, for the audience to remember what is being said, it must be clear, simple, and restated several times, in different ways. After the main points are made, feel comfortable in discussing whatever is brought up or additional points that may be of interest.

Wardrobe is important since first appearances are crucial in all forms of the media. Don't wear anything so flashy that your clothes draw attention away from you. Don't overdress or underdress. Clothing you would expect to see on a bank vice president or TV newscaster will be good at any hour (1).

On television the color and print of an outfit are important. Try to avoid stark white or black in lieu of more muted colors: gray, darker blue, yellow, and beige. Patterned items, if they are worn, should be quiet, very small, and only one at a time. Avoid wearing herringbone and too busy-looking clothing.

Jewelry can be a problem on television because it can reflect into the camera or keep hitting a lapel microphone as you are interviewed. Wedding rings and watches are usually fine, but bracelets, pins, necklaces, or chains may have to be taken off. Eyeglasses, especially with metal frames, can also reflect the light. However, if you can't see without them and you don't wear contacts, don't take them off. They may ask questions about the slide they are showing on the monitor or a cameraperson may try to signal to you.

The Interview

When an interviewer meets a knowledgeable guest, the guest is usually given more freedom to carry the conversation. But this is not always the case, especially when the interviewer feels loss of control. So be aware and empathetic to needs other than just your own.

Try to be relaxed and don't forget to smile. Hold something in your hands if you like, but don't play with it or mutilate it as you are interviewed.

Before an interview on radio or television begins, it's usually possible to take a few minutes with the host to mention the items you feel are most important to discuss. If you have props, slides, charts, or whatever, be sure that the host is aware of them and when they are to be used. It is also appropriate to ask if the host is familiar with the topic you plan to speak on. If he or she is not, offer several key points that might be of interest. Be careful not to explain everything ahead of time because the host may unintentionally make *your* points in his introduction and cause you to momentarily panic.

There are interviewers in all forms of the media who enjoy controversy and antagonizing guests, but this is not usually the case. The best way to handle this type of person is to be well prepared and to remain calm. In radio and television the audience will usually side with the person they like and respect the most. At a newspaper writers will write whatever they want anyway. So, keep the discussion lively, but keep to the facts as you know them. Try not to be drawn into emotional controversies that have no satisfactory answers. Don't be afraid to have an opinion, however. Sometimes the best answer is to say that you don't have an answer to the problem. When telephone calls are taken over the air from the public, there again is risk involved, but remaining calm and logical is the best defense along with a sense of humor and being well prepared.

Be very aware of time limitations. Make your answers interesting and to the point. Unless it is the only appropriate answer, don't just answer with a yes or no. Use examples to make your point. And, it's very important that you *listen* to questions and conversation instead of just thinking about your next statement because you may be caught off guard with a simple, "What do you think about that, Ms. Jones?"

Bridging is a conversation tool that is used by anyone who wants to change the direction of questioning. The best guests don't evade the difficult questions —they restructure them. Before answering a question you don't like or that doesn't fit your needs, volunteer additional or different information introduced by a lead-in clause such as: "Let us consider the larger issue here . . .", or "Instead of that, you should be aware that . . .", or "Another issue the public is even more upset about is . . ." (1).

Trained guests volunteer much more than the required information when they like a question. No question is sacred, and none need be answered slavishly. It is possible, through bridging, to bring up more interesting issues than you are being asked by the interviewer (1).

The A or B Dilemma is where the interviewer asks a question and only gives two or so answers to choose from, both of which put you on the spot. An example would be, "Why do dietitians have such unrealistic ideas about what people eat? Is it because of poor training or aren't they observant?" What would you say? Probably, the best answer would be to either disagree with the original statement or avoid the trap by offering an alternative not given by the interviewer.

Whenever you are on the premises of a media interview be cautious of the things you might say or do. When in a radio or television studio always be aware that a "live" microphone or panning camera may be picking you up. On the premises is not the time to mention to a colleague or friend that the hospital kitchen was just closed by the Health Department or that a patient is suing you for malpractice.

After the interview

Obviously, after interviews take a moment to thank interviewers for their time and express a desire to do it again sometime. If no offer is forthcoming, offer to be a resource person, leave your card, and plan to call again in a month or two.

REFERENCES

1. Hilton, Jack: *On Television!: A Survival Guide For Media Interviews,* Amacom, New York, 1980.
2. Lant, Jeffrey: *The Unabashed Self-Promoter's Guide: What Every Man, Woman, Child, and Organization in America Needs to Know About Getting Ahead by Exploiting the Media,* JLA Publications, 1983.

chapter 23

The "Write" Way to Get Published

Susan Tornetta Magrann, M.S., R.D.

Don't skip this chapter because you *think* you don't have the skills to be a writer.

Writing talent is not something you are born with like curly hair or brown eyes. Learning how to write is like mastering any new skill whether it is skiing or developing healthy eating habits. It is the mark of a truly educated person, a necessary communication tool for the professional practitioner. You need motivation, guidance, and practice, practice, practice.

WHY WRITE?

The abundance of inaccurate nutrition articles and books written by pseudonutritionists should motivate dietitians to pick up their pencils or learn to use word processing by computer. Complaining about nutrition misinformation will not solve the problem. Even instructing patients in a one-to-one situation won't have a tremendous impact. But dietitians writing interesting articles and books about sensible nutrition will. Just think how many people you can reach with one article —probably more people than you could counsel in a lifetime.

A second motivational factor is the self-satisfaction you will experience when you see your name and work in print. It is what will spur you on to write additional pieces.

Writing gives you a chance to be creative. It is like painting a beautiful picture or sewing a gorgeous outfit. You start out with a few basics—paper, pen, and an idea—and you can create a masterpiece.

And you can't overlook the financial rewards. But don't spend the money yet. The publications most likely to print your first articles will probably pay poorly. But they do provide the opportunity to get established and perfect your writing skill. Besides, many of these initial contacts can serve as a network to meet the right people from bigger—and better paying—publications.

Having had the experience of writing for a variety of publications helped me convince a large supermarket chain that I was the person best qualified to write a monthly nutrition newsletter for their approximately 200 stores.

There also are other financial gains from getting published. Most publishers —especially those that don't pay well—are willing to print a brief statement about your background and the location of your private practice. This can attract potential clients or business contacts. You could also include information about nutrition materials you developed and how they can be purchased. This is how one dietitian is marketing her self-published book.

THE RIGHT START

Ready to dust off the old typewriter? Good. But before you begin, you should *polish your writing skills.* Attend a publishing workshop, hire a tutor, or take a writing course at a local college. Or at least check out library books on the topic such as *Writing with Precision* by Jefferson Bates. Two major national writer's magazines—*The Writer* and *Writer's Digest*—also offer invaluable writing tips.

Reading newspapers, magazines, and books also can advance your writing education. Scrutinize what you read. Take a close look at the lead and the format of the article. Analyze what techniques the writer uses to capture your interest. If you spot a poorly written article, think about how you could improve it.

A writer whose style is worth particular study is Barbara Gibbons. Check if your newspaper carries her syndicated column the *Slim Gourmet.*

WHAT TO WRITE ABOUT

Now that your fingers are itching to write, you must focus on an idea. It is easy to come up with good ideas if you keep your eyes and ears open. Nutrition is an "in" topic. Listen to what people are talking about. Read a variety of newspapers, magazines, and books. Watch the news.

Once you have an idea, you must make it uniquely yours by giving it a different slant. Editors want articles that are timely, and your slant can help update any nutrition subject. For example, more career women are waiting to become mothers. Why not slant your piece toward nutrition during pregnancy for the woman over 30.

Major news stories can make a nutrition topic timely. Karen Carpenter's death made anorexia nervosa a topic people wanted to read about. A recession makes food budgeting especially pertinent to the consumer.

Use your calendar to help inspire timely ideas. Waistline survival tips for holiday partying would be perfect for the December issue of a magazine. But you better think about Christmas in July since editors plan months in advance.

In developing your idea, keep in mind who your readers will be and what would interest them. For example, the majority of senior citizens do not care about basic nutrition for infants. But they may enjoy a story on healthy snacks for visiting grandchildren.

You should be able to state your idea in one sentence. Make it specific. General ideas don't sell. You are more likely to spark an editor's interest with "Ten Tips for Looking Great in a Swimsuit" than a general article covering weight reduction principles.

People love to clip recipes and editors know it. So consider developing recipes to sell your message. Don't just write about the need to use less salt but include recipes that show how delicious low sodium dishes can be.

Make sure you choose a topic that is of personal interest to you. This will keep you motivated to do the research and survive numerous revisions.

THE COMPUTER AND WRITING

With the growth in popularity of the personal computer, a discussion on writing would not be complete without mentioning how one can be used. Software such as Word Star or Multimate or Easy Writer can allow you to use the computer as a word processor. This gives you the capability to compose directly onto the computer screen, correct or reword the manuscript as necessary, and then print it when you are happy with it. The manuscript can be stored on software, later recalled on the screen, and revised by the word, sentence, or paragraph. Time-consuming handwritten or typed manuscripts that must be completely redone when changes are made become problems of the past. Software such as the Dictionary can correct spelling in your manuscript. It cannot, however, check for incorrect word usage or poor grammar.

A modem device and your telephone can allow your computer to access stored information in larger computer databases. This would allow you to conduct literature, newspaper, or scientific journal searches for the most current information and could greatly reduce the amount of time needed for research. For practitioners who do not live close to a good medical or research library this capability for accessing information would be especially invaluable.

As computers become more popular, it will no doubt be possible to have an editor check and revise your manuscript on their computer and send it back to your computer—all without either of you leaving your home or office. See Chapter 10 for more information on computer usage.

FINDING A PUBLISHER

After your idea is clearly defined, your next step is to find a publisher. You can start by referring to a writer's directory book which should be available in your local library. *Writer's Market, Writer's Yearbook,* and *Literary Market Place* are the best known books. (See Recommended Readings at the end of the chapter.) They are updated yearly and contain the names of thousands of newspapers, magazines, and book publishers.

In addition, there are market listings in *Writer's Digest* and *The Writer.*

You can also write directly to a magazine and ask if it accepts material from freelance writers; also ask them to send "spec sheets" or Writer's Guidelines.

The following is a sample of the information listed in the directories for magazines and newspapers.

1.   Name and address of the magazine or newspaper and the editor's name Your letter is more likely to be read if you send it to a specific editor. Since editors change frequently, check the masthead of a current issue of the publication.

2.   Type of magazine   If your idea is about nutrition during pregnancy, you would focus on a magazine geared to women in their twenties and thirties. Obviously magazines aimed at senior citizens or men won't be interested.

3.   Date established   Recently established magazines are more likely to accept your material since they have not built up a list of regular contributors. At the same time, they are more likely to fold before you ever receive payment.

4.   Circulation   Generally, the higher the circulation, the higher the pay rate—but this will also mean more competition.

5.   Pay rates and preferred length of articles   Editors work with a fairly set budget so there is not much room for negotiating fees unless you're well known or have a really "hot" story.

6.   Terms of payment   "Payment on acceptance" means that the magazine will pay you as soon as the editors agree to buy your article. "Payment on publication" means they will pay you when your article appears in the magazine. This could be several months or longer after you submit the article. "Kill fee" is a portion of the agreed-on price for an article that was assigned but the editor decided not to use. You are still free to sell your article to another magazine.

7.   Rights purchased   When you sell your article, you are selling the publisher the rights to reprint these words: "First serial rights." First serial rights means the newspaper or magazine has the right to publish your article for the first time in their periodical. "Second serial rights" gives a newspaper or magazine the right to print your article after it has already appeared in some other newspaper or magazine. This term also refers to the sale of part of a published book to a newspaper or magazine. "All rights" means the writer forfeits the right to use his material again in its present form. This is also true for "work-for-hire" agreements because the writer has signed away all rights to the company making the assignment.

8.   By-line   This means your name will appear on your article.

9.   SASE   (Self-Addressed Stamped Envelope) If you do not include one, and most request it, the editor will probably not reply to your letter.

10.   Lead time   Many editors request that seasonal material be submitted a specific number of months in advance. Editors have a lead time of several months so they don't want to see ideas for a Christmas holiday article in October.

If you're interested in having a book published, the market listing will tell you what types of books a company publishes, how they want the material submitted, and what terms to expect if you're offered a book contract. The author's payment is called a royalty and is usually calculated as a percentage of the retail price of copies sold. For hardbacks, 10 percent is the usual base rate and 7½ to 8 percent for paperbacks. Generally, the percentage will increase if your book sells over a certain number.

You also can find a potential publisher by looking at books that cover a topic similar to the one you intend to write about. Check in the front of the book for the name of the publishing house.

SELLING YOUR IDEA

Now that you have pinpointed which publishers are most likely to be interested in your work, you must sell them your idea.

A Query Letter

Before you write your article, you should send the editor a query letter (see Figure 23.1). Most editors prefer that you do not telephone or send the complete article.

The query letter is your sales tool. Since editors will formulate their impressions of you from this letter, it is wise to use quality 8½" × 11" stationery and to change your typewriter ribbon often enough so you get crisp, black impressions or use film ribbon.

A query letter should contain these basic components:

1. Description of your idea, why it is timely, and your slant. Include an abstract of how you plan to develop your idea and a suggested length and deadline.
2. An explanation of why the editor's readers would want to read the article.
3. Why you are qualified to write the article and resource people you plan to interview. Include a statement about your professional background as well as one or two samples of published works. If you haven't been published, you need not mention this fact.

The ideal query runs one to two single-spaced pages—just long enough to develop your idea but short enough to be read quickly by the editor.

Enclose a SASE and your phone number in case the editor wants to contact you. You should receive a reply in four to six weeks. If you have not heard by that time, drop the editor a note or telephone asking whether a decision has been made about your query.

You can send simultaneous queries and even get the assignment from two

Figure 23.1 Sample Query Letter

Susan Magrann, M.S., R.D.

CONSULTING NUTRITIONIST

5252 LINCOLN AVENUE
CYPRESS, CA 90630
PHONE: (714)

June 20, 1987

John Smith, Editor
Today's Family
1410 First Street
Morristown, NJ 07960

Dear Mr. Smith:

Are your readers buying what they think they are buying when they go to the supermarket? Shopping today is fraught with mysterious codes and language.

Do fruit drinks or fruit-flavored drinks contain more fruit juice?

Does the term "lite" mean low in calories?

Is instant breakfast a nutritious meal?

Does white bread contain any nutrients?

The answers are all there on the products' labels.

I would like to take the mystery out of label reading by writing a 1000-word article covering the following points:

1. HOW TO INTERPRET A PRODUCT'S NAME. Included would be a chart of the legal meaning for various terms. For example:

If the Label Says . . .	It Means . . .
Fruit juice	100% real fruit juice
Juice drink	35 to 69% real juice
Fruit drink	10 to 34% juice
Fruit-flavored drink	less than 10% juice

Your readers will probably be surprised to learn that the term "lite" can refer to other properties of the food besides calories. "Lite" corn chips aren't lower in calories; they're thinner.

2. INGREDIENT LISTING. You can learn a great deal about the product's composition since ingredients are listed in descending order by weight. Included will be a description of hidden sources of sugar, salt, and saturated fats. If your readers check the ingredients for instant breakfast, they will find that in addition to sugar, corn syrup solids, another form of sugar, is also listed.

3. NUTRITION LABELING. The article will have a detailed explanation of what every line means on the nutrition label and will define the term "U.S. RDA."

As for white bread, the nutrition label shows that it does contain some nutrients, although less than what is found in whole wheat bread.

Figure 23.1 *(Continued)*

I hope I will have the opportunity to help your readers become better-informed consumers.

Besides being a registered dietitian, my nutrition articles have appeared in several publications including *The Jogger.* I also write a monthly nutrition newsletter for a large supermarket chain on the West Coast. Enclosed are two samples of my work plus my curriculum vitae.

Sincerely,

Susan Magrann, M.S., R.D.

---

or more editors. You can accept more than one assignment for a topic as long as you write different articles. This may be frowned upon however if the magazines are in direct competition.

To increase your chances of acceptance, *you should become familiar with the magazine before sending a query.* Either get copies from the library or purchase sample issues from the editor.

Take a close look at the magazine's format, style of writing, and length of articles. Even study the advertisements. They can provide a good insight about what type of people read the periodical. If there are advertisements for children's toys and baby food, this will clue you that the audience is mainly young parents.

A Book Proposal

If you're working on a book, you would send the prospective publisher a proposal. The proposal should be about five to ten single-spaced pages and contain all the elements of a good query letter as well as a synopsis or outline of the chapters. Most publishers would also like at least two good sample chapters. For additional tips, refer to *How To Write "How-To" Books and Articles* as well as the *Writer's Handbook.*

Since your proposal can remain under consideration for many months, it is reasonable to send it to two to three editors at the same time but you must inform them that others are reviewing the same material.

Don't get discouraged when selling your book idea. Published dietitians tell stories about the numerous proposals they submitted before a publisher showed an interest.

Using A Literary Agent

You don't have to have a literary agent in order to sell your book. Many dietitians have sold their book ideas directly to the publisher. Besides, unless you're an established writer, it will be difficult to find an agent. Since agents' fees are usually about 10 percent of your royalties, they want to feel certain you will earn enough money to be worth their time and effort.

If you decide to pursue getting a literary agent, you can start by asking for suggestions from editors you have worked with. Or, if you know other writers, they may have some leads. *The Literary Market Place* contains a comprehensive listing of literary agencies.

Self-publishing

If you or your agent cannot find an interested publisher, you can always publish the book yourself. Of course, you have to invest your own money. But if you don't have confidence that the book will sell why should a publisher?

Ellen Coleman, a dietitian from California, self-published her book, *Eating For Endurance,* and it has done so well it is already in its second printing. She decided to self-publish because editors felt the topic did not have a wide appeal and wanted her to dilute the material.

If you're interested in self-publishing, read *The Publish-It-Yourself Handbook.* There is also an excellent article in the March, 1983, issue of the magazine *Writer's Digest* entitled, "The Complete Guide To Selling Your Self-Published Book." The article contains names of distributors who are willing to market your book.

Illustrations

Don't overlook the value of good illustrations in your book to increase sales. Unless you are talented, your best bet is to find a freelance professional artist and/or photographer. Contact other writers who have used local illustrators and get their recommendations. Or look in the Yellow Pages under "Artists—Commercial" and "Photographers—Commercial." There is also lots of good young talent at local universities and art schools.

WRITING YOUR MASTERPIECE

Congratulations. You sold your idea. Now you only have a *deadline* to worry about. This can cause panic—and an illness called "writer's block." Don't worry, it need not be terminal. There are measures to overcome the condition.

First, find a location—either at home, work, or at the library—where you can work without interruptions. If the phone is a problem, consider investing in an answering machine.

Second, select the best time for you to write and force yourself to stick to it. Most people have a specific time of the day they feel most creative. You will be more productive by spending whatever amount of time you can spare every day at your "peak creative time" than trying to cram the assignment into a couple of 8-hour days.

Third, break your writing into small parts. This will keep you from feeling overwhelmed by the project.

Outline

Maybe the first day will be spent on your outline. It is essential to have some type of outline since it makes the next step—research—much easier. An outline helps you gather and organize all the pertinent information you need. While doing your research, you may decide to revise your outline.

Research

Begin your research by reviewing materials you have at home or work. Then you'll want to expand your information by going to a local library and/or medical library or by a computer search.

Interview dietitians and other professionals who are experts in the topic you're writing about. In addition to providing valuable information, they can direct you to reference books and articles.

Don't let the term *interview* scare you. It's just a fancy name for talking to someone. Most people will be flattered that you value their opinion. In order not to waste the expert's time, prepare a list of questions before contacting him.

Writing

After research comes the hardest step for most people—writing. Some would-be authors are guilty of research overkill to delay the inevitable.

It is easier to write your first draft if you don't worry about its being perfect at this point. Just sit at your desk and put your thoughts on paper. Don't stop for any corrections or even crossing out words. Once you force yourself to do the first draft, your work will become easier.

Next, revise and fine tune your piece. The first revision will probably be the most extensive. Keep in mind you want your work to be clear, concise, accurate, and interesting.

Check that your lead sentence is a grabber. Unless you capture the audience's attention, they won't continue to read on. It can take a good deal of time to develop your lead but it's definitely worth the effort.

Next, take a close look at each word. Specific and short words crowd more meaning into a small space. Cross out unnecessary words and check for spelling.

Avoid overusing a particular word especially within the same paragraph. This is when a thesaurus or a dictionary of synonyms and antonyms is invaluable.

Now you're ready to study sentences. Do they flow smoothly? Is the length of your sentences varied? Generally, shorter sentences are easier for the reader to understand.

After sentences comes paragraphs. Each paragraph should contain a main idea. Avoid paragraphs that are too long. You can even slip in some single sentence paragraphs for a change of pace.

Look for a snappy ending. The reader will then leave the story with a favorable impression.

After your first revision, put your work away for a few days so you will be able to take a fresh look at it. Now you're ready to do your second, third, or however many additional revisions it takes to make it perfect.

Editing

If you lack confidence about your writing and feel it is never perfect, pay a professional writer to edit it. You can find someone by contacting a college that has a journalism program. There may be an instructor or a senior student who could help.

Depending on your subject, you also may want an expert in that area to check your work for accuracy.

Final Copy

The end is almost near. You are ready to type your final copy. Don't forget to follow the guidelines the publisher sent you. After you've cleaned up all those typos, you're ready to mail off your masterpiece.

Since you've invested so much time and energy creating this literary work, you don't want someone to steal your material. If you're not familiar with copyright laws, refer to Chapter 14, protecting your ideas and interest.

The last step: relax.

You'll need to gather strength before you start your next writing project.

One final piece of advice. Resist spending all of your writer's fee on buying copies of your work for friends and relatives.

On second thought, why not? You should be proud of your accomplishment.

And you thought you couldn't be a writer!!!

RECOMMENDED READINGS

Magazines

The Writer. Published Monthly by The Writer, Inc.
Writer's Digest. Published Monthly by Writer's Digest.

Books

Marketing Information
Literary Market Place. Bowker, Annual.
Writer's Market. Writer's Digest, Cincinnati, OH, Annual.
Writer's Yearbook. Writer's Digest, Cincinnati, OH, Annual.

Writing and Publishing
Getting Published: A Guide for Businesspeople and Other Professionals by Gary Bellien. New York, John Wiley and Sons, 1984.
How To Get Happily Published by Judith Appelbaum and Nancy Evans. New York, Harper & Row, 1978.

How to Write "How-To" Books and Articles by Raymond Hull. New York, Writer's Digest Books, 1981.

How to Write and Publish a Scientific Paper, 2nd ed., by Robert Day. Philadelphia, ISI Press, 1983.

Magazine Article Writing by Betsy P. Graham. New York, Holt, Rinehart and Winston, 1980.

The Publish-It-Yourself Handbook edited by Bill Henderson. Weinscott, NY, Pushcart Press, 1973.

The Writer's Handbook edited by Sylvia K. Burack. The Writer, 1982.

The Writer's Survival Manual by Carol Meyer. New York, Crown Publishers, 1982.

Style

A Dictionary of Modern English Usage by H. W. Fowler. Oxford University Press, 1965.

The Elements of Style by W. Strunk and E. B. White. Macmillan Publishing Co., 1978.

The Most Common Mistakes in English Usage by Thomas E. Berry, McGraw-Hill Book Co., 1971.

chapter 24

Continued Competency

The fact that we should stay current with new advances in the field of nutrition is often just taken for granted. However, staying up to date is not a task that can be accomplished by attending a meeting or two a year and skimming a journal monthly. The rate of change in nutrition and its related specialties is happening faster than we have ever experienced before, and it may continue that way for some time.

Money is finally starting to be earmarked for research in nutrition, thus generating new information regularly. Government changes in regulations and payments for patient services are demanding that changes be made in nutrition documentation and expected output. "Outside" competition to nutrition practice demands that our expertise and practice improve to stay ahead. The use of high technology, the computer in particular, will require that we have an appreciation and working knowledge of new systems that should free our time and give us the opportunity to better use our expertise. New techniques and human behavior skills need to be employed to be more effective in our roles as counselors. The public expects and is demanding that we take stands on the issues and that we provide information. Maintaining the status quo will drop us behind. Every dietetic professional will be challenged.

It is well known that merely getting 75 hours of continuing education credit every 5 years will keep a dietitian registered. But, depending upon the quality of the programs and the subjects chosen to attend, a practitioner may or may not learn anything new. A practitioner's goal should not be to merely stay registered, but instead to become an expert and remain one.

As the marketplaces continue to change, especially for entrepreneurs, it is imperative that a dietitian gain nondietetic experience and attend seminars. Also, lay literature and world and economy periodicals should be regularly reviewed. Nutrition can no longer be seen as a narrow field of study. It is an element of life intertwined and influenced by many other constituent parts.

In business the practitioner is again greatly affected by nondietetic influences. The local and national economies, consumer trends, insurance coverage, competition, and available financing are just a few of the concerns. The more knowledgeable an entrepreneur is about these items, the more prepared the person will be to handle business life.

Educators tell us that the mark of an educated person is one who knows where to look something up. If you subscribe to several newsletters and take the time to read the Periodical Reviews in the back of the *Journal of The American Dietetic Association,* scanning nutrition literature is relatively simple. It is not necessary to purchase all of the most expensive resource books as long as you have several available to you. World and economic news can be found encapsulated in the daily newspapers or weekly and monthly publications. Business news can be found in magazines, trade journals, newspapers, and newsletters.

The following list of references is not meant to be a complete list or an endorsement. Practitioners have shared the names of references and resources that have been beneficial to them. You may have additional ones that fit your needs better. Before subscribing to the periodicals buy a few issues at the newsstand and look up journals in the library to see if you like them. Many publishers will also agree to trial subscriptions for shorter periods than one year. Newsletter editors often offer to refund a partial subscription price, if you are not satisfied with the publication. Take advantage of these offers and don't hesitate to stop publications that do not fit your needs or interests. Staying current can be costly both in time and money, so evaluate your references carefully. See Figure 24.1 for James C. Rose's article on the new dietetics.

REFERENCES AND RESOURCES

Local Resources

Adult education classes
Bank seminars
Chambers of Commerce
College and university courses, especially the Extension Division
Executive (professional) clubs and organizations
Internal Revenue Service (tax classes)
Local newspapers, newsletters, and magazines
Local private practitioners

American Dietetic Association

Audio Cassette Series

Includes tape(s), study guide and continuing education credit application

Figure 24.1 **The New Dietetics**

(*Source: Hospital Food & Nutrition Focus,* July 1985. Reprinted with permission of Aspen Publishers, Inc. Copyright © 1985.)

THE NEW DIETETICS

For over 50 years, a few basic diet therapy regimens have consumed the majority of our labor hours. Calorie control, diet for diabetes mellitus, carbohydrate control, sodium control, and fat modifications have taken the front seat in terms of interest and deployment of resources. Our menus are devised in accord with the premises of these diets; our very world has depended upon providing services to those patients who require these types of services—patients with diagnoses of heart disease, diabetes, renal disease, and many others.

In the last decade we have become more sophisticated in our provision of nutritional care. We now focus more closely on laboratory values, on protein (nitrogen) and calorie ratios, and on measuring the relative risk of malnutrition. But the content of the diets we provide has really not changed. There are still low sodium products, controlled fat products, and "magic" mixtures that emanate from the nourishment control centers. The nutrients in favor may differ from setting to setting, but our basic approach to treatment has been static. . . .

America is in the bionic age. Artificial organs, transplants, and other such medical wonders are becoming commonplace in some settings. Few deny that soon the lifelong behavior modification requirements for diabetes mellitus clients will no longer be necessary—an artificial pancreas will eliminate the need for diet control. Artificial kidneys and new methods for treatment have revolutionized our basic theories of protein, electrolyte, and fluid controls in renal disease. Liberality in treatment of the aged and increasing knowledgeability of consumers concerning nutrition have altered the requirements for our services. Sodium and fat modifications are no longer universally viewed as the treatment of choice for hypertension and coronary artery disease. Our crackers and butter theories are not now held in high esteem in all medical circles.

The implications for our industry are clear. Recognizing that many of our staff have insufficient current knowledge to bridge the gap from the old to the new dietetics, we have a responsibility to provide meaningful continuing education for the seasoned—not just the novice—practitioner. If we bury our noses in current staffing configurations and fail to look to the future promised by new research, we will be poorly equipped to have a role in the new dietetics. . . .

Certainly, our entire future does not rest on research in the nutrient-brain matrix, but how many of our dietitians have even heard of the research? How many of us have enough familiarity with these activities to respond to the questions of consumers or physicians? If we are acquainted with the research, are we discounting it as "not yet proven" rather than preparing ourselves for potential opportunities?

Though it is true there may be no long-term future for dietetics in this particular area of research—drug therapy may replace diet therapy—are we ready and willing to look beyond our old realm, our old world? Are we prepared to adapt our entrepreneurial approach to the new reality of medical advances?

James C. Rose, RD, DHCFA, LD
Editor

Q & A

Becoming a Consultant

I don't want to start a clinical private practice, but I would like to become a consultant. I think I can make just as much money. How do I begin?

Becoming a consultant in any practice area of dietetics is a growing career alternative for dietitians. It is not necessary to be in a clinical private practice to be successful in business. In fact you may find that you can generate a larger income sooner by pursuing contracts as a consultant.

Several factors influence your chances of becoming a consultant who is in demand. First, you need specialized experience and/or training to be considered an "expert" in a field. Being a Registered Dietitian will open many doors, but top consultant positions will require more years and work. Second, it helps to be published and/or a known speaker on the specialty area. This will distinguish you and extend your reputation and presumably your credibility. Finally, you need good personal qualities and interesting ideas and programs that are unique and set you apart from your competition.

Successful consultants learn to work well with their clients so that the client feels he is getting the best service available for the money. Good consultants are careful to discuss with clients the expected outcomes before and during a project. Communication is open and frequent with possible problems being top agenda items. It is imperative that clients be satisfied.

To begin as a consultant, conduct a market survey (as discussed earlier) to see if your defined services fit the needs of your target market. If you are satisfied with your market survey results, organize your marketing strategies (determine how you plan to sell and promote your services). Then organize, refine and attractively "package" any program materials you plan to use. Finally, contact prospective clients by phone or letter to request an appointment to discuss what you offer.

On a local basis, dietitians often consult with food services, restaurants, wellness programs, HMOs and PPOs, hospital based programs, nutrition assessment teams, renal units, school systems, live-in institutions, police and fire departments, government programs and so on. The services consultants offer range from program development, in-service training, computer assessment of menus, recipe development, systems analysis and kitchen layout design, writing, one to one or group counseling to marketing, management or sales.

On a national scale consulting is especially suited to experienced practitioners with established professional networks and contacts, and with recognized reputations as experts in their field. Consultant positions on this scale could include program development for spa chains, government, hospital and business agencies, the food or pharmaceutical industries, national or state health-related services and so on.

As formerly stable positons in dietetics are cut due to budgetary or philosophical changes, many dietitians are rethinking what they have to offer and how their services could benefit their former employers. It is not unusual today to see dietitians acting as consultants for more money per hour, but for fewer hours to hospitals, government agencies and other institutions.

Study Kits

Includes tapes and binder with study guide, articles and workbook, plus continuing education credit application

Video Cassette Series

Includes video, study guide, and continuing education credit application
Programs can be rented or purchased

Publications

Exchange lists for meal planning
Family Cookbook
Handbook: Interactions of Selected Drugs and Nutrients in Patients
Handbook of Clinical Dietetics
Nutrition Services for Older Americans: Foodservice Systems and Technologies
Sports Nutrition
The Manual of Clinical Nutrition and Clinical Nutrition Supplement
Vitamin-Mineral Safety, Toxicity, and Misuse

Small Business Administration

ACE (Active Corps Executives): working business people who volunteer their time to consult with entrepreneurs and conduct seminars
SCORE (Service Corps of Retired Executives): retired business people who volunteer their time to consult with entrepreneurs
SBI (Small Business Institute): training and classes for entrepreneurs
Publications (topics):
    Accounting
    Advertising and public relations
    Borrowing/Raising equity
    Budgeting

Computers
Credit and collections
Financial management
Form of business (legal)
Incorporating a business
Insurance
Management techniques
Marketing
Patents
Recordkeeping
Starting a business
Taxes
Venture Capital

Small Business Administration offices are located in each state. Look in the telephone book under "U.S. Government" and ask for the address and telephone number of the nearest office.

Private Practices

Bitz, Peggy, R.D., and D. Derelian, R.D.: "Changing Dietitians' Attitudes Toward Client Counseling," *JADA,* Sept. 1978.

Consulting Nutritionists in Private Practice, Newsletters, CN Dietetic Practice Group of ADA, 1976–1987.

Hunerlach, Carol, R.D.: "Private Practice: Nutrition Counseling," *JADA,* Nov. 1975.

King, Kathy, R.D.: "Private Preventive Nutrition Clinic," *JADA,* April 1975.

King, Kathy, R.D.: "Marketing Your Services," *The Community Nutritionist* 1, May–June 1982.

Kunis, Beila Simon, R.D.: "Entering Private Practice in Dietetics," *JADA,* Aug. 1978.

Leonard, Rodney: "Private Practice: On Your Own," *The Community Nutritionist,* 2 July–Aug. 1982.

McCoy, Barbara: "Private Practice: Starting from Scratch," *JADA* 81:65, 1982.

McCoy, Barbara: "Private Practice: Continuing from Scratch," *JADA* 84:78, 1984.

Mills, Marcia, R.D.: "The Private Practice of Dietetics: A Resource for Physicians," in *Nutritional Support of Medical Practice,* Schneider, Anderson, and Coursin, eds., Harper & Row, NY, 1977.

Realities in Private Practice, 3rd ed., Nutrition Plus, Inc., 10 Congress Street, Suite 320, Pasadena, CA 91105, 1981.

Reidy, Elizabeth, R.D., and D. Reidy, J.D.: "Malpractice Law and the Dietitian," *JADA,* Oct. 1975.

The No-Nonsense Guide to Starting Your Own Business, Starmark, Chicago, IL, 1980.

Trihart, Eleanor, R.D., and M.B. Noel, R.D.: "New Dimensions: The Dietitian in Private Practice," *JADA,* July 1978.

Business References

Belkin, Gary S.: *Getting Published: A Guide for Businesspeople and Other Professionals,* John Wiley, New York, 1984.

Chenevert, Melodie: *STAT Special Techniques in Assertiveness Training for Women in Health Professions,* Mosby, St. Louis, MO, 1983.

Cohen, Herb: *You Can Negotiate Anything,* Lyle Stuart, NY, 1980.

Curtin, Richard T.: *Running Your Own Show,* John Wiley, NY, 1982.

Dible, Donald M.: *Business Startup Basics,* The Entrepreneur Press, 3422 Astoria Circle, Fairfield, CA 94533, 1978.

Fisher, Roger, and W. Vry: *Getting to Yes: Negotiating Agreement Without Giving in,* Houghton Mifflin, Boston, MA, 1981.

Hayes, Rick Stephan, and C. R. Baker: *Simplified Accounting for Non-accountants,* John Wiley, NY, 1980.

Ilich, John and, B. S. Jones: *Successful Negotiating Skills for Women,* Playboy Paperbacks, NY, 1981.

Kelly, Kate: *How To Set Your Fees and Get Them,* Visibility Enterprises, NY, 1984.

Kleinman, Carol, *Women's Networks,* Lippincott and Crowell, Philadelphia, PA, 1984.

Lane, Marc J., *Taxation for Small Business,* Ronald Press, NY, 1982.

Mancuso, Joseph R.: *How to Start, Finance, and Manage Your Own Small Business,* Prentice-Hall, Englewood Cliffs, NJ, 1978.

McCay, James T.: *The Management of Time,* Prentice-Hall, 1959. (classic)

McConnell, Charles R.: "From Idea to Print: Writing and Publishing A Journal Article," *Health Care Supervisor,* 2:78–94, 1984.

McCormack, Mark H.: *What They Don't Teach You At Harvard Business School,* Bantam, NY, 1984.

Pooley, James, *Trade Secrets,* Osborne/McGraw-Hill, Berkeley, CA, 1982.

Questions and Answers About Trademarks, U.S. Dept. of Commerce Patent and Trademark Office, Aug. 1979.

Ragan, Robert C., and J. Zwick: *Fundamentals of Recordkeeping and Finance for the Small Business,* The Entrepreneur Press, NY, 1978.

Shaffer, Martin, *Life After Stress,* Plenum, NY, 1982.

Shook, Robert L., *Why Didn't I Think of That!,* New American Library, NY, 1982.

Tepper, Terri and N. D. Tepper, *New Entrepreneurs,* Universe Books.

Zinsser, William: *On Writing Well,* 3rd. ed., Harper & Row, NY, 1980.

Zinsser, William: *Writing with a Word Processor,* Harper & Row, NY, 1983.

Support Organization, Membership Helpful

The Center for Entrepreneural Management, Inc., 83 Spring Street, New York, NY 10012, (212) 925-7304, CEM headquarters office director, Dr. Joseph R. Muncuso. CEM began as a division of American Management Association, but is now a nonprofit professional organization, with a number of regional centers, particularly aimed at help for the small businessperson.

Nutrition Reference Books

Altschule, Mark: *Nutritional Factors in General Medicine,* Charles C. Thomas, Springfield, IL, 1978.

Goodhart, R., and M. Shils (eds): *Modern Nutrition in Health and Disease: Dietotherapy,* Lea and Febiger, Philadelphia, PA, 1979.

Halpern, Seymour: *Quick Reference to Clinical Nutrition,* J. B. Lippincott, Philadelphia, PA, 1979.

Handbook of Clinical Dietetics, The American Dietetic Association, 1980.

Hess, Mary Abbott, and A. E. Hunt: *Pickles and Ice Cream,* McGraw-Hill, New York, 1982.

Hodges, Richard: *Nutrition in Medical Practice,* W. B. Saunders, Philadelphia, PA, 1980.

Katch, Frank, and W. D. McArdle: *Nutrition, Weight Control and Exercise,* Lea and Febiger, Philadelphia, PA, 1983.

Mahan, Kathleen, and J. M. Rees: *Nutrition in Adolescence,* C. V. Mosby, St. Louis, MO, 1984.

Mason, Wenberg, and Welsch: *The Dynamics of Clinical Dietetics,* John Wiley, NY, 1977.

McArdle, William, F. I. Katch, and V. L. Katch: *Exercise Physiology,* Lea and Febiger, Philadelphia, PA, 1981.

Nutrition References and Book Reviews, 5th Ed., NRBR Comm., Chicago Nutrition Assoc., 8158 S. Kedzie Ave., Chicago, IL 60652, 1981.

Nutritive Value of Convenience Foods, West Suburban Dietetic Association, P.O. Box 1103, Hines, IL 60141.

Pediatric Nutrition Handbook, American Academy of Pediatrics, P.O. Box 1034, Evanston, IL 60204, 1979.

C. Pemberton, and C. Gastineau, eds. *Mayo Clinic Diet Manual,* W. B. Saunders Co., PA, 1981.

Powers, Dorothy, and A. O. Moore: *Food-Medication Interactions,* 4th ed., F-MI Publishing, P.O. Box 26464, Tempe, AZ 85282.

Roe, Daphne A.: *Drug-Induced Nutritional Deficiencies,* AVI, Westport, CT, 1976.

Roe, Daphne A.: *Alcohol and the Diet,* AVI, Westport, CT, 1979.

Rose, James C.: *Handbook for Health Care Food Service Management,* Aspen Systems Corp., Gaithersburg, MD, 1984.

Simko, Margaret, C. Cowell, and J. Gilbride: *Nutrition Assessment,* Aspen Systems Corp., Gaithersburg, MD, 1984.

Williams, Melvin: *Nutritional Aspects of Human Physical and Athletic Performance,* Charles Thomas, Springfield, IL, 1982.

Zohman, Lenore: *Beyond Diet . . . Exercise Your Way to Fitness and Heart Health,* Best Foods Info Service, Box 307, Conventry, CT.

Newspapers and Periodicals

Newspapers

Wall Street Journal
USA Today
Local daily papers
Local weekly papers

Periodicals

American Health
Business Week
Forbes
Fortune
Harvard Business Review
Health (American)
Inc.

Newsweek
Prevention (check it out occasionally)
Savvy
Self
Success
Time
Venture
Working Woman

Newsletters and Journals

American Journal of Clinical Nutrition, 9650 Rockville Pike, Bethesda, MD 20014

Clinical Consultation in Nutritional Support, Medical Directions, Inc., 625 N. Michigan Ave., Chicago, IL 60611

CNI Weekly Report, 1146 19th St., N.W., Washington, DC 20036

Community Nutritionist (The), CNI Magazine, 1146 19th St., N.W., Washington, DC 20036.

Consulting Nutritionist in Private Practice Newsletter, ADA Practice Group Newsletter

Consumer Reports, 256 Washington St., Mt. Vernon, NY 10550

Contemporary Nutrition, General Mills, Inc., P.O. Box 1113, Minneapolis, MN 55440

Current Dietetics, Ross Labs, 625 Cleveland Ave., Columbus, OH 43216

Dairy Council Digest, National Dairy Council, 6300 N. River Rd., Rosemont, IL 60018

Environmental Nutrition, 52 Riverside Dr., Suite 15-A, New York, NY 10024

FDA Consumer, 5600 Fishers Lane, Rockville, MD 20857

Harvard Medical School Health Letter (The), 79 Garden St., Cambridge, MA 02138

Healthline, 1320 Bayport Ave., San Carlos, CA 94070

Hospital Food & Nutrition Focus, Aspen Systems Corp., 1600 Research Blvd., Rockville, MD 20850

Journal of American Dietetic Association (check Publication Review Section)

Journal of Nutrition Education, 2140 Shattuck Ave., Berkeley, CA 94704

Journal of Nutrition For the Elderly, The Haworth Press, 28 E. 22 St., New York, NY 10010.

Kiplinger Washington Letter, 1729 H St., N.W., Washington, D.C. 20006

Legislative Newsletter, The American Dietetic Association, 430 N. Michigan Ave., Chicago, IL 60611

Nutrition Action, The Center For Science In the Public Interest, 1755 "S" St., N.W., Washington, DC 20009

Nutrition and Health, Institute of Human Nutrition, Columbia University, 701 W. 168th St., New York, NY 10032

Nutrition and the M.D., P.O. Box 2160, Van Nuys, CA 91405

Nutrition Today, 101 Ridgley Ave., Annapolis, MD 21401

Nutritional Support Service, Journal of Practical Application in Clinical Nutrition, 12849 Magnolia Blvd., North Hollywood, CA 91607

Obesity and Bariatric Medicine, 333 W. Hampden Ave., Englewood, CO 80110

Sports Medicine Digest, P.O. Box 2160, Van Nuys, CA 91405

Sports-Nutrition News, P.O. Box 986, Evanston, IL 60204

Topics in Clinical Nutrition, Aspen Systems, 16792 Oakmont Ave., Gaithersburg, MD 20877

Tufts University Diet & Nutrition Letter, Box 34T, 322 W. 57 St., NY, NY 10019

Wellness/Health Promotion

Resource Organizations

American Alliance for Health, Physical Education, Recreation and Dance (AAHPERD), 1900 Association Dr., Reston, VA 22091
Association for Fitness in Business (AFB), 95 Hope St., Stamford, CT 06907
American College of Sports Medicine, P.O. Box 1440, Indianapolis, IN 46206
Institute for Aerobics Research, 11811 Preston Rd., Dallas, TX 75230
National Health Information Clearinghouse, P.O. Box 1133, Washington, DC 20013–1133
President's Council on Physical Fitness and Sports, 400 Sixth St., S.W., Room 3030, Washington, DC 20201

Newsletters

"Current Awareness in Health Education," Center for Health Promotion and Education, Centers for Disease Control, Atlanta, GA 30333
"National Library of Medicine News," Public Health Service, National Institutes of Health, 8600 Rockville Pike, Bethesda, MD 20209
"PROmoting HEALTH," American Hospital Association, Center for Health Promotion, 840 N. Lake Shore Dr., Chicago, IL 60611, Att: Sharyn Bills
"Employee Health and Fitness," American Health Consultants, 67 Peachtree Drive, N.E., Atlanta, GA 30304
"University of California, Berkeley Wellness Newsletter," P.O. Box 10922, Des Moines, IA 50340

Publications

Allen, Robert F., and L. Shirley: *Lifegain,* Appleton-Century-Crofts, NY, 1981
Ardell, Donald B.: *High Level Wellness,* Bantam Books, NY, 1979
Bauer, Katherine: *Improving the Chances for Health: Lifestyle Change and Health Evaluation,* National Center for Health Education 211 Sutter St., San Francisco, 1981
Berry, Charles A.: *Good Health for Employees and Reduced Health Care Costs for Industry,* Health Insurance Association of America, Washington, DC, 1981
Cunningham, R. M.: *Wellness At Work,* Inquiry Book, Chicago, 1982
Farquhar, John W.: *The American Way of Life Need Not be Hazardous to Your Health,* W. W. Norton, NY, 1978
Healthy People: The Surgeon General's Report on Health Promotion and Disease Prevention, Superintendent of Documents, Government Printing Office, Washington, DC, 1979
Ryan, Regina S. and J. W. Travis: *Wellness Workbook,* Ten Speed Press, Berkeley, CA, 1981
Somers, Anne R., ed.: *Promoting Health: Consumer Education and National Policy,* Aspen Systems, Germantown, MD

Consumer Awareness

Barrett, Stephen: *Health Robbers,* G. F. Stickley, Philadelphia, PA, 1976
California Council Against Health Fraud, "Newsletter," P.O. Box 1276, Loma Linda, CA 92354
Consumer Information Center, Dept. G, Pueblo, CO 81009
Cunningham, John: *Controversies in Clinical Nutrition,* G. F. Stickley, Philadelphia, PA, 1980
Deutsch, Ronald: *New Nuts Among the Berries,* Bull Pub., Palo Alto, CA, 1977
FDA Consumer (order from Consumer Information Center)
Gussow, Joan: *The Feeding Web,* Bull Pub., Palo Alto, CA, 1978
Herbert, Victor, and S. Barrett: *Vitamins and "Health" Foods,* G. F. Stickley, Philadelphia, PA, 1982
Herbert, Victor: *Nutrition Cultism,* G. F. Stickley, Philadelphia, PA, 1980
Los Angeles District—CA Dietetic Association, P.O. Box 3506, Santa Monica, CA 90403
Marshall, Charles W.: *Vitamins and Minerals,* G. F. Stickley, Philadelphia, PA, 1983
"Nutrition References and Book Reviews," Chicago Nutrition Association, 8158 S. Kedzie Ave., Chicago, IL 60652

Counseling and Eating Behavior References

Aronson, Virginia, and B. D. Fitzgerald: *Guidebook for Nutrition Counselsors,* The Christopher Publishing House, North Quincy, MA, 1980
Bailey, Covert: *Fit or Fat?,* Houghton Mifflin, Boston, MA, 1978
Bandler, Richard and J. Grinder, *Frogs Into Princes* (Neuro Linguistic Programming), Real People Press, Moab, UT, 1979
Bruch, H.: *The Golden Cage: The Enigma of Anorexia Nervosa,* Harvard University, 1978, and Vintage Books, 1979
Cordell, Franklin, D., and G. R. Giebler: *Psychological War on Fat,* Argus Communications, Niles, IL, 1977
Dusek, Dorothy E.: *Thin and Fit: Your Personal Lifestyle* (Wellness Approach to Weight Loss), Wadsworth Pub., Belmont, CA, 1982
Ferguson, James M.: *Habits, Not Diets,* Bull Pub., Palo Alto, CA, 1976
Ferguson, James M.: *Learning to Eat,* Bull Pub., Palo Alto, CA, 1975
Ikeda, Joanne: *For Teenagers Only: Change Your Habits to Change Your Shape,* Bull Pub., Palo Alto, CA, 1978
Jeffrey, D. Balfour, and R. C. Katz: *Take It Off and Keep It Off: A Behavioral Program for Weight-Loss and Healthy Living,* Prentice-Hall, Englewood Cliffs, NJ, 1977
Jordan, H. A., L. S. Levitz, and G. M. Kimbrell: *Eating Is Okay,* Rawson Associates, New York, 1976
Mellin, Laurel: *Shapedown* (Weight Management Program for Adolescents), Balboa Pub., San Francisco, CA, 1983
Nash, Joyce D., and L. O. Long: *Taking Charge of Your Weight and Well-Being,* Bull Pub., Palo Alto, CA, 1978
Remington, Dennis, G. Fisher, and E. Parent: *How to Lower Your Fat Thermostat,* Vitality House International, Provo, UT, 1983
Schwartz, Lawrence H., and J. L. Schwartz: *The Psychodynamics of Patient Care,* Prentice-Hall, Englewood Cliffs, NJ, 1972

Snetselaar, Linda G.: *Nutrition Counseling Skills,* Aspen Publications, Gaithersburg, MD, 1983

Stuart, Richard B., and B. Davis: *Slim Chance in a Fat World: Behavioral Control of Obesity,* Research Press, Champaign, IL, 1978

Teaching Tools and Handouts

American Diabetes Association, 2 Park Ave., New York, NY 10020

American Dietetic Association, 430 N. Michigan Ave., Chicago, IL 60611

American Heart Association, 7320 Greenville Ave., Dallas, TX 75231

American Institute of Nutrition, 9650 Rockville Pike, Bethesda, MD 20014

American Medical Association, 535 N. Dearborn St., Chicago, IL 60610

American Society for Parental and Enteral Nutrition, 428 E. Preston St., Baltimore, MD 21202

Best Foods, Box 8000, International Plaza, Englewood Cliffs, NJ 07632

Cambridge Scientific Industries, P.O. Box 265, Cambridge, MD 21613 (Lange Skinfold Caliper)

Consumer Information Center, Health Services Administration, Rockville, MD 20857

Doyle Pharmaceutical Co., 5320 W. 23rd St., Minneapolis, MN 55416

General Mills Nutrition Department, Dept. 45, P.O. Box 1112, Minneapolis, MN 55440

Hurley Medical Center, Health Education Dept., One Hurley Plaza, Flint, MI 48502

Illinois Nutrition Educators, Inc., P.O. Box 1386, Evanston IL 60204

Los Angeles District California Dietetic Association, P.O. Box 3506, Santa Monica, CA 90403

McGaw Laboratories, P.O. Box 11887, Santa Anna, CA 92714

Mead Johnson, 2404 Pennsylvania Ave., Evansville, IN 47721

Nasco Plastic Food Models, P.O. Box 3837, Modesto, CA 95352

National Dairy Council, 6300 N. River Rd., Rosemont, IL 60018

National Heart, Lung and Blood Institute, 9000 Rockville Pike, Bethesda, MD 20014

NEW-TRITION News Releases, Emily Smart, M.A., R.D., Mercy Hospital and Medical Center, 4077 Fifth Ave., San Diego, CA 92103–2180

Nourishing Thoughts Enterprises, P.O. Box 1402, Hudson, OH 44236

Nutri-Art, 6210 Ridge Manor Dr., Memphis, TN 38115

Nutrition Consultant Services of Houston, University Bank Plaza, 5615 Kirby Dr., Suite 512, Houston, TX 77005

Nutrition Education Center, Capitol Federal Bldg., 9500 Nall Ave., Suite 304, Overland Park, KS 66212

Nutrition Graphics, 336 N.W. 29th St., Corvallis, OR 97330

Nutrition in the Life Cycle, P.O. Box 513, Verdugo, CA 91046

Oryx Press, 2214 N. Central at Encanto, Phoenix, AZ 85004, "Directory of Food and Nutrition Information Services and Resources"

Pelouze Scale Co., 1218 Chicago Ave., Evanston, IL 60202 (small food scales)

Positive Eating Patterns, P.O. Box 31711, Omaha, NE 68131

RJL Systems Inc., 9930 Whittier, Detroit, MI 48224 (Impedance method to evaluate body composition)

Ross Laboratories, 625 Cleveland Ave., Columbus, OH 43216

SKYNDEX (electronic body fat calculator), Skyndex Bio-Medical Systems, Inc., P.O. Box 520, Fayetteville, AR 72702

Society for Nutrition Education, 1736 Franklin St., Suite 900, Oakland, CA 94612

Third Party Billing Forms, CN of CA, 10 Congress St., Suite 320, Pasadena, CA 91105

Winding Your Weigh Down, Nutrition Consultant Services of Houston, 5615 Kirby Drive, Suite #512, Houston, TX 77005

Audiovisuals

American Diabetes Association, 2 Park Ave., New York, NY 10016

American Dietetic Association, 430 N. Michigan Ave., Chicago, IL 60611 (Check "Film Festival" and abstract book from each national meeting also.)

"Audiovisuals For Nutrition Education," Society for Nutrition Education, 2140 Shattuck Ave., Suite 1110, Berkeley, CA 94704

Churchill Films, 662 N. Robertson Blvd., Los Angeles, CA 90069

Dairy Council, Inc., 12450 N. Washington, Thornton, CO 80241

Dietary Films, Ltd., Ronnie Korschum, R.D., 9380 S.W. Sunset Dr., Suite B-150, Miami, FL 33173

Doyle Pharmaceutical Co., Nutrition Dept., 5320 W. 23rd St., Minneapolis, MN 55416

General Mills, Inc., P.O. Box 1113, Minneapolis, MN 55440

Harvard University, School of Public Health, Dept. of Nutrition, 665 Huntington Ave., Boston, MA 02115

Info Medix, 12800 Garden Grove Blvd., Suite E, Garden Grove, CA 92643–2043

Journal Films, Inc., 930 Pitner Ave., Evanston, IL 60202

Oryx Press, 2214 N. Central at Encanto, Phoenix, AZ 85004, "Audiovisual Resources in Food Nutrition"

Society for Nutrition Education, 1736 Franklin St., Suite 900, Oakland, CA 94612

Spectrum Films, 2785 Roosevelt St., Carlsbad, CA 92008

The Polished Apple, 3742 Seahorn Dr., Malibu, CA 90265

Tupperware Educational Services, Dept. EFC80/P.O. Box 2353, Orlando, FL 32802

Walt Disney Educational Media Co., 500 S. Buena Vista St., Burbank, CA 91521

Index